William N. Kelly, PharmD, ISPE

Prescribed Medications
and the Public Health
Laying the Foundation
for Risk Reduction

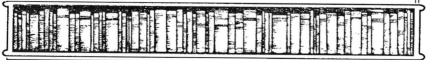

"The release of the IOM's *To Err Is Human* in 1999 brought the issue of medication error into the forefront of both health care systems as well as the public. Since this report, health care systems have implemented safer medication practices based on recommendations and goals from agencies such as JCAHO. However, these goals and recommendations may be just a beginning to improving medication safety, as there are many other facets of medication error and adverse drug reaction prevention that are revealed in *Prescribed Medications and the Public Health*.

This very timely and definitive book not only focuses on types of errors that are also targeted in the JCAHO National Patient Safety Goals, but exposes the reader to areas of error that were not recognized as such. When most think of medication error, medication errors of commission come to mind. These are errors that occur by direct, yet unintentional action of those involved. Dr. Kelly also exposes the reader to forms of error know as errors of omission, an adverse drug event that may cause harm to a patient based on the lack of something being performed.

I have long believed that adverse drug events that are directly related to the pharmacologic action of the drug are in most instances a form of medication error, usually one of omission. Dr. Kelly's text has much devoted to this very important aspect of drug safety, identifying factors that lead up to such drug misadventures. In addition to this, the text is truly a complete read on all aspects of error, including the nature and scope of the problem, detecting, documenting, and reporting of adverse drug events, liability for these events, and what I think is most important, evidence that supports methods to prevent and reduce injury from adverse drug events.

Prescribed Medications and the Public Health should prove an enlightening read for physicians, pharmacists, nurses, health care administrators, medical legal professionals, and others who have a valid interest in medication safety and adverse drug event prevention. As a pharmacy educator, I look forward to introducing this text to my students in order to increase their awareness of the scope of medication error problems and provide them with tools to lessen their severity or prevent them altogether."

Patrick J. McDonnell, PharmD
*Associate Professor
of Clinical Pharmacy,
Temple University
School of Pharmacy*

More pre-publication
REVIEWS, COMMENTARIES, EVALUATIONS . . .

"**D**r. William Kelly has written a text that is more than timely. It summarizes the work that has occurred in just over the five years since the IOM's astonishing report *To Err Is Human* (1999), and notes where some incremental improvement has occurred, but also acknowledges that there is a long way to go. Since that time, the academic and professional literature has been replete with valuable science, technical and health policy reports about the extent and nature of health-system errors that put patients at risk. A subset of these errors relate to medication use and are confounded to some extent by known and unknown adverse events that may be reasonably associated with the use of medicine. Dr. Kelly provides a broad overview of a highly complex topic involving many actors and institutions.

Many features of this text merit attention. First, it is the product of a single author and thus presents a consistent tone and approach throughout. Second, it is adroitly written to serve the needs of health care practitioners, patients/consumers, health policy experts, risk managers, and others. Third, its scope is broad, moving through a clearly delineated series of topics that end in specific recommendations and solutions for practitioners, patients, and health policy experts. I highly recommend this text to all who care about promoting risk-reduction strategies to promote patients' safety and safe medication use."

Roger L. Williams, MD
*Executive Vice President
and Chief Executive Officer,
United States Pharmacopeia (USP)*

Pharmaceutical Products Press®
An Imprint of The Haworth Press, Inc.
New York • London • Oxford

Prescribed Medications and the Public Health
Laying the Foundation for Risk Reduction

PHARMACEUTICAL PRODUCTS PRESS®
Titles of Related Interest

Pharmacy Ethics edited by Mickey Smith, Steven Strauss, H. John Baldwin, and Kelly T. Alberts

Advancing Prescription Medicine Compliance: New Paradigms, New Practices edited by Jack E. Fincham

A History of Nonprescription Product Regulation by W. Steven Pray

Pharmacy and the U.S. Health Care System, Third Edition edited by Michael Ira Smith, Albert I. Wertheimer, and *Jack E. Fincham*

Taking Your Medicine: A Guide to Medication Regimens and Compliance for Patients and Caregivers by Jack E. Fincham

Prescribed Medications and the Public Health
Laying the Foundation for Risk Reduction

William N. Kelly, PharmD, ISPE

Pharmaceutical Products Press®
An Imprint of The Haworth Press, Inc.
New York • London • Oxford

428240

FEB 1 2 2008

For more information on this book or to order, visit
http://www.haworthpress.com/store/product.asp?sku=5688
or call 1-800-HAWORTH (800-429-6784) in the United States and Canada
or (607) 722-5857 outside the United States and Canada
or contact orders@HaworthPress.com

Published by

Pharmaceutical Products Press®, an imprint of The Haworth Press, Inc., 10 Alice Street, Binghamton, NY 13904-1580.

PUBLISHER'S NOTE

The development, preparation, and publication of this work has been undertaken with great care. However, the Publisher, employees, editors, and agents of The Haworth Press are not responsible for any errors contained herein or for consequences that may ensue from use of materials or information contained in this work. The Haworth Press is committed to the dissemination of ideas and information according to the highest standards of intellectual freedom and the free exchange of ideas. Statements made and opinions expressed in this publication do not necessarily reflect the views of the Publisher, Directors, management, or staff of The Haworth Press, Inc., or an endorsement by them.

This book has been published solely for educational purposes and is not intended to substitute for the medical advice of a treating physician. Medicine is an ever-changing science. As new research and clinical experience broaden our knowledge, changes in treatment may be required. While many potential treatment options are made herein, some or all of the options may not be applicable to a particular individual. Therefore, the author, editor and publisher do not accept responsibility in the event of negative consequences incurred as a result of the information presented in this book. We do not claim that this information is necessarily accurate by the rigid scientific and regulatory standards applied for medical treatment. **No warranty, express or implied, is furnished with respect to the material contained in this book. The reader is urged to consult with his/her personal physician with respect to the treatment of any medical condition.**

Cover design by Marylouise E. Doyle.

Library of Congress Cataloging-in-Publication Data

Kelly, William N.
    Prescribed medications and the public health : laying the foundation for risk reduction / William N. Kelly.
        p. cm.
    Includes bibliographical references and index.
    ISBN-13: 978-0-7890-2360-5 (hc. : alk. paper)
    ISBN-10: 0-7890-2360-1 (hc. : alk. paper)
    ISBN-13: 978-0-7890-2361-2 (pbk. : alk. paper)
    ISBN-10: 0-7890-2361-X (pbk. : alk. paper)
    1. Medication abuse. 2. Medication abuse—United States.
[DNLM: 1. Medication Errors—prevention & control—United States. 2. Drug Therapy—adverse effects—United States. 3. Health Policy—United States. 4. Safety Management—methods—United States. QZ 42 K29p 2006] I. Title.

RM146.5.K45 2006
362.29'9—dc22

                                                                                    2005029487

To T. Donald Rucker, PhD,
productive scholar, mentor, and friend.

ABOUT THE AUTHOR

William N. Kelly, PharmD, is President of William N. Kelly Consulting, Inc., a company devoted to the advancement of medication safety, health care education, and pharmacy practice. Previous to starting his company in January of 2005, Dr. Kelly was a tenured Professor at the Mercer University School of Pharmacy and a Guest Researcher at the Immunization Safety Branch of the Centers for Disease Control and Prevention (CDC), both in Atlanta.

Dr. Kelly has published over 60 peer-reviewed manuscripts, ten chapters in books, and has presented his work nationally and internationally. He is the author of *Pharmacy: What It Is and How It Works.*

Dr. Kelly is past Chair and a member of the United States Pharmacopeia's (USP's) Expert Committee on Safe Medication Use and a past member of the National Coordinating Council on Medication Errors and Prevention. He is also a member of the Research Advisory Panel for the American Society of Health-System Foundation for Education and Research.

Dr. Kelly holds a BS degree in pharmacy from Ferris State University, a doctor of pharmacy (PharmD) degree and residency certificate in clinical pharmacy from the University of Michigan, and has completed a Fellowship in Executive Management at the Leonard Davis Institute of Health Economics at the University of Pennsylvania. He has also completed graduate work in pharmacoepidemiology and biostatistics at McGill and Emory Universities, and is a fellow of the International Society for Pharmacoepidemiology (ISPE).

CONTENTS

Foreword

Drugs are enormously beneficial in the aggregate, but they can also cause substantial harm, as has become increasingly clear in recent years. To gain approval for a new agent, the pharmaceutical industry must clear a high bar, showing that the medication is safe and effective in controlled trials. However, these trials only include hundreds to thousands of patients, and many side effects are not detected until the drugs are exposed to larger populations, which generally include people underrepresented in early trials, such as the old and young, and the sick. A series of recent studies have demonstrated that medications cause many adverse effects, generally more than reported in trials, and some new associations have become apparent, for example the reports of complications with use of Vioxx and myocardial infarction. However, many of the adverse effects, or adverse drug events, occur with "old" drugs, those that have been used for decades. Many of these are predictable, and preventable, or associated with errors in care.

The Institute of Medicine's report *To Err Is Human: Building a Safer Health System,* issued in 1999, pointed out that health care in the United States is not as safe as it should be, and that many patients are injured unnecessarily by the health care that is intended to help people. It went on to suggest that medications cause many of these injuries, and that delivering safe care depends on the systems by which care is delivered. Although this groundbreaking report caused waves, seven years later the industry has been slow to change. The public, however, has become more concerned about medications, and in many instances unjustifiably so, and often either reject or stop taking medications that are known to be beneficial and even lifesaving. Both the issues of risk and benefit are extremely important from the public health perspective, in part because of the extraordinary amount of medication use in our society today, and also because we have so many drugs that work.

Prescribed Medications and the Public Health
© 2006 by The Haworth Press, Inc. All rights reserved.
doi:10.1300/5688_a

In this sweeping book, Bill Kelly takes on these and other questions about medications and their effects on health. For example, how can drugs cause so much good, and at the same time so much harm? Are there ways to improve the likelihood that less harm will ensue? How can the dream of the *To Err Is Human* report be realized? What should individual health care organizations do to improve their medication safety? What needs to be done at other levels, for example in manufacturing, regulation, and distribution of medications?

Kelly is eminently qualified to discuss these issues. For many years, he served as professor and chairman of the School of Pharmacy at Mercer University in Atlanta. Subsequently, he moved to the Centers for Disease Control and Prevention, and most recently he has worked as an independent consultant, which has given him more time to reflect and take on projects such as this effort. He has long been an acute observer and thought leader in this important area; I got to know him through his service as chair of the U.S. Pharmacopeia's Safe Medication Use expert committee.

A part of the solution is technology. If physicians begin to use electronic health records and prescribe electronically, that will represent a major positive step. A number of studies have demonstrated that, at least in the hospital setting, this method improves medication safety. Other technology such as barcoding will likely prove useful in dispensing and administration. Yet none of these technologies are being adopted as fast as they might be. Kelly discusses what the barriers are, and how they might be overcome.

However, technology alone is insufficient, and it must be used judiciously. For any technological solution to be used effectively, it is important that a culture of safety be present. Many nontechnological solutions can result in important benefits. In particular, the skills of pharmacists must be much better leveraged. Technology should make it possible to relieve pharmacists of many menial tasks, and free them to interact more with patients.

As Kelly describes, the stakes are enormous, and the atmosphere is often highly charged. Drug companies represent some of the most innovative and profitable in industry and they have contributed a tremendous amount to America's health and well-being. Yet at the same time the drug safety problem—which the pharmaceutical industry has minimized—causes substantial morbidity and mortality, and must be addressed more effectively. At the same time, if we could more effectively address issues around compliance, especially for chronic conditions such as coronary artery disease, that might provide the greatest public health benefit of all. Although there is no easy way out of this conundrum, Kelly does a wonderful job of presenting it and some of the potential solutions.

David W. Bates, MD, MSc
Chief, Division of General Internal Medicine,
Brigham and Women's Hospital;
Medical Director of Clinical and Quality Analysis,
Partners Healthcare;
Professor of Medicine,
Harvard Medical School;
and Professor of Health Policy and Management,
Harvard School of Public Health, Boston, MA

Preface

Considering the extent of medication use—millions of doses taken each day—drugs are remarkably safe. However, for a small percentage of patients, the legitimate use of medication results in a threat to life, permanent disability, or even death. Much of this morbidity and mortality is preventable—it simply should not happen!

In 1999, the Institute of Medicine (IOM) of the National Academy of Science issued a galvanizing report titled *To Err Is Human: Building a Safer Health System*. Few publications have received such lasting attention from the media and health professions. This report dealt with the extent of medical errors in the United States. The study estimated that 44,000 to 98,000 Americans die each year because of medical errors. At least 7,000 of these deaths can be traced to medication errors. Furthermore, medical errors in general may rank as the eighth leading cause of death in the United States. The estimated cost for these tragic events is $17 to $29 billion a year. However, if the nation possessed a more comprehensive medical reporting and standardized patient record system, the true incidence of untoward consequences seems likely to be even higher.

Much of the morbidity and mortality cited in the IOM report focuses on medication errors. Yet this aspect of the drug usage problem illustrates only tip of the iceberg. Lurking beneath the surface are additional adverse drug consequences manifest in factors such as drug reactions, drug-drug interactions, and allergic drug reactions. Until the IOM report, most health care practitioners accepted medication safety problems as an inherent side effect of using medications. Hence the full scope of the problem remained largely hidden from public scrutiny.

Medication safety problems, however, have been occurring for a long time. Perceptive analysts and thoughtful citizens alike would be forced to raise the basic question—why has the problem not been self-correcting? For example, since 1979, at least twelve books have

Prescribed Medications and the Public Health
© 2006 by The Haworth Press, Inc. All rights reserved.
doi:10.1300/5688_b

been published alerting the public and health care administrators to selected dimensions of the drug use problem. Various dangers associated with use of each medication are found either while researching patient risks and benefits during clinical trials or after the medication has been prescribed for some time. Yet most medication-related problems can be prevented by improving the quality of technical information, enhancing system design to take advantage of computerized record keeping, as well as monitoring of prescribing practices and patient outcomes.

Then, why do medication errors and other adverse drug events persist? The short answer seems to be because the medication use process is too complex and has been broken for a long time—one might argue that we have been accustomed to certain levels of risk. The long answer may stem from the fact that the dysfunctional medication use system is but a fragment of a larger problem—a broken health care system that often is "fixed" more with Band-Aids than optimizing adjustments. Thus, reform efforts are confronted with a fundamental dilemma: Should patients and health professionals wait for the health care system to be revamped while allowing many medication safety problems to continue, or should the nation strive to repair the medication use system first and hope that the larger health care system will be fixed eventually? Some evidence suggests that the last approach has been chosen more by default than systematic review of health policy.

Selected examples of a broken medication use system include: patients receiving the wrong drug because look-alike and sound-alike names led to product confusion; look-alike drug packaging; the prescribing of drug-drug interactions overlooked by inadequate pharmacy computer systems; lack of bar coding of medication administered to patients; drugs prescribed in excess amounts or actually contraindicated for particular patients; and, drugs administered to patients when the individual had indicated a previous allergic reaction to the same medication. Other major issues include: lack of centralized, electronic medical records, no national center on patient safety, lack of mandatory reporting of fatal adverse medication events, and a pharmaceutical industry in need of reform and greater regulatory control.

This book provides a snapshot in time to depict the nature and extent of medication safety issues in the United States. Although medication safety is America's other drug problem, our predicament is not confined to this country. Other advanced nations seem to experience similar levels of morbidity and mortality associated with medication use.

Hence the medication safety issues discussed in this book encompass a deeper and broader model that those identified by the IOM reports. This book offers micro and macro solutions to the general problem and is intended for both health practitioners and health policy specialists interested in mitigating instances in which patients are placed at risk when medication therapy is involved. The first few chapters deal with the nature and scope of the problem and why patients are harmed by medication. The middle chapters treat the discovery, assessment, and reporting of medication injury. The later chapters chart courses on how medication safety problems could be reduced and controlled.

It has been seven years since the first IOM report, and from most viewpoints, a great effort has taken place to improve medication safety. However, our ability to document reduced harm to patients is less tangible. This deficiency may be traced to the fact that medication safety has not yet reached a tipping point where medication safety is widely recognized as a major health problem. Perhaps the only real gains in medication safety will occur via concerted leadership of health care practitioners as supported by patients and their employers. Conversely, sustained progress seems less likely to the extent that the nation relies on efforts by elected government officials, health insurance executives, or the pharmaceutical industry.

The author's goal for this book has been singular—to help stimulate society to come to grips with a pandemic problem that results in harm to many patients. Most of these medication-related problems are preventable. Sooner or later, most citizens will find it essential to balance the beneficial results associated with appropriate drug therapy while simultaneously minimizing any concomitant risks. I hope that this book will provide guidance for developing your contribution to this worthwhile effort.

Acknowledgments

I could not have written this book without the help of my wife Trudy, a superb reference librarian. She retrieved references needed for this project, helped edit the contents, and gained copyright permissions when appropriate.

The idea for this book originated with my editor, Dennis B. Worthen, PhD, Lloyd Scholar at the Lloyd Library in Cincinnati. As we both believe, there is an overwhelming need for a basic reference such as this one.

Most of all I want to express my gratitude to T. Donald Rucker, PhD, to whom this book is dedicated. Dr. Rucker is Professor Emeritus, the College of Pharmacy, University of Illinois at Chicago, a well-known health care economist, and a longtime student and critic of the medication use process. This book came to completion through his continuing encouragement. During preparation of this book, Rucker received the 2003 Avedis Donabedian Quality Award from the American Pubic Health Association in November, 2003 when he presented a paper: "Improving Quality Improvement in Health Care: Foundations and Frontiers." Dr. Donabedian was a premier scholar at the University of Michigan and an internationally recognized authority in public health.

Finally, I would like to thank Mercer University, my Dean, Hewitt W. (Ted) Matthews, PhD, and Robert T. Chen, MD, MA, FISPE, Chief of the Vaccine Safety Branch of the Centers for Disease Control (CDC) where I was a guest researcher. Drs. Matthews and Chen have served as role models as I endeavored to pursue scholarly activities.

Prescribed Medications and the Public Health
© 2006 by The Haworth Press, Inc. All rights reserved.
doi:10.1300/5688_c

Chapter 1

America's Drug Problems

"America's drug problem" is a familiar phrase. When asked what this means, most people would say it refers to the drug abuse problem in the United States—using and abusing drugs for the purpose of "getting high."

There is no question the United States has a drug abuse problem. The U.S. Department of Health and Human Services performs a survey of roughly 67,500 people each year to describe the epidemiology of illicit drug, alcohol, and tobacco use by the civilian, noninstitutionalized population of the United States aged 12 years and older.[1] The 2002 National Survey on Drug Use and Health reveals that "an estimated 19.5 million Americans, or 8 percent of the population aged 12 or older, were current illicit drug users." Current use was defined as use of an illicit drug during the month before the survey interview. The most commonly abused drugs in the United States are listed in Table 1.1.

Information from the Drug Abuse Warning Network (DAWN) for the year 2000 shows there were "601,776 estimated drug-related emergency department (ED) episodes in 2000 and among these, there were 1,100,539 drug mentions (more than one drug may be in a person's system at admission)."[2] ED visits involving the club drug Ecstasy (MDMA) increased 58 percent, heroin and morphine increased 15 percent, and oxycodone increased 68 percent from the previous year.

The results of a study prepared by the Lewin Group for the National Institute on Drug Abuse estimated the total economic cost of drug abuse was $97.7 billion in 1992.[3] This figure represents a 50 percent increase over the cost estimate from 1985 data. "More than half of the estimated costs of drug abuse were associated with drug-related crime." These figures are much different today—probably much higher.

Prescribed Medications and the Public Health
© 2006 by The Haworth Press, Inc. All rights reserved.
doi:10.1300/5688_01

TABLE 1.1 The Most Common Drugs Used Illicitly in the United States, 2002

Drug	Abusers	U.S. Population
Marijuana	14,600,000	6.2%
Psychotherapeutic drugs[a]	6,200,000	2.6%
Cocaine[b]	2,000,000	0.9%
OxyContin[a]	1,900,000	0.9%
Hallucinogens[c]	1,200,000	0.5%
Heroin	166,000	0.1%

Source: The U.S. Department of Health and Human Services. *Results from the 2002 National Survey on Drug Use and Health: National Findings.* Substance Abuse and Mental Health Services Administration. http://www.samhsa.gov/oas/nhsda/2k2nsduh/Results/2k2results.htm. Accessed 10/6/2003.

[a]Nonmedical use
[b]Of these, 567,000 used crack
[c]Of these, 676,000 used Ecstasy

AMERICA'S "OTHER" DRUG PROBLEM

Beneath the mantle of America's drug abuse problem lies an equally insidious, equally harmful, and prevalent, but less well-known, drug problem—the unsafe use and harmful effects of medications legally approved for use in the United States.

Although drugs often relieve and sometimes cure various ailments and vaccines prevent some diseases, neither of these are totally safe. They have a dark side and can cause side effects, adverse drug reactions, and allergic reactions, and can be prescribed, dispensed, or administered in error. Although a rare event, drugs can be made, labeled, or packaged incorrectly by the manufacturer. Furthermore, one prescribed drug or substance can interact with another prescribed drug or illicit substance.

It is easy to dismiss statements in a prescription drug's package insert, e.g., "1 percent of patients may experience [a side effect such as] syncope [sudden fainting]." However, this serious adverse effect can result in an accident if the syncope occurs when driving a car. The 1 percent figure sounds so small when read, but looms large when it affects you or someone you love.

The 1 percent adverse reaction rate blossoms to large numbers of patients when put into the context of how much medication is used in the United States. As shown in Table 1.2, the number of outpatient prescriptions rose dramatically from 1997 to 2000.[4] It is expected that nearly $4 billion outpatient prescriptions will be dispensed in the United States by 2005.[5]

Reasons for this rapid growth in prescription use in the United States include heavy promotional efforts by drug manufacturers such as "direct-to-consumer advertising," overprescribing by doctors, cost pressures to discharge patients early, and the "graying" of America. Older Americans take more medications than those under 65 and physiological changes often make them more vulnerable to the negative effects of the drugs they take. The overprescribing (sometimes called "polypharmacy") is of particular concern as it results in millions of avoidable side effects, adverse reactions, drug interactions, and errors.

These figures do not include the use of over-the-counter medications (OTCs), herbal products, or medication used in hospitals, managed care organizations, and nursing homes, all of which are increasing each year. Table 1.3 lists the top-ten drug products in the United States, based on sales dollars during 2003.[6] The three top commonly used herbal preparations were ginseng (3.3 percent of the population), *Gingko biloba* extract (2.2 percent of the population), and *Allium sativum* (garlic) (1.9 percent of the population).[7]

TABLE 1.2. Total Utilization and Expenditures for Outpatient Prescription Medications, 1997-2000

Year	Prescriptions[a]	Expenditures[a]
1997	1.9	$72.3
1998	2.0	$78.0
1999	2.1	$94.2
2000	2.2	$103.0

Source: USDHHS. Agency for Healthcare Research and Quality. (2003). Statistical Brief #21: Trends in Outpatient Prescription Drug Utilization and Expenditures: 1997-2000. www.meps.ahrq.gov/papers/st21/stat21.htm.

[a]In billions

TABLE 1.3. Top Ten Drug Products in the United States (2003 – Total Market by Sales Dollars)

Rank/Drug	Company	Primary Use	U.S. Sales (US $Billions)
1. Lipitor	Pfizer US Pharm	cholesterol	$6.30
2. Zocor	MSD	cholesterol	$5.10
3. Prevacid	Tap Pharm	ulcers	$4.40
4. Procrit	Ortho	anemia	$3.20
5. Nexium	AstraZeneca	acid reflux disease	$2.90
6. Zyprexa	Lilly	psychosis	$2.80
7. Zoloft	Pfizer US Pharm	depression	$2.80
8. Celebrex	Pharmacia/Upjohn	pain	$2.50
9. Epogen	Amgen	anemia	$2.50
10. Neurontin	Pfizer US Pharm	seizures	$2.40

Source: NDCHealth, NDC PHAST, 3/2005. Adapted from NDCH. http://rxlist. com/top200sales2003.htm. Accessed July 10, 2004.

Note: The information contained in this report was derived using NDCHealth proprietary methodologies and is based on prescription data and wholesale acquisition cost (WAC) prices for retail, mail order, clinics, hospitals, long-term care and home health care organizations and other non-retail channels.

DRUG MISADVENTURES

The rising use of medication comes with a rising number of adverse drug reactions, drug interactions, allergic drug reactions, and medication errors. Together these unfortunate happenings are called "adverse drug events" (ADEs). A *drug misadventure* is the clinical outcome of an ADE.[8]

"Drug misadventuring in the United States is a serious public health problem whose extent cannot be accurately described and whose outcomes are not well known."[9] Thus, drug misadventuring can be described as an iceberg—what we don't know is submerged below the waterline. Unfortunately, what we do know is that drug misadventures are the single most frequent and deadliest cause of adverse medical events.

The mechanisms of drug misadventures include inherent adverse drug reactions (ADRs) and medication errors. Some experts believe allergic drug reactions and harm from drug-drug interactions are an ADR. The clinical outcomes from drug misadventures range from mild discomfort to death, and are annoying, inconvenient, and costly. Unlike side effects, these mechanisms are always unexpected and unwanted. Side effects are mild, expected nuisances associated with the drug that are known based on the pharmacology of the drug, and experienced by many people taking the drug.

How Big a Problem Are Drug Misadventures?

Drug misadventuring is widespread and is a serious problem. Yet the problem is largely unknown by the public and has been denied or not recognized by many health care workers. This all changed in 1999 when the Institute of Medicine (IOM)—a part of the U.S. National Academy of Sciences—produced an attention-grabbing, 300-plus page report titled *To Err Is Human: Building a Safer Health System.*[10] Few publications have received such lasting attention by the media and within the health professions. This report dealt with the extent of medical errors in the United States.

The IOM report noted that adverse medical events resulted in 2.9 to 3.7 percent of all hospitalizations and that this resulted in more than 33 million admissions to hospitals in 1997. The report estimated that 44,000 to 98,000 Americans die each year because of medical errors (at least 7,000 from medication error), and that this may be the eighth leading cause of death in the United States. The estimated cost for these tragic events was $17 to $29 billion a year.

The IOM expert panel for this report quoted one study that "found that two out of every 100 hospital admissions experienced a preventable ADE, resulting in an average increased hospital cost of $4,700 for an admission or about $2.8 million yearly for a 700-bed teaching hospital." The IOM figures are "a very modest estimate of the magnitude of the problem since hospital patients represent only a small proportion of the total population at risk, and direct hospital costs are only a fraction of total costs."[10]

In 1995, researchers at the University of Arizona, using a cost-of-illness model, estimated the cost of drug-related morbidity and mortality resulting from drug-related problems (DRPs) in the ambulatory setting at $76.6 billion yearly.[11] This model was subsequently updated to estimate that in 2000, the cost of drug-related morbidity and mortality in the ambulatory environment was $177.4 billion.[12]

The IOM was amazed by the silence on this important public health issue, stating, "For the most part, consumers believe they are protected. Media coverage has been limited to reporting of anecdotal cases."[10] The IOM also went on to state that these medical errors occur as a result of a decentralized and fragmented health care delivery system, and, some health providers believe, the medical liability system is a serious impediment to systematic efforts to uncover and learn from errors.

The response to the IOM report from the medical community varied. Some believe the rates of medical and medication errors are unacceptable in a medical system that promises "first to do no harm," to beliefs that the figures in the IOM report were exaggerated.[13,14] The response by the pharmacy community was muted, the response by the nursing community was almost not audible, and the response by hospital administrators was nonexistent.[15]

Although the media coverage of the report was extensive, it is difficult to judge the lasting impact on a public that often exhibits a short memory. The greatest impact and response to the IOM report was shown by the policymakers of the government and various health care agencies. Within two weeks of the report's release, the United States Congress held hearings and the president ordered a federal study to discover the feasibility of carrying out the reports recommendations.

Future Shock Is Now

The IOM report is not new news, so it is difficult to understand why the report has had such a big impact. Health care workers (doctors, nurses, and pharmacists) are well aware of how often medical and medication errors occur in the inpatient hospital environment, but are less sure of the prevalence of errors and adverse treatment effects that occur in the ambulatory (outpatient) environment.

A parade of prophets has warned about this problem for years. In 1979, Robert S. Mendelsohn, MD, in his book *Confessions of a Medical Heretic,* said "the greatest danger to your health is usually your own doctor."[16] Mendelsohn goes on to say that "drugs are now being so over-prescribed that more illnesses are being caused by their side effects—which doctors neglect to tell their patients about—than are being cured."

In 1984, Charles Medawar wrote a book titled *The Wrong Kind of Medicine?*[17] In it, he describes over 800 ineffective, or inappropriately or extravagantly prescribed drugs. Although these inferior prescribed nostrums were used in the United Kingdom, many are still used in the United States. Medawar feels these drugs were made available because the drug companies need to survive. He goes on to say the drugs are prescribed because doctors are under pressure to do so because of "clinical freedom" and a natural response to the demands on them to heal. In the United States, an inferior drug may be the only one on the formulary, or the only drug reimbursed by the patient's insurance company.

In 1985, professor Ron Stewart, of the University of Florida, authored a revealing book titled *Tragedies from Drug Therapy.*[18] Stewart presented ten examples in which drugs caused tragedies. He went on to explain why these events occurred (between 1937 and 1982) and what could be done to prevent them from occurring in the future. Unfortunately, many of Stewart's suggestions have gone unheeded.

Medawar wrote another book in 1992 titled *Power and Dependence.*[19] The subtitle of this book is *A Social Audit on the Safety of Medicines.* The book focuses on the conduct of the medical profession, government agencies, and the drug companies. He compares the extent of drug injury to the extent of injury due to car accidents. He says drug injury is often avoidable, and that "most of it can be traced to misconduct of some kind."

Worst Pills—Best Pills was published in 1999 by Sidney M. Wolfe, MD.[20] Wolfe cites 160 pills no one should use, and asks "why are these drugs available?"

THE MEDICATION USE SYSTEM

At the core of drug misadventures is a broken medication use system (MUS), or at least one that needs more support and more checks and balances. One of the problems is that the medication use system is too complex. The MUS includes: drug discovery and approval; marketing, production and distribution; and prescribing, dispensing, administration, monitoring, and treating adverse effects.

The complexity and some key problems with the MUS were first identified in 1987 in a convincing monograph by T. Donald Rucker, PhD, titled "Prescribed medications: system control or therapeutic roulette?"[21] Qualitative and quantitative evidence strongly suggest that Rucker was correct. The MUS was broken in 1987 and continues to be broken today.

Not only is the MUS too complex for a drug traveling through it, but it is also complex for the multitude of people and organizations involved in it. The MUS includes: drug manufacturers, the Food and Drug Administration, marketing and advertising agencies, drug wholesalers, doctors, pharmacists, nurses, health care students, professional licensing boards, companies making drug distribution equipment and software, hospitals, managed care organizations, home health agencies, nursing homes, buyers of health care including the government and private companies, pharmacy benefit organizations and health insurers, and, finally, the patient, who often gets lost and forgotten.

In 2003, Hepler and Segal wrote "the MUS is an interplay of issues including access, cost, and quality, complicated by drug law and health insurance provisions."[22] Furthermore, "medication use is further complicated by the interplay of clinical and personal values and the need for patients to cooperate in their own care."

If It Ain't Broke, Don't Fix It

A large part of the problem has been lack of acknowledgment that a problem exists by those who work in the health care system. Until the IOM report, it was "business as usual" (this may be a classic case of "not seeing the forest for the trees). Doctors, pharmacists, and nurses have all been trained to "first, do no harm." However, until the IOM report, safety improvements to the MUS were minimal. The following is only a small sample of "symptoms" contributing to the "diagnosis" of a broken MUS. The balance of this book will provide many other examples.

DRUG SUPPLY PROBLEMS

Approving Drugs for Use That Should Not Be Approved

The U.S. Food and Drug Administration sometimes approve drugs for use that should not be approved, such as ticrynafen (Selacryn), a diuretic and antihypertensive drug. It was approved for use and promoted in April of 1979, then removed from the market nine months later in January 1980.[18] The FDA has come under pressure as more drugs are being removed from the market for safety reasons. For example, nine drugs were withdrawn between September 1997 and June 2000 (less than four years), but only 20 were withdrawn between December 1971 and December 31, 2001 (30 years).[23] Some people feel this problem is because of pressures from the drug companies and some members of Congress to approve drugs more quickly. Other reasons given are the agency does not always follow the advice of its advisory panels, and the FDA is undermanned and underfunded.[24]

Drug Defects

Although drug companies have a high level of quality control in their manufacturing process, drug defects occur. For example, several years ago a public notice in major newspapers alerted "women who used the Nortel 7/7/7 birth control pill should closely examine 28-day packs of the contraceptive because color-coded pills may be out of order, putting users at risk of pregnancy." The company recalled 470,000 packs of pills from pharmacies.

Internet Prescriptions

Over 1,400 Web sites provide access to prescription medication. As shown on a recent episode of *The Montel Williams Show*, it is easy to buy medication without a prescription.[25] On the show, parents of a teenaged boy told how he had been able to order drugs over the Internet without prescriptions (and without their knowledge) and died.

Splitting Pills

More and more people are cutting their medication in half—some because they have to do this, and some because it saves money. A friend explains, "I am now taking Sotalol in the reduced dose of forty milligrams twice a day. Since the smallest strength available is eighty milligrams, I must cut the tablet in half." He goes on to ask—"Is this an example of prudent initial prescribing by my cardiologist to see if I can tolerate this agent?" This practice may increase the risk of non-compliance (not taking the drug) because one cannot assume 100 percent of the patients will correctly split and take the medication as indicated. If it does represent prudent prescribing, is the manufacturer refusing to produce the 40 mg tablet simply to serve corporate rather than patient purposes? Authors of one study "concluded that tablet splitting does not generally produce uniform and equal half tablet doses, and that split tablets should be evaluated using weight variation criteria before tablet splitting programs are initiated."[26] The U.S. Department of Veterans Affairs is so concerned about the potential problems with splitting tablets that it has a written policy.[27]

Counterfeit Drugs

On an episode of *The Montel Williams Show,* which aired on October 16, 2003, a guest on the program discovered that the growth hormone drug he was taking for HIV was counterfeit. How could this happen? The recent escalation of drug prices for patients in the United States and cheaper prices for the same drugs in other countries has caused patients and some Internet-based businesses to buy drugs from foreign sources.

Although importing drugs is considered illegal by the FDA, the importing of drugs by patients in the United States was $300 million in 2003.[28] The drug makers are fighting this problem for economic reasons while the FDA is fighting it because it is illegal and they can no longer guarantee the safety of the drug supply in the United States.[29]

The counterfeit drugs and packaging are so much like the real drugs and packaging that your pharmacist doesn't even know they are bogus.[30] Counterfeit drugs may have no active ingredient, have a lower dose of the real drug, or include another substance. The FDA has seen a fourfold increase in the number of counterfeiting cases since the 1990s.[31] The FDA reports that 90 percent of the drugs intercepted at the borders are potentially dangerous. They include drugs that have been withdrawn from the U.S. market, animal drugs never approved for human use, counterfeit drugs, drugs with dangerous interactions, drugs with dangerous side effects, and narcotics.[32]

In a four-part series of articles titled "U.S. Prescription Drug System Under Attack," *The Washington Post* reports that the Internet distribution of prescription medication is a "vast, unregulated shadow market" that is generating multibillions of dollars and is growing stronger.[33] This shadow market, run by criminal profiteers, unscrupulous wholesalers, rogue Internet sites, and foreign pharmacies, is exploiting gaps in state and federal regulations causing "pharmaceutical roulette" for many unsuspecting Americans. The *Post* article goes on to report "stretching from Florida to California, the Internet pipeline has left a trail of deaths, overdoses, addictions and emotionally devastated families." Examples cited include cancer patients receiving watered-down drugs, teenagers overdosing on narcotics ordered online, and AIDS clinics receiving fake HIV drugs.

The FDA's counterfeit drug task force gathers drug wholesaler "best practices" information before making recommendations for changes that might reduce the risk of counterfeit drugs entering the system.[34] The agency is also studying the use of radio frequency identification (RFI) technologies incorporated into drug products that would track the distribution of drugs and help reduce the risk of counterfeit drugs.[35]

POOR PRESCRIBING, DISPENSING, AND ADMINISTRATION OF DRUGS

Poor Prescribing

Reasons patients sometimes are prescribed the wrong drug or poor drug therapy include: poor medical school training on the proper use of drugs, overworked doctors, drug company sales representatives that overstate the value of their drugs, poor drug formularies, overuse of abbreviations, reliance on manual systems (such as writing prescriptions by hand), lack of an electronic medical record, poor monitoring once the drug is started, no linkage between pharmacy and laboratory data, and lack of decision support when prescribing. In addition is the prescribing of marginal products, which should be removed from the market.

Another area of concern is the use and misuse of drugs by older people. This will probably intensify with the rapid growth of this age group. Many drugs should not be used by the elderly. Some older people need less dosage of some drugs, and people 65 years or older need to receive more details about their drugs.[36] Also, there is the problem of the senescent drug "abuser" or "spaced-out grandma syndrome."[37] Dr. Wendell R. Lipscomb has described this problem in grand fashion.[38]

This syndrome is a collection of signs and symptoms one might expect in the youthful hippie drug experimenter of the 1960s. I have increasingly been called on to consult on cases of "spaced-out" grandmas who owe their status to the good intentions of their family doctors. Usually in their seventies, these grandmas have been overtreated for multiple conditions, e.g., arthritis, hypertension, periodic headaches, occasional sleeplessness, and mood swings. Each complaint is dealt with on a pragmatic basis of one symptom, one drug. Somehow the total effect of the therapeutic cocktail is never considered.

Another problem is the number of people prescribed painkillers who became addicted to the medication. A recent example of someone having this problem is talk radio host Rush Limbaugh who took prescribed narcotics for acute back pain.[39]

Yet another problem is the overprescribing of drugs for "unapproved (off-label) uses." There was a Web site that provided prescribers information on a vast array of "off-label" uses of drugs and assures that Medicaid will cover it. To be fair, there are some exceptions to using a few drugs for off-label purposes and the practice is not illegal. However, the prescriber needs to be careful when selecting a drug for an off-label use, have good justification, and take extra precautions.

Poor Dispensing

As with poor prescribing, the reasons for poor dispensing are multiple and include: sound-alike drug names, look-alike drug names, look-alike drug packaging, use of manual systems, not enough pharmacists, poor drug-drug interaction screening programs, limits on pharmacy technician-to-pharmacist ratios, excessively expensive automation, and not counseling patients about their medication.

Poor Administration

Some of the reasons patients receive the wrong drugs when hospitalized and in nursing homes include: a shortage of nurses, nonuse of bar coding, too much paperwork, and not enough double checks and balances. When patients are ambulatory and on their own, all sorts of problems can occur including not taking the medication as directed, or not taking it at all.

POOR PATIENT COMMUNICATION

Busy Doctors, Nurses, and Pharmacists

Patients often get lost in the shuffle and must fend for themselves in a health care system in which many doctors, nurses, and pharmacists are always in a hurry to take care of the next patient. In fact, there is a documented shortage of nurses and pharmacists. However, the problem may lie at a deeper level. Some doctors, nurses, and pharmacists don't want to talk with patients, and when they do, they often use confusing words, and can be paternalistic and condescending. Because of these problems, patients sometimes do not take their medication as prescribed, don't take it at all, or use the drugs inappropriately, ending in treatment failure or an adverse outcome.

Confusing Patient Package Inserts

Some prescription medications must be dispensed with a patient package insert (PPI) approved by the FDA. However, PPIs can be confusing to patients because of the types of words used or conflicting information. For example, the top of one PPI reads "this agent is a beta-blocker for treating an irregular heartbeat." However, at the bottom of the PPI under "side effects" it says, "check with your doctor immediately if you experience an irregular or fast heartbeat." Where is the safety when patients are given conflicting drug information?

DRUG COMPANIES' CONTRIBUTIONS
TO THE PROBLEM

Pressure to Make Prescription-Only Drugs
Over-the-Counter Drugs

The drug companies have discovered that if they convert older drugs to over-the-counter medication when the patent is about to expire, that they make more money. Yet, how safe is this practice? The FDA oversees this process and makes the drug companies jump through a series of hoops before letting the companies switch their products to OTC status. What is the safety record associated with these relaxed rules?

Compromising Safety for Profits?

A friend recently complained that as director of quality assurance for a large drug company he had only a $2 million dollar budget to control the safety and purity of product X, but the marketing department had a $20 million budget to unload the same product. Maybe the real reason for many recalls is that drug companies put their scarce budget money into promotion, and quality assurance gets what is left over.

Overdose?

Jay S. Cohen, MD, an associate professor of family and preventive medicine at the University of California in San Diego, has been a well-spoken critic of the drug companies. In his 2001 book *Overdose—The Case Against the Drug Companies,* Cohen accuses drug companies of many poor practices.[40] Some of these include poor research methods, deliberate efforts to create easy, one-size-fits-all dosages, and recommended doses that cause many side effects which could be avoided with lower, effective doses. Cohen also says "drug companies slant research, skew reported findings, hide unfavorable results, manipulate the publishing process, threaten researchers planning to publish negative findings, and spend billions [of dollars] to influence doctors." Although drug companies have produced many new and wonderful drugs and vaccines they can do better.

The Food and Drug Administration

Cohen states that the FDA approves drugs and improper dosages, and that the monitoring of newly approved drugs is inadequate.[40] The FDA has its hands full dealing with an industry that has plenty of economic and political clout. It is dealing with many heavy-duty issues such as drug counterfeiting and illegal Internet sales, and is limited in its resources by the federal budget process and the laws that give it its power.

A BROKEN PART OF A LARGER BROKEN SYSTEM

The broken MUS, however, is part of something larger that is also broken—the entire health care system. As pointed out by the IOM, "the health care system is decentralized and fragmented."[10] Many readers probably missed this key point in the report because of the many statistics about medical errors in the report.

Fortunately, the IOM authored a follow-up report.[41] In this report, the IOM called the current health system poorly organized, too complex, uncoordinated, with too many patient "hand offs" that slow down care and decrease, rather than improve, safety. "These cumbersome processes waste resources; leave unaccountable voids in coverage; lead to loss of information; and fail to build on the strengths of all health professionals involved to ensure that care is proper, timely, and safe."

An example of this broken system is a recent report that some leading hospitals have "dropped the ball" and made mistakes.[42] Children's Hospital of Boston, a Harvard-affiliated teaching hospital, was sharply criticized for its handling of four cases in which patients died. In one case, a five-year-old boy having an epileptic seizure died after the doctors treating him thought someone else was in charge. In another case, at Duke University Medical Center in North Carolina, a 17-year old young woman died after a transplant operation in February after she was given the organs that did not match her blood type.

As with drug misadventures, critics have cited this problem for a long time. One recent example is Michael L. Millenson. Although Millenson is not a health care provider, he does a scholarly job of describing a health care system in disarray in his book titled *Demanding*

Medical Excellence.[43] This book, published before the first IOM report, describes common examples to show the serious flaws in contemporary medical practice. His suggestions for improvement are useful.

More recently, Donald M. Berwick, MD, a respected authority on health care and the founder, president, and CEO of the Institute for Healthcare Improvement, provided an extraordinary address at the 11th Annual National Forum on Quality Improvement in Health Care.[44] The title of the address was "Escape Fire." In it, he describes the health care system on the verge of its own conflagration. Berwick describes the failings of the health care system in treating his wife for a serious illness. "Only by abandoning many of the traditional tools of health care delivery, only by opening the system to the patients it serves and creating a standard of excellence . . . will the health care system be transformed."

SUMMARY

Medication safety is a major public health problem, and it qualifies as America's "other" drug problem. Drug misadventures in the form of adverse reactions, drug interaction, allergic reactions, and medication errors cause harm, are costly, and lessen patient satisfaction and faith in the health care system. Recent problems with counterfeit drugs and ready access to drugs via the Internet provide cogent examples of why our current drug market may be unsafe.

In some respects, we have not made much progress from the days of patent medicines and caveat emptor. Counterfeit drugs provided via Internet Web sites are modern-day surrogates for the secret remedies described in 1909 by the British Medical Association, and by Cook in 1957.[45,46] Unfortunately, much of the public is unaware of the problem.

The examples of drug misadventuring in this chapter are the tip of an iceberg. Many examples will follow. Because of the sub-rosa nature of many of these problems, and the resulting consumption of health services, much of the social cost lies below the threshold of understanding, thus the true scope of the problem is difficult to discover. The economist might say the implicit dimensions of the problem could easily outweigh the explicit perception. The etiology of the medication safety issue lies within a broken health care system.

Since the IOM rang the bell in 1999 about medical errors, there has been a flurry of activity to improve medication safety. We now know more than we did before the IOM report, however, great strides are yet to be made to reduce death and injury from medication.[47]

The following relevant questions remain: (1) What are the major constraints that have weakened the efforts of health professionals to minimize medication safety problems? and (2) What social pressures can be applied to help make control possible? These questions and other related issues are explored in the following chapters.

Chapter 2

The Nature and Scope
of the Medication Safety Problem

The first chapter discussed the problem of drug misadventuring. This chapter defines the nature and scope of the problem.

THE NATURE OF THE PROBLEM

Every drug has the potential for problems associated with its use. That is why the FDA approves drugs as "generally safe and effective in most patients." This implies the drug may not be 100 percent safe or 100 percent effective in all patients. If the benefits of a drug outweigh its risks, the drug receives approval.

Adverse drug reactions (ADRs) happen because of something inherent in the drug, something inherent in the patient (the host), or a combination of factors between the drug and the host. The FDA requires study of a drug by its manufacturer before it is approved for use. However, the number of patients receiving the drug before it is FDA approved may be no more than a few thousand people.[1] Once the drug is approved for use, it is used by thousands of culturally diverse patients of all ages and by a much broader group than in the pre-approval trials. Thus, it is common for problems, not known to the drug's manufacturer and the FDA, to occur after the drug is approved.

Another variable the FDA cannot control is how the drug will be used in practice. The FDA recommends how the drug should be used through its requirements for labeling (a term used to describe what

Prescribed Medications and the Public Health
© 2006 by The Haworth Press, Inc. All rights reserved.
doi:10.1300/5688_02

the FDA requires in a drug's package insert). Although this allows doctors flexibility in treating patients, it also allows prescribing the drug for *off-label* uses that may be unproven or unsafe. A regulation cannot prevent a doctor from ordering the wrong dose of a drug, the wrong drug, two drugs that interact causing one drug to act more prominently, or ordering a drug when the patient has pointed out that he or she is allergic to that drug or class of drugs.

What Can Go Wrong

When something goes wrong with a drug, the event is called a "drug misadventure" or an adverse drug event (ADE). A drug misadventure, or an iatrogenic hazard or incident occurs because:

- there is an inherent risk when drug therapy is indicated
- the omission or commission by administering a drug or drugs during which a patient is harmed, with effects ranging from mild discomfort to fatality
- the outcome may be independent of preexisting pathology or disease process
- there is error (human or system, or both), immunological response, or idiosyncratic response
- it is always unexpected and thus unacceptable to patient and prescriber[2]

The risks of using drugs include inherent adverse effects, product quality defects, and not using the drug correctly, all of which can result in an ADE. In 2002, the FDA recalled 354 prescription drug products and 83 over-the-counter (OTC) drug products because of problems in the manufacturing or distribution.[3]

The mechanisms and relationships of ADEs to one another are shown in Figure 2.1. Some ADRs and errors cause no harm and thus are potential ADEs. Some ADRs and errors cause harm and thus are ADEs. Some ADEs are preventable and some are not. Some experts feel some ADRs, all medication errors, all known drug interactions, and drug misadventures from known drug allergies are preventable (the latter is also probably an error). Some ADRs, drug allergies unknown to the patient, and unknown drug interactions (for newly approved drugs) are not preventable.

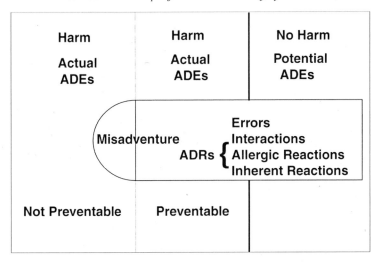

FIGURE 2.1. ADE Mechanisms and Relationships

Case Examples

The following cases will help clarify some of the definitions used previously.

Case 1: A Side Effect

Carol Smith, a 16-year-old high school student, has been waking up lately with a "raw throat," she has been sneezing, and her eyes have been watering a lot. She sees her family doctor and is diagnosed with seasonal allergies. Her doctor prescribes an antihistamine. After taking several doses, Carol notices the medication makes her drowsy and gives her a dry mouth.

Case 2: An Adverse Drug Reaction

Doug Jones, a 54-year-old salesperson, recently experienced a myocardial infarction (heart attack). To prevent a second heart attack, his doctor recommends that Doug take one baby aspirin every day. Doug doesn't hear the part about "baby" and takes one adult aspirin every day for a week. He notices that his gums bleed a lot after he brushes his teeth. After two weeks of taking the aspirin, Doug notices he has black, tarry stools. In a follow-up visit, his doctor tells him to stop taking the aspirin as it is causing gastrointestinal bleeding. Doug says, "is taking one adult aspirin too much?" This was a case of an ADR and an error.

Case 3: A Drug Interaction

Dorothy McKane is the 35-year-old mother of Stacey (seven years old) and Billy (three years old). Dorothy has had asthma for ten years and takes theophylline prescribed by her pulmonary doctor to help her breathe better. She develops what she thinks is a bad cold and goes to see her family doctor. Dorothy is diagnosed as having an upper respiratory infection. Her family doctor prescribes an antibiotic called erythromycin. Because she is in a hurry, Dorothy goes to the pharmacy next to the doctor's office rather than to her regular pharmacy. After taking the erythromycin for three days, Dorothy has nausea and vomiting and feels like she has an irregular heartbeat. She returns to her family doctor who takes a blood sample. The test shows that Dorothy has theophylline toxicity due to an interaction between the theophylline and the erythromycin.

Case 4: An Allergic Drug Reaction

Sam Ellis is a 24-year-old college student who is allergic to penicillin. Sam knows this because his grandmother, who cared for Sam when he was a child, told him that he got a bad rash when he was seven years old when he was given a penicillin shot. Sam goes to the health clinic at his college because he has a sore ear and a fever. The doctor examines Sam, discovers an ear infection, and prescribes ampicillin. Sam does not think that this is penicillin and takes the prescription to a pharmacy. When paying for the prescription, Sam asks the clerk (a high school student) whether his prescription is penicillin. The clerk says, "I don't think so." Sam goes home and takes the first dose of medication. Within an hour, Sam gets a red, itchy rash on his arms and trunk.

Case 5: A Medication Error

Julie Parsons is a 62-year-old secretary for a law firm. Julie has trouble sleeping because of leg cramps. She goes to her family doctor who prescribes quinine. Julie goes to her neighborhood pharmacy and has the prescription filled. After several days of taking the medication, Julie is still having leg cramps at night, and now feels like her heart is skipping beats and she feels terrible. She returns to her doctor with her medication container and tells the doctor "this stuff is hurting me more than helping me." The doctor looks at the medication container and sees that it is labeled quinidine rather than quinine.

THE SCOPE OF THE PROBLEM

ADEs happen in various environments including hospitals, long-term care facilities, and in patients' homes. Someone experiencing an ADE tries to suffer though it, sees the doctor, or goes to an emergency room. There have been several studies to discover how often ADEs occur (see Table 2.1).

ADEs in Hospitals

Two studies using statewide samples provide some of the best evidence of ADEs in hospitals. In a study of Colorado and Utah, the ADE rates for every 100 patients admitted to a hospital was 0.56.[4] A similar study performed in New York found a rate of 0.72.[5] Other studies with less restrictive definitions of adverse drug events found rates of 2.4 to 6.5 ADEs for every 100 patients.[6,7] However, the Government Accounting Office (GAO), in a report to Congress, cautions that the true extent of the health risk with adverse drug events is uncertain because of the limited amount of incidence data.[8]

Emergency Room Visits Because of ADEs

Several studies have been conducted to discover the number of emergency room (ER) visits because of ADEs. In 1996, a study was performed in the ER of a 560-bed hospital.[9] During one month, 3.9 percent of patient visits to the ER were associated with a drug-related illness. Counting only those patients who were taking medication before the ER visit, 8.6 percent visited the ER for a drug-related illness. Reasons for the drug-related illnesses included not taking the drug as prescribed (58 percent), inappropriate prescribing (32 percent), and ADRs (10 percent). Sixteen percent (16 percent) of these patients were hospitalized because of an ADE. In another study, 1.7 percent of patients were in the ER because of an ADE, and of these, 14.1 percent resulted in admission to the hospital.[10] A study in 2002 showed that as many as 28 percent of all emergency room visits were drug-related.[11] Of these, 70 percent were probably preventable, and 24 percent resulted in hospitalization.

TABLE 2.1. The Prevalence and Preventability of Drug-Related Illness by Setting

Setting	Drug-Related Illness	Prevalence	Preventable
While in hospital	ADEs[a,b]	0.6-0.73/100 admissions	NR
	ADEs[c,d]	2.4-6.5/100 admissions	26-76%
	ADEs[e]	1 in 20 treatments	NR
	ADEs[f]	10/1000 patients days	26%
	Potential ADEs[d]	5.5/100 admissions	100%
ICUs	ADEs[f]	19/1000 patient days	27%
Emergency room visits	ADEs[g,h,i]	1.7- 3.9%	66%
	Drug-related visits[j]	28%	70%
Hospitalization	ADEs[h]	14.1-16%	NR
	Drug toxicity[e]	3% of admissions	NR
Nursing homes	ADEs[k]	1.9/resident months	NR
	Potential ADEs[k]	0.7/resident months	100%

Note: Potential ADEs while in hospital were intercepted before patient was harmed; NR = not reported.

[a] Thomas EJ, Studdet DM. Newhouse JP, Peterson LA, Small SD, Servi D, Laffel G, Sweitzer BJ, Shea BF, Hallisey R, et al. (2000). Incidence and types of adverse events and negligent care in Utah and Colorado. *Med Care* 38:261-271.

[b] Brennan TA, Leape LL, Laird NM, Hebert L, Localio AR, Lawthers AG, Newhouse JP, Weiler PC, and Hiatt HH. (1991). Incidence of adverse events and negligence in hospitalized patients: results of the Harvard Medical Practice Study 1. *N Engl J Med* 324(6):370-376.

[c] Classen DC, Pestotnik SL, Evans RS, Lloyd JF and Burke, JP. (1997). Adverse drug events in hospitalized patients. Excess length of stay, extra costs, and attributable mortality. *JAMA* 277(4):341-342.

[d] Bates DW, Cullen DJ, Laird N, Peterson LA, Small SD, Servi D, Laffel G, Sweitzer BJ, Shea BF, Hallsey R, et. al. (1995). Incidence of adverse drug events and potential adverse drug events. *JAMA* 274(1):29-34.

[e] Jick H. (1984). Adverse drug reactions: the magnitude of the problem. *J Allergy and Clin. Immunology* 74:555-557.

[f] Cullen DJ, Sweitzer BJ, Bates DW, Burdick E, Edmonson A, and Leape LL. (1997). Preventable adverse drug events in hospitalized patients: A comparable study of intensive care and general care units. *Crit Care Med* 25(8):1289-1297.

[g] Dennehy CE, Kishi DT, and Louie C. (1996). Drug-related illness in emergency department patients. *Am J Health-Syst Pharm* 53:1422-1426.

[h] Schneitman-McIntire O, Farnen TA, Gordon N, Chan J, and Toy WA. (1996). Medication misadventures resulting in emergency department visits at an HMO medical center. *Am J Health-Syst Pharm* 53:1416-1422.

[i] Hafner JW, Belknap SM, Squillante MD, and Bucheit KA. (2002). Adverse drug events in emergency department patients. *Ann Emergency Med* 39(3):258-267.

[j] Patel P, and Zed PJ. (2002). Drug-related visits to the emergency department: how big is the problem? *Pharmacotherapy* 22:915-923.

[k] Gurwitz J, Field S, Avorn J, McCormick D, Jain S, Eckler M, Benser M, Edmondson A, and Bates DW. (2000). Incidence and preventability of adverse drug events in nursing homes *Am J Med* 109:87-94.

ADEs in Nursing Home Patients

In 2000, Gurwitz and colleagues reported the most comprehensive study of ADEs in nursing homes to date.[12] The incidence of ADEs was 1.9 for each resident month.

ADEs in Older Adults

For various reasons (further explored in Chapter 14), adults 65 years old and older experience more ADEs than those in any other age group. For example, a 2003 study found that the incidence rate of preventable drug-related morbidity in Medicare enrollees in a hospital-based health care plan in Florida was 28.8/1,000 enrollees.[13] Rothschild and Leape explore this issue.[14]

ADEs in ambulatory patients are covered in Chapter 9.

ADEs in Other Settings

People may be getting harmed in other settings by the legitimate use of medication, but there are little or no data. Examples include: poison control centers, free clinics, military bases, school health programs, social service agencies, employer-sponsored health clinics, public health clinics, prisons (federal/state/local), HMO clinics that run without claim forms, and patients buying medications from Canada.

ADVERSE DRUG EVENT SEVERITY

In 1974 a well-known pharmacoepidemiologist (Jick) wrote an article titled "Drugs—Remarkably Nontoxic."[15] Jick stated, "the rates and severity of adverse reactions to individual drugs are remarkably low in view of their pharmacologic properties." He went on to say that "the high prevalence of drug-induced morbidity and mortality mainly reflects extensive drug use rather than the intrinsic toxic potential of particular drugs." During the next ten years, more quantitative information on the adverse effects of drugs increased. In 1984, Jick stated, "about 10 percent of adverse [drug] reactions are regarded as life-threatening" and "virtually all organ systems have been involved with adverse drug effects."[16]

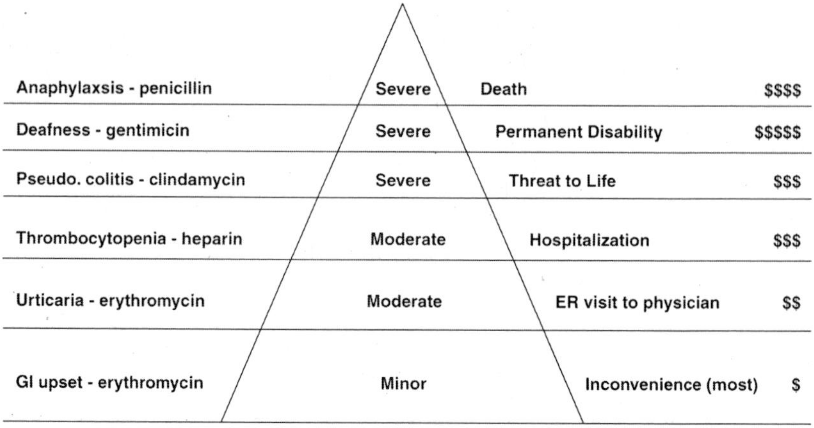

Anaphylaxsis - penicillin	Severe	Death	$$$$
Deafness - gentimicin	Severe	Permanent Disability	$$$$$
Pseudo. colitis - clindamycin	Severe	Threat to Life	$$$
Thrombocytopenia - heparin	Moderate	Hospitalization	$$$
Urticaria - erythromycin	Moderate	ER visit to physician	$$
GI upset - erythromycin	Minor	Inconvenience (most)	$

FIGURE 2.2. The Range, Severity, Consequences, and Cost of ADEs

As shown in Figure 2.2, the severity of ADEs varies from minor to severe, and the effects vary from inconvenience to death. Hafner and colleagues reported that patients with ADEs in emergency rooms most commonly had hypoglycemia, bleeding, or a rash from the drugs they were taking.[17] Bates and colleagues reported in their hospital study that 1 percent of ADEs were fatal, 12 percent were life-threatening, 30 percent were serious, and 57 percent were significant.[7] These investigators also found that the rate of ADEs was highest in medical ICUs, followed by surgical general care units, then medical general care units, and was lowest in surgical ICUs after adjustments for the number of drugs used. Classen and colleagues reported the extra stay for patients in the hospital because of ADEs was 1.74 days.[6]

Drug-Induced Death

The incidence of death because of the legitimate use of drugs is illusive and a matter of debate. Estimates have been as high as 140,000 and as low as 7,000 people a year in the United States.[18] However, these estimates have been extrapolated from poorly designed studies or from studies of medical inpatients prescribed more drugs than other inpatients, far more than ambulatory patients. A well-designed study is yet to be performed to discover the true incidence of drug-induced death. The problems in discovering an accurate incidence rate for drug-induced death are well described.[18]

Although drug-induced fatal ADEs are rare, they are tragic if they happen to a family member, a friend, or someone you love. A comprehensive description is available of over 447 published case reports of fatal ADEs published over a 20-year period.[19] Many of the suspected drugs could have been monitored with blood level tests but were not. The most common ADEs were hepatitis, hepatic failure, cardiopulmonary arrests, and overdose. The author estimates that 68 percent of these cases could have been prevented.

Drug-Induced Threats to Life

Less rare than death is when someone experiences a life-threatening reaction because of measures applied to save his or her life.[20] A study in 2001 described 846 case reports published over a 20-year period. As with drug-induced fatalities, many of the drugs incriminated could have been monitored by blood tests, but were not. Half of the drug-induced events were judged preventable.

Drug-Induced Permanent Disability

Drugs can also damage vital organs. According to one report, the most common drug-induced permanent disabilities are brain damage, blindness, tardive dyskinesia, deafness, quadriplegia, and hearing loss.[21] The disabling effects of some medications may be subtle, and some elderly patients are more sensitive to the effects of drugs such as sedatives and tranquilizers. One study found that 15 percent of patients ages 25 to 75 living at home were restricted in one or more areas of their lives, and that some of the disabling symptoms in these patients were similar to the adverse effects of drugs.[22]

COST OF THE PROBLEM

Extra medical expenses are incurred anytime someone experiences a harmful ADE. For example, the mean cost of ADE visits to an emergency room in a 2002 study was $1,764 versus $1,133 for a non-

ADE visit.[17] One 2001 study found the hospital admission cost $6,685.[23] Patients experiencing an ADE after being hospitalized increased costs $2,162 to $3,244.[6,23,24] Moore and colleagues estimate that 5 to 9 percent of hospital costs are related to adverse drug reactions (ADRs).[25] One study in nursing homes ended with a shocking statement that "for every dollar spent on drugs in nursing facilities, $1.33 in health care resources are consumed in treating drug-related problems."[26]

The total annual cost of drug-related morbidity and mortality in the ambulatory environment was first estimated to be $76.6 billion in 1995 by Johnson and Bootman.[27] Five years later (2000), their cost estimate was revised to exceed $177.4 billion.[28]

Patients sometimes bring lawsuits against hospitals, care givers, and drug companies when they feel there is negligence or a product defect associated with the harm they received from a drug. A recent series of studies showed that between the mid-1970s and the mid-1990s, the average settlement or judgment for a drug-induced fatality case was $1.1 million (range of $35,000 to $9 million); for a case of drug-induced life threats, $1.2 million (range of $32,000 to $8 million); and for cases of drug-induced permanent disability, $4.3 million (range $20,000 to $127 million).[19,20,21]

DRUGS COMMONLY ASSOCIATED WITH ADVERSE DRUG EVENTS

Most drugs have side effects, and many have the potential to cause an ADE. However, some drugs cause more ADEs than others. The drugs commonly associated with ADEs are shown in Table 2.2. The classes of drugs that produce the most ADEs are: pain relievers, antibiotics (and other microbial drugs), cardiovascular agents, cancer drugs, and anticoagulants. Individual agents identified in most ADE studies include: insulin, warfarin, phenytoin, digoxin, morphine, trimethoprim-sulfamethoxazole, theophylline, methotrexate, and valproic acid. ADE drugs may differ by setting because each setting uses a different mix of drugs to treat patients. Whether a drug is commonly associated with an ADE is a factor of a drug's potential toxicity, how often it is used, how much it used, and patient risk factors.

TABLE 2.2. Drugs Commonly Associated with ADEs by Setting

Emergency Room Patients	Hospitalized Patients	Nursing Home Patients	Patients in all Settings
1996[a] (n = 50)	1995[b] (n = 247)	2000[c] (n = 546)	2001[d] (n = 1520)
albuterol (asthma)	pain relievers	antipsychotics	methotrexate (cancer)
insulin (diabetes)	antibiotics	antibiotics	heparin (clotting)
warfarin (clotting)	sleeping pills	antidepressants	trimethoprim-sulfa
phenytoin (seizures)	cancer drugs	sedatives/hypnotics	methoxazole (infection)
prendisone (steroid)	cardiac drugs	anticlotting drugs	valproic acid (seizures)
			phenytoin (seizures)
			trimethoprim-sulfamethoxazole
			oxycodone-acetaminophen
1996[e] (n = 1074)	1997[f] (n = 2227)		
trimethoprim-sulfa	morphine (pain)		
methoxazole (infection)	digoxin (heart)		
erythromycin (infection)	meperidine (pain)		
proclorperazine (nausea)	oxycodone-acetamophen (pain)		
theophylline (asthma)	impenem (infection)		
aspirin (pain)			
2002[g] (n = 338)	1997[h] (n = 264)		
insulin (diabetes)	antibiotics		
warfarin (clotting)	pain relievers		
furosemide (fluid)	electrolyte conc.		
chemotherapy (cancer)	peptic ulcer drugs		
digoxin (heart)	cardiac drugs		
	2001[i] (n = 155)		
	antimicrobials		
	antipsychotics		
	narcotics		
	antidepressants		
	anticlotting drugs		

[a] Dennehy CE, Kishi DT, and Louie C. (1996). Drug-related illness in emergency department patients. *Am J Health-Syst Pharm* 53:1422-1426.

[b] Bates DW, Cullen DJ, Laird N, Peterson LA, Small SD, Servi D, Laffel G, Sweitzer BJ, Shea BF, Hallsey R, et al. (1995). Incidence of adverse drug events and potential adverse drug events. *JAMA* 274(1):29-34.

[c] Gurwitz J, Field S, Avorn J, McCormick D, Jain S, Eckler M, Benser M, Edmondson A, and Bates DW. (2000). Incidence and preventability of adverse drug events in nursing homes. *Am J Med* 109:87-94.

[d] Kelly WN. (2001). Potential risks and prevention, part 1: Fatal adverse drug events. *Am J Health-Sys Pharm* 58(14):1317-1324.

[e] Schneitman-McIntire O, Farnen TA, Gordon N, Chan J and Toy WA. (1996). Medication misadventures resulting in emergency department visits at an HMO medical center. *Am J Health-Syst Pharm* 53:1416-1422.

[f] Classen DC, Pestotnik SL, Evans RS, Lloyd JF and Burke JD. (1997). Adverse drug events in hospitalized patients. Excess length of stay, extra costs, and attributable mortality. *JAMA* 277(4):341-342.

[g] Patel P and Zed PJ. (2002). Drug-related visits to the emergency department: how big is the problem? *Pharmacotherapy* 22:915-923.

[h] Cullen DJ, Sweitzer BJ, Bates DW, Burdick E, Edmondson A and Leape LL. (1997). Preventable adverse drug events in hospitalized patients: A comparable study of intensive care and general care units. *Crit Care Med* 25(8):1289-1297.

[i] Senst BL, Achusim LE, Genest RP, Cosentino LA, Ford CC, Little JA, Raybon SJ and Bates DW. (2001). Practical approach to determining costs and frequency of adverse drug events in a health care network. *Am J Health-Sys Pharm* 58:1126-1132.

Drugs and Lethal ADEs

Several studies have listed drugs where it was more likely than not that a drug was associated with a death. The most common drug categories in one hospital study and incident ADR rates were: antitumor drugs (0.18 percent), anticlotting drugs (0.036 percent), diabetic drugs (0.032 percent), steroids (0.017 percent), pain relievers (0.013 percent), cardiac glycosides (0.006 percent), sleeping pills (0.002 percent), and antibacterial and antiviral agents (0.001 percent).[29] Another study reviewed 447 published case reports of fatal ADEs from 1976 to 1995.[19] The most common drugs thought to be responsible for these fatal events were: valproic acid, cyclophosphamide, bleomycin, trimethoprim-sulfamethoxazole, and diatrizoate.

Drugs and Life Threats

The drugs most commonly reported in 846 published case reports of drug-induced threats to life from 1978 to 1997 were: heparin, methotrexate, vancomycin, phenytoin, and cyclosporine.[20]

Drugs and Permanent Disability

The drugs most commonly reported in 227 published case reports of drug-induced permanent disability from 1977 to 1997 were: diphtheria, tetanus toxoid, and pertussis vaccine, theophylline, gentimicin, cisplatin, and methothrexate.[21]

SUMMARY

Drugs represent a double-edged sword—mostly they help, but sometimes they harm. Drugs can harm due to their inherent toxicity or because they are poorly prescribed, dispensed, or administered. The mechanisms of the harm are adverse drug reactions, allergic drug reactions, drug interactions, or medication errors. These harmful drug misadventures occur in all settings and the severity ranges from inconvenience, moderate distress, permanent disability, threat to life, or death.

Chapter 3

How Medication Harms Patients

Drug misadventures happen for a reason. Sometimes they occur because of a drug, sometimes because of a patient, and sometimes because of an interaction between a drug and a patient. Sometimes they happen for no reason at all. Some drug misadventures are preventable while others are not. This chapter will explore the reasons for adverse drug events (ADEs) and how they sometimes can be prevented.

PATIENT FACTORS THAT CONTRIBUTE TO ADVERSE DRUG EVENTS

Physiologic Factors

Patient factors can cause ADEs. One is age. Children under the age of two years old and those 65 years and older are more vulnerable to the negative effects of drugs. The young, such as newborns and neonates, have immature organs that are important in detoxifying (mainly the liver) and removing (mainly the kidney) drugs from the body.

Decreased Capacity to Detoxify and Eliminate Drugs

As people age, their liver and kidneys slow down. If the liver is unable to metabolize certain drugs, they build up in the system, even when usual doses of the medication are given. The dose needs to be reduced or given less often. The same is true of the kidneys, the organs that eliminate drugs from the body. If the usual dose of the drug is not reduced, and the kidneys are not eliminating the drugs, the drug

Prescribed Medications and the Public Health
© 2006 by The Haworth Press, Inc. All rights reserved.
doi:10.1300/5688_03

can build up in the system and become toxic. It is not unusual for kidney function to be reduced by 50 percent by age 75.[1] Drugs that build up in the system are usually toxic to a certain organ, for example the eyes, ears, heart, lungs, kidneys, and liver.

To prevent drug toxicity, patients taking drugs chiefly detoxified by the liver or removed by the kidneys and known to cause problems, need to have their liver and renal function checked before these drugs are prescribed. If these drugs are taken regularly, then liver and kidney function tests need to be done routinely.

Altered Drug Absorption

The drug absorption function can be altered in an aging patient. Because of reduced gastric acidity, drugs spend increased time in the stomach, or reduced intestinal blood flow can also be present. Thus, the rate and extent of drug absorption into the blood can be altered.

Altered Drug Distribution

Some drugs distribute to lean body tissue, whereas others distribute to fat. As a person ages, there is less lean body mass and more fatty tissue. There is also less total body water and less serum albumin. Using normal adult doses without considering lean body mass and total body water can result in too much or too little drug being sent to the site of action.

Increased Sensitivity to the Harmful Effects of Drugs

Some believe elderly patients are more susceptible to the effects of drugs, while others believe this sensitivity may be because older patients take more medication. Evidence suggests that older patients are more susceptible to the drugs that affect the central nervous system such as analgesics, tranquilizers, and antidepressants. The following drugs should not be used in the elderly.[2]

> *Antihistamines*
>> Blood products/modifiers/volume expanders
>> Platelet aggregation inhibitors
> *Cardiovascular agents*
>> Antihypertensives

    Peripheral vasodilators
    Antiarrhythmics
Central nervous system agents
    Narcotics
    Sedatives and hypnotics
    Antidepressants
Gastric Agents
    Antiemetics
    Anticholinergics/antispasmodics
    Antidiarrheas
Genitourinary Agents
    Antispasmodics
Hormones/Synthetic/Modifiers
    Hypoglycemic agents
Musculoskeletal Agents
    Nonsalicylate nonsteroidal anti-inflammatory drugs
    Skeletal muscle relaxants (modified with permission)

Functional Decline

Other risk factors for ADE are an increased severity of illness, and functional decline such as confusion, incontinence, loss of appetite, and a tendency to fall.

Gender Differences

More ADEs are reported in females than males. Although some suspect hormones as the cause of this difference, the true reason is unknown.

Patient Understanding and Active Involvement

Patients who do not understand or do not want to understand their drug therapy are more likely to experience problems with the use of their medication. On the other hand, the more patients know about their drugs—what they are, how they are to be taken, and what may go wrong—the more likely they are to avoid an ADE. Questions patients should ask their doctor or pharmacist are:

1. What is the name of this drug?
2. Why am I taking it?
3. How do I take it?
4. What should I expect?
5. How long should I take it?
6. How will I know if it is working?
7. What common negative effects does this drug cause?
8. What should I do if I think I am experiencing an adverse effect?

DRUG FACTORS THAT CONTRIBUTE
TO ADVERSE DRUG EVENTS

Problems with the Drugs Themselves

Various problems are directly related to the drug product.

Adverse Effects

Some adverse effects happen based on a drug's pharmacology and are dose related—the higher the dose, the more pronounced the effect. An example would be the use of morphine. In smaller doses, the drug achieves pain relief, but in higher doses the drug reduces respiration, and can eventually stop a person from breathing. These effects are dose related and preventable, and can be controlled by not using the drug in certain types of patients or conditions, customizing the dose, and carefully monitoring the patient.

Other adverse drug reactions have no correlation with the drug's pharmacology and are not dose related. These drug reactions are classified as "bizarre," or "idiosyncratic." An example would be taking dimenhydramine (a common antihistamine) and having one's hair turn green.

The Drug Should Not Have Been Approved
in the First Place

Some ADEs occur because the drug should never have been approved for use. The reasons for approving drugs that should not have been approved are poorly understood and require further investigation. Between September 1997 and April 2000, the FDA withdrew nine drugs from the market. Columnist Thomas J. Moore reported, "In March [2000], the FDA withdrew Rezulin after it was implicated in 63 reported deaths and 27 cases of life-threatening disability caused by liver damage."[3] Moore goes on to say "two days later, the agency withdrew the heartburn drug Propulsid after 80 deaths from cardiac arrest and 347 life-threatening cardiac emergencies."

When the Public Citizen Health Research Group polled FDA medical officers who perform the reviews of new drug applications, 34 said, "the pressure to approve new drugs had increased since 1995, and 19 officers named specific drugs they believed should not have been approved."[3]

Manufacturing Defects

Drug products can occasionally have manufacturing problems such as physical defects, product malfunctions, inaccurate or incomplete product labeling, foreign objects or materials in the product or container, and therapeutic failure or subpotency.[4] Fortunately, these problems are rare. The United States Pharmacopeia (USP), the organization in the United States that sets drug standards, has an active system for reporting drug product defects.

Overpromotion

Overpromotion of drug products by manufacturers is a way of life. The drug industry spends millions of dollars to influence doctors through journal advertising. Drug salespeople will do most anything to have their product used. They influence consumers through direct-to-consumer advertising on television and in magazines. The FDA should be the first line of defense against overpromotion of prescription drug products, "but asking the FDA to rein in the pharmaceutical industry is a bit like sending someone out to catch Niagara Falls in a bucket."[5]

Poor Research Methods

Jay S. Cohen, MD, has accused the pharmaceutical industry of poor research methods and deliberate efforts to make easy, one-size-fits-all dosages.[6] Cohen goes on to say that many drugs approved by the FDA have recommended doses higher than needed. These higher doses cause more ADEs.

Generic Drugs

Although generic drugs are less expensive than brand-name drug products, some feel that these drugs are not as effective or as safe as brand-name products. However, the adverse drug reaction rates for brand-name and generic equivalents are not different.[7]

OTC Drugs

Over 100,000 over-the-counter (OTC) products include more than 800 active ingredients and cover more than 100 therapeutic categories of drugs.[8] The biggest question about the use of OTC drug products has been whether they work. Although some OTC products may relieve some symptoms, they can mask symptoms of a disease that needs diagnosis and definitive treatment.

Under the FDA's working regulations, drugs that can be used safely and effectively without professional guidance may be sold OTC. These drugs gain approval under provisions of the OTC Drug Review or are approved to switch from a prescription drug to an OTC drug. The FDA has standards for the effectiveness, labeling, and safety of OTCs. Safety means a low incidence of adverse reactions or a low number of significant side effects under satisfactory directions for use. OTC products can be toxic, depending on the age of the patient, dosage, duration, what acute and chronic diseases are present, and other drugs the patient may be taking.

Many OTC products contain multiple substances that are used in a "shotgun" approach, that is, hoping that one of the ingredients help. For example, many OTC cold preparations contain decongestants, cough suppressants, antihistamines, and an analgesic. Some OTC products contain substances that work against one another. Common cold preparations often contain ephedrine or pseudoephedrine to reduce nasal congestion. These substances can cause central nervous system (CNS) stimulation, hypertension, and an increased heart rate. Phenylpropanolamine, another nasal decongestant in some OTC preparations, can cause slowing of the heart. Case reports show toxicity and death when some of these cough and cold preparations have been used in children.[9]

When changing prescription-only drugs to OTC drugs, the FDA considers safety, effectiveness, the benefit-to-risk ratio, and whether understandable labeling can be written for the use of the drug without medical supervision. However, these changes have become more frequent. A recent switch of an prescription-only antihistamine to OTC status was promoted and welcomed by the insurance industry. Such a move shifts the burden of payment from the insurance company to the patient.

The FDA is systematically reviewing the active ingredients in OTC products and has put in place national uniformity guidelines for labeling. However, there is no formal monitoring of safety once a prescription drug switches to OTC status.

Another concern is the unsupervised nature of OTC use—patients are left to fend for themselves. Doctors and pharmacists rarely ask patients about their use of OTCs and patients often do not perceive OTCs as medications. Go into any pharmacy and you will see people wandering up and down the OTC aisles looking for something that will help them with some ailment. They pick up bottles and read labels, but most are not sure what is best, and they may choose the wrong product. Pharmacists, often only a few feet away, are busy behind the prescription counter, oblivious to patients who need help with OTC selection and counseling.

Pharmacists are well trained to help decide if an OTC is what is needed or whether the condition needs to be diagnosed by a doctor. They also know which products work better than others. Unfortunately, many pharmacists are too busy filling prescriptions. The FDA provides an easy-to-understand guide for consumers on the use of OTCs on its Web site (www.fda.gov).[10]

Counterfeit Drugs

Chapter 1 covered some of the issues of counterfeit drugs. These drugs represent a major threat to the U.S.'s drug supply and are a potential way for terrorists to harm U.S. citizens. Although the FDA has seized some counterfeit drugs harm from these drugs is yet to be reported.

UNSAFE PRACTICES THAT CONTRIBUTE TO ADVERSE DRUG EVENTS

In addition to the inherent ability drugs have to cause harm, the improper use of a safe drug can also cause harm. The mechanisms of unsafe practice are improper prescribing, dispensing, administering, and monitoring. In hospitals, 49 percent of these problems occur during the prescribing and monitoring stages, 11 percent when a medication order is transcribed, 14 percent during dispensing, and 26 percent when the drug is administered to the patient.[11] The nature and extent of unsafe medication practices in the ambulatory environment are less clear, and are discussed in Chapter 9.

Prescribing

As shown in Exhibit 3.1, some unsafe prescribing practices by health care professionals can contribute to a patient experiencing an ADE.

Most doctors properly prescribe drugs—some do it all the time, and some do it most of the time. Many system failures contribute to the problem.[12] More and more medication is being used, and overuse is becoming a significant health risk, especially for people age 65 and older. This age group has two to three times as many adverse reactions.

Dispensing

ADRs can occur even if the medication is dispensed correctly. However, as shown in Exhibit 3.1, there are actions pharmacists do or don't do that allows these events to occur.[13] For instance, not personally offering to counsel ambulatory patients about their medication cannot be excused as it is the last chance to help patients avoid problems, and it is required by law. Community pharmacists (and the companies they work for) who think they are fulfilling the law by having patients "sign here" are deluding themselves. OBRA 90 says the pharmacist must *personally* offer to counsel patients about their medication. If a pharmacist allows a clerk to make the offer, then the pharmacist is shirking his or her professional responsibility.

EXHIBIT 3.1.
Practices by Health Care Professionals
That Can Contribute to ADEs

Prescribing by Doctors

- Prescribing a drug that works as well as another drug, but has more adverse effects
- Prescribing a drug that is contraindicated for the patient
- Ordering too much of a drug or prescribing it to be given too often
- Ordering two or more drugs together that interact
- Prescribing a drug the patient has said he or she is allergic to
- Prescribing a drug too long a time period
- Not reducing the dose when the patient has reduced kidney function
- Not reducing the dose when the patient has reduced liver function
- Leaving patients on parenteral drug therapy when oral therapy would do
- Prescribing too many drugs for the patient (polypharmacy)[a]
- Routinely prescribing drugs for "off-label" purposes[b]
- Not educating the patient about the drug

Dispensing by Pharmacists

- Not interviewing and documenting clinical information on new patients
- Not recording allergy and ADR information on patients
- Not clarifying poorly written prescriptions or drug orders
- Overriding drug interaction alerts
- Not affixing warning stickers to medication containers
- Not counseling patients about their medication

Drug Administration by Nurses

- Not confirming that a patient has a history of allergy
- Not documenting what happens when the patient has an allergic reaction
- Not checking wristbands before administering medication

Monitoring the Patient

- In general, patients are not actively monitored for ADEs

[a]Jacoby S. (2003, November). Overmedicating America. *AARP Bulletin.*
[b]Young A and Adam C. (2003, November 2). Off-label drug usage routine but dangerous. Part 1 of "Risky Prescriptions." *The Charlotte Observer*, p. 1A.

Most patients have no idea why they are signing for their medication.[14] When patients ask pharmacy clerks this question, some clerks have been overheard to say "it is to document that you picked up the prescription," or "it is for insurance." The real reason for the signing is that corporately owned pharmacies have statements for patients to sign which waive the patients' rights to counseling about their medication by their pharmacist. Most of the time, patients have no idea what they signed, and were never offered counseling by the pharmacist. Corporate pharmacies do this so they don't have to hire more pharmacists.

Administration

Nurses contribute to ADEs, mostly through errors of omission.[15] The nurse, as the last check in the inpatient area, needs to follow up and find out if the patient has a medication allergy. The nurse should document the name of the drug and what happens when the patient receives the drug on the patient's medical record cover, the patient's wristband, and in the nurse's notes.

Monitoring the Therapy

In general, patients are not monitored closely enough to see if they are in the early stages of an ADE. Actions are post-ADE, rather than being proactive to prevent the events or to catch them early. One study showed that most patients who were prescribed relatively toxic drugs and experienced serious ADEs could have been monitored by measuring levels in the blood, but did not have these levels ordered by their doctor.[16]

In general, pharmacists need to become more active in monitoring for ADEs. Community pharmacists need to ask patients on the first refill of the medication two questions: (1) How is the medication working for you? and (2) Are you having any problems with the medication?

Nurses also need to be aware of the common adverse reactions for the drugs they administer, and be vigilant for any signs of an ADE. In general, nurses need better training in ADE prevention and monitoring.

WHY UNSAFE MEDICATION PRACTICES HAPPEN

No doctor, pharmacist, nurse, or other health care worker wants to harm patients. This is the opposite of what they want, and is contrary to the oaths they take as health care practitioners. When patients are harmed by what health care professionals do or not do, there is a double insult—they came for help and did not get it. Instead they were harmed.

Except for ADRs that are bizarre and unpredictable, ADEs occur for the following reasons: (1) poor systems that lack enough checks and balances, (2) workload and staffing problems, and (3) human error.

Poor Systems

Although health professionals have a well-learned, well-engrained way of prescribing, dispensing, administering, and monitoring drug therapy, it simply is not working—there is too much drug morbidity and mortality. One academic scholar pointed out the complexity of the drug use system as early as 1987.[17] The medication use system was broken then and remains broken today. Doctors, pharmacists, and nurses have too much to remember, too much to do, and are constantly interrupted in their work. Procedures are often being cut short, and checks and balances eliminated.

Workload, Staffing, and Fatigue

In general, doctors, pharmacists, and nurses are a tired lot. There simply are not enough of them to take care of the rising number of patients. As the baby boomers retire and become elderly, the system is going to be chaotic and unsafe unless something drastic is done. At this writing, there are major shortages of nurses and pharmacists. Medical residents are working up to 80 hours a week routinely. (It was more hours until work rules were put into place.) This is only going to get worse. Hospitals are hiring many "temporary" nurses and pharmacists to fill the gaps, however, many of these replacements have been out of the workforce for some time, and many are not trained well enough.

Community pharmacies are especially suffering from shortages of pharmacists, however, the reasons are more complex than simply a supply issue. Pharmacists in chain stores, food stores, and mass merchandiser pharmacies complain that they do not have enough help and many are afraid they will make an error that will harm someone.[18]

Some pharmacists say they do not have enough time during the day to get lunch or take a break. Common sense dictates that the more prescriptions a pharmacist prepares and dispenses in an hour the more chance that an error will result. However, studies to prove this are difficult to get approved from an investigational review board (IRB) for ethical and safety reasons, and study designs suffer from observer bias. Some would say that pharmacists should leave if they feel they are working under unsafe conditions, however, corporate pharmacies pay the best wages and usually have the best benefits.

Even though they know many pharmacists are working under extreme conditions, most state boards of pharmacy (not Florida, New Hampshire, or North Carolina) fear interfering with the employer-employee relationship, and leave these pharmacists and patients at risk. Boards expect pharmacists to take whatever time is necessary in processing prescriptions so the safety of the public is not risked. However, many pharmacists are expected and pressured to fill many prescriptions in an hour. If they cannot keep up the pace, they are let go.

Nurses and pharmacists are simply not given enough support to do their jobs safely in the form of more help and more automation. Profits in corporate pharmacy companies, and brick and mortar in hospitals are higher priorities than patient safety.

Human Error

No one wants to make an error, but it happens. Human error is a fact of life. We make errors, thus "to err is human." Yet is it forgivable? *Human error* is any human action or lack of it that exceeds the tolerances defined by the system with which the human interacts. Examples are a pharmacist filling a prescription incorrectly, a nurse forgetting to give a medication to a patient, and a doctor forgetting that a patient is allergic to a drug they are about to prescribe.

There are two kinds of human error—knowledge deficit errors and performance deficit errors. *Knowledge deficit errors* occur when the person does not possess the knowledge needed to carry out the function correctly. In *performance deficit errors,* the person performing the error knows better, but fails to do what they should. Performance deficit errors occur in higher abundance in health care, and usually occur during heavy or light workloads, when there are interruptions, or when the health care professionals "cut corners" and do not follow the proper procedure.

Human Factor Engineering

Knowledge about how people process information can be used to improve medication-use safety. This practice is called *human factor engineering*—"an applied science of system design that evaluates human strengths and compensates for human limitations. Thus, knowledge of how humans process information is essential to design such a system."[19] Human factors (HF) can be used to analyze errors that have already occurred through a root cause analysis (RCA), or to discover the points at which failure may occur (failure modes) in the future.

PREDICTING WHO MAKES MEDICATION ERRORS

Medication errors can be predicted by focusing on humans. Human engineering is not only possible, but is necessary. Prefrontal factors are the most important in predicting behaviors and performance of individuals. A battery of tests predicts performance outcomes.

A recent demographic study compared a group of pharmacists who often misfilled prescriptions with a control group of pharmacists with low error rates.[20] The misfill group of pharmacists had deficits on measures of executive functioning. For example, they were older, had more years of experience, and filled fewer prescriptions daily than the control group. Their working memory, associative learning processes, verbal organization, attentional control, and adaptive flexibility all scored lower than the control group. However, they scored higher in pleasant personality traits. For this group, change was possible by manipulating their environment or altering the systems they employed.

The take-away message is that people vulnerable to committing medication errors can be identified, can be helped to know where their weaknesses are, and can decrease their likelihood of making errors.

MANAGING BEHAVIOR TO REDUCE MEDICATION ERRORS

Since the IOM report, organized health care settings such as hospitals, and to a much lesser extent, community pharmacies, have been working on improving the existing medication-use system.[21] Although this is good, the one area where they are most vulnerable—human behavior—remains their weakest link. Most managers have only a common sense understanding of behavior. A point to ponder is—the behavior you see in your workplace is exactly the behavior your management systems, procedures, and supervision are designed to produce.[21] Thus, if there are too many medication errors (one is too many), then something needs to change in the management system, procedures, or supervision.

Behavior is a function of its consequence.[21] Events that follow our behavior and don't matter to the performer don't matter. Any behavior that doesn't matter comes to a stop. Most corrective action plans for medication errors focus on the precursor events to behavior rather than on the consequences of behavior. We typically retrain, retell, and remind people of the correct procedures. All of these steps may be necessary, but they are hardly enough. The only way to error proof any process is to manage the consequences of error-free performance.

BLAMING HEALTH PROFESSIONALS FOR ERRORS

Blaming health care professionals for making errors, especially if it is their first one, does more harm than good. Again, no health professional wants to make an error or harm a patient. Second, despite a goal of zero errors in health care, humans make errors. Third, no amount of blame will change any harm that has been done. Last, health professionals who make serious errors are devastated and usually punish themselves more than any outside force because they take their oaths seriously.

Taking away a health professional's license and livelihood because he or she made one serious error is also not the answer. Hospital administrators and professional licensing organizations are starting to get this message, but the media and public "still cry for a pound of flesh" when a health professional makes an error and someone is seriously harmed. Health professionals are victims in these situations as well—victims of poor systems. Most medication errors are associated with multiple reasons as to why they occurred.

Punishing health care professionals for serious errors also creates an environment in which errors will be hidden rather than reported, documented, and investigated for ways to prevent them in the future. A culture of mistrust prevails and no one wants to report an error they have made or someone else made.

ADVERSE DRUG EVENTS
DUE TO HOST-DRUG INTERACTION

Many ADEs occur because of an interaction between the drug and the patient. Patients who normally do not experience an adverse reaction when taking a drug may do so when they have a certain disease process. As the number of diseases increase, so do the number of drugs being used, and thus the increased likelihood of drug-disease interaction. In this case, a drug used in one condition worsens another condition. An example of this is when a beta-blocker drug such as propranalol is used to treat a heart problem in a patient with asthma. The propranolol may take care of the heart problem but it also reduces breathing in a patient already experiencing breathing problems. In addition, the presence of certain diseases together may dramatically reduce the effectiveness of some drugs. As the number of coexisting diseases increase, the predictability of how a drug will work decreases.

Another drug-disease interaction that can occur is when the patient is genetically predisposed to the drug. In these cases, the patient, because of genetics, may not possess the enzyme, or not enough of the enzyme, responsible for metabolizing the drug. As more dosing takes place, the drug builds up in the blood and becomes toxic. Various ethnic groups lack certain enzymes that metabolize certain drugs.

WHAT IS PREVENTABLE?

Some ADEs are preventable and some are not. For example, adverse drug reactions that have no basis for their development—the bizarre or idiocyncratic—are not preventable. However, all ADRs based on pharmacology that are an extension of their pharmacologic effect are preventable. So are all known drug interactions, all known medication allergies, and all medication errors. None of these should ever happen.

SOLUTIONS TO PREVENTING
ADVERSE DRUG EVENTS

Preventing ADEs is not easy. Since the IOM report, there has been a flurry of activity to reduce the drug morbidity and mortality associated with medication errors. Some of this activity is coordinated, such as that of the United States Pharmacopeia. It helped create a National Coordinating Council for Medication Error Reporting and Prevention (NCC MERP) which is composed of many interdisciplinary professional and consumer groups. The Agency for Healthcare Research and Quality (AHRQ) is also working to fulfill the recommendations on medical errors by the IOM. However, the entire medication-use system is broken and will not be adequately repaired by the usual approach—haphazard incrementalism (i.e., applying Band-Aids, when a whole new body is needed). Yet no one is taking a "zero-based" approach to the problem.

SUMMARY

ADEs happen because of inherent toxicity in certain drugs, unsafe practice by some health care professionals, human error, and most of all, because of deficiencies in the medication-use system. Until this system is reengineered by health care professionals, safety engineers, and behaviorial scientists by taking a "zero-based" approach, ADEs will continue to be a major public health problem.

Chapter 4

The Problem of Adverse Drug Reactions

The previous chapter dealt with adverse drug events, a term that encompasses a multitude of drug misadventures which include adverse drug reactions, drug interactions, allergic drug reactions, and medication errors. This chapter will explore adverse drug reactions (ADRs).

DEFINITIONS

"ADRs are generally considered to be any effects or reactions of drugs that are undesirable from the perspective that they lead to increased morbidity and mortality."[1] The World Health Organization (WHO) defines an ADR as "any response to a drug which is noxious and unintended, and which occurs at doses commonly used in man for prophylaxis, diagnosis, or therapy of disease, or for the modification of physiological function."[2] The difference between a side effect and an ADR is that a side effect is a dose-related, expected, and mild negative effect of a drug.

After a drug is approved for use, the FDA wants information of any unexpected ADRs. The Code of Regulations [21 CFR 314.80(a)] defines "unexpected" as a reaction that is not listed in the current labeling for the drug and includes an event that may be symptomatically and pathophysiologically related to an event listed in the labeling, but differs from the event because of greater severity or specificity.

Prescribed Medications and the Public Health
© 2006 by The Haworth Press, Inc. All rights reserved.
doi:10.1300/5688_04

TYPES OF ADVERSE DRUG REACTIONS

Two types of ADRs have been identified. Type A ADRs are an extension of the drug's pharmacology, are dose-related, and therefore are preventable. Type B ADRs are not pharmacologic, not dose related, and therefore, are not predictable nor preventable. Type B ADRs are often classified as bizarre or idiosyncratic. The basis of Type B ADRs may be genetic or immunologic.[3]

CASE EXAMPLES

Type A ADR

Sally is a 34-year-old working mother. She is under stress, both at home and at her law firm, and there is no end in sight. Her stress causes her to be irritated and unable to sleep. After seeing her doctor, she is told to exercise more and to use stress-reduction exercises daily. Sally tries these suggestions, but is just too busy. Sally's friend Sue has had similar problems, so Sue gives Sally a few tranquilizers to try. The drug helps, so Sally pressures her doctor to prescribe a tranquilizer, 5 mg three times a day. As the days get more stressful, Sally starts taking the drug three times during the day and once at bedtime. Sometimes during the day she gets drowsy and sometimes forgets if she has taken the drug. She drives home one day and almost falls asleep at the wheel. She wakes up just in time to keep from hitting a car in front of her. When she goes to get a refill of her prescription, the pharmacist tells her that she should still have a week's worth of the drugs left, but she only has two tablets.

Type B ADR

Tom, a 41-year-old construction worker, is having more and more headaches and does not know why. His wife makes him an appointment to see a doctor. It is discovered that Tom has high blood pressure. His doctor prescribes an ACE inhibitor to lower his blood pressure. Tom starts taking the drug and after a few days his headaches start to disappear. He takes the drug once a day and is compliant. After two weeks of taking the drug, Tom develops a tickle in his throat and needs to cough to clear the tickle. The problem will not go away. He goes to his pharmacy looking for a cough syrup, but can't figure out which one to use—there are so many different ones. Fortunately, a pharmacist sees Tom wandering around the over-the-counter section of the pharmacy and asks Tom what he needs. Tom explains the tickle in his throat and the pharmacist asks what other drugs Tom is taking. Tom can't remember the name of the drug, but says that it is for blood pressure. The pharmacist looks up Tom's prescriptions and sees that he is taking an ACE inhibitor that can cause a chronic cough in 5 to 15 percent of patients. The pharmacist calls Tom's doctor about this problem. The doctor switches Tom to another blood pressure medicine and the cough immediately goes away.

RECOGNIZING AND REPORTING ADVERSE DRUG REACTIONS

Doctors, nurses, pharmacists, and patients need to be continually vigilant to detect ADRs in the early stages of development. Unfortunately, this rarely happens. In fact ADRs can happen for some time before they are detected. Patients should be counseled on what can commonly go wrong with a drug they are taking, what to look for, and what to do if they think they are experiencing an ADR. However, this is rarely done. They are usually told to call their doctor if they have a problem with a drug but are never told what to look for.

New, serious, or unusual ADRs can be reported by anyone (including patients) to the FDA through the agency's MedWatch program, available on the Internet (www.fda.gov), or published by health care practitioners as case reports in medical or pharmacy journals. However, there is no law requiring practitioners to do this, even if it involves a death. Thus, only a tiny portion of serious ADRs are reported from practitioners, probably because they are "too busy." Pharmaceutical manufacturers are mandated to report all ADRs reported to them to the MedWatch program. The Joint Commission on the Accreditation of Healthcare Organizations (JCAHO) requires hospitals to have written policies and procedures for monitoring, documenting, and reporting ADRs.

Because ADR reports often make their way slowly to the FDA, months may go by, and many patients harmed, before the FDA recognizes that there is a major problem with a drug. The FDA needs a quicker system to identify ADRs associated with newly approved drugs, especially for those used in the ambulatory environment.

EPIDEMIOLOGY OF ADVERSE DRUG REACTIONS

Incidence and Prevalence

The incidence of ADRs in the public is unknown. However, what is known is that about 8 percent of emergency room (ER) patients are there because of an ADR, and that 3 to 8 percent of patients admitted to the hospital are admitted because of an ADR.[4] Also, about 7 out of every 100 patients in the hospital will experience a serious ADR, and roughly 3 patients out of every 1,000 patients in a hospital may die of an ADR.[5] Based on these figures, more than 2 million Americans may experience an ADR and 106,000 may die of an ADR every year while in the hospital. Based on autopsy reports of patients who have died in the hospital, 8.3 percent had a drug-associated event.[6]

The incidence of adverse drug events (ADEs), many of which are ADRs, may be as high as 350,000 yearly.[7] Overall, in the hospital environment, serious ADRs may occur in 7 percent of patients, and 37.5 percent of these patients are 65 years or older.[8] Fifty-two percent of ADEs are ADRs, and 19 percent of these are Type A ADRs and 81 percent are Type B ADRs.[9]

Patient Variables

ADRs are reported more for females (54 percent) than for males (46 percent).[9] Why females are more susceptible is unknown. It may be that they take more medication or there may be a hormonal component. Some people believe the very young and the very old incur more ADRs. Others believe that ADRs are evenly distributed over all age groups when the data are adjusted for the medication used. Some also believe there is a relationship between the degree of illness and the likelihood of experiencing an ADR because of compromise from disease.

Drug Variables

Over a 20-year period, the most common categories of drugs responsible for serious, reported ADRs were: central nervous system (CNS) agents, antimicrobial agents, cancer drugs, cardiovascular agents, and blood formation and coagulation drugs.[9] The most common drugs reported to cause serious ADRs (during that 20-year period) were: valproic acid (seizures), trimethoprim-sulfamethoxazole (antimicrobial), vancomycin (antimicrobial), methotrexate (cancer), and immune serum globulin (serum antibodies).[9]

The oral route of administration is the most common (63.4 percent) reported in ADR reports, followed by the parenteral (delivered by needle) route (9.5 percent). One-third of ADRs occur on the first day of therapy, and another 19 percent on days 1 to 7.[10]

Severity

The most common ADRs are: headaches, rashes, application site reactions, and diarrhea. Fortunately, these events are usually mild. The most common body systems affected are: the body as a whole, the skin and appendages, the nervous system, and the digestive system.[10]

Target Organs and Serious Drug-Induced Diseases

Serious ADRs most often affect the digestive, liver, and biliary systems, the blood and blood-making components, and the cardiovascular system. The most common serious ADR events are: hepatic failure, hepatitis, cardiopulmonary arrest, agranulocytosis (clinical signs of an abrupt onset of low white cell counts), and toxic epidermal necrolysis (a severe, sometimes fatal skin condition).[9]

Outcomes

Most ADR outcomes cause little more than annoyance or inconvenience, and most of these problems are readily treated. Of the serious ADR outcomes reported to the FDA, the most common were hospitalization (24.1 percent), death (7.2 percent), and threats to life (6.1 percent).[10]

POOR PRACTICES THAT CONTRIBUTE TO ADVERSE DRUG REACTIONS

Since Type A ADRs are dose related and an extension of the drug's pharmacology, dosing the drug correctly can prevent many of these reactions. Dosing correctly means knowing the patient. Knowing the patient means considering the patient's age, weight, renal and liver functions, what other drugs are being used, and any history of previous reactions. It also means starting with a low dose and going slow.

Most doctors know this, but often overlook at least one of these factors because they are too busy. Pharmacists are the double check in the system, but often are too busy filling prescriptions or drug orders. Too often, doctors get blamed for doing something wrong when it comes to medication. The pharmacist should double check the system.

Most experts believe Type B ADRs are not preventable as they are not foreseeable. However, some of these reactions take advantage of already compromised body systems, and these systems should be checked before a drug, especially one that is known to damage a certain body system, is prescribed. Good medicine dictates that baseline monitoring take place before a drug is prescribed. For example, if a drug is toxic to the kidneys, then a renal function test should be ordered before prescribing it. However, this sometimes does not happen.

BLACK-BOX WARNINGS

When the FDA discovers new safety data on an already marketed drug, it places a "black-box warning" on the drug's package insert.[10] Black-box warnings typically list adverse drug events, drug interactions, and limits for use (see Exhibit 4.1). These are useful, however, most doctors and pharmacists do not read package inserts. If the warning is highly significant, the FDA sends out a "Dear Doctor letter" and sometimes (but not often enough) a "Dear Pharmacist letter." This is an improvement, but doctors and pharmacists usually do not read these letters. Warnings are also posted on the FDA's Web site, but most doctors and pharmacists do not look there either. Only recently has a compendium of black-box warnings been available.[11]

Since black-box warnings are unknown or ignored, there needs to be a better way to make sure these warnings are followed. Suggestions include: (1) making sure all health care practitioners know these warnings, (2) making sure computerized physician warning systems are in place in all emergency and acute care settings, and (3) making pharmacists more accountable so that they double-check the warnings in the ambulatory and long-term care environments.

EXHIBIT 4.1.
An Example of a Black-Box Warning
for Fentanyl Transdermal

Indication: only for chronic pain in patients who are already receiving continuous opioid therapy and cannot be managed by lesser means.

Risk of potentially fatal hypoventilation: contraindicates use in acute or postoperative pain, or intermittent pain responsive to prn or non-opioid therapy.

Initial doses: <25 mcg/hr

Contraindicated: in children <12 yrs or <18 yrs and <50 kg (unless in investigational research setting).

Dosage forms: 50, 75, and 100 mcg/hr dosages for use ONLY in opioid-tolerant patients.

Source: From product labeling.

RECOGNIZING AND ASSESSING ADVERSE DRUG REACTIONS

Since recent epidemiologic evidence estimates that ADRs represent the fourth to the sixth leading causes of death in the United States, increased diligence is needed to recognize and assess these potentially life-threatening events.

Recognition

Early recognition can often prevent the event from being severe. For some reason, many patients do not connect an adverse reaction with the use of a drug. They often look for other causes of the problem. To have a reaction, the person must have touched, breathed, or swallowed it, and the exposure must have occurred before the adverse event occurred, usually within a few hours of taking the drug.

Probability Assessment

Just because an adverse effect occurs after taking a drug, it does not mean the drug caused the event. An analogy is if it rains and you go outside and there are frogs on the sidewalk, it does not mean that it rained frogs.

Making a definite connection between drug exposure and causality is difficult. Using clinical judgment alone to decide whether a drug is the cause of an adverse event has shown poor correlation.[12] Sir Austin Hill was the first to develop objective criteria for determining the strength of an association between an exposure (like a drug) and an outcome.[13] Since then, many tools have been developed to test the probability for cases. Most tools have been tested for reliability, but many are cumbersome to use.

The Naranjo algorithm is a validated and readily accepted way to assign the likelihood of a drug causing an untoward event.[14] The Naranjo algorithm uses a simple ten-item questionnaire with specifically assigned numerical values to discover an overall total score for probability (Exhibit 4.2). Naranjo scores of 9 or 10 indicate an ADR was *definite;* scores of 5 to 8 *probable;* scores of 1 to 4 *possible;* and scores of less than 1 *doubtful.*

Although useful and commonly accepted, the Naranjo algorithm has its limitations. For example, for someone who dies or is permanently disabled, withdrawing or readministering the drug is not going to reveal any clues on whether the drug was associated with the outcome. Another limitation is that dosages are not mentioned in any of the questions. Other ADR probability methods have been developed to forgo these limitations.[15, 16, 17] Despite having reasonable reliability, many of these other methods take longer to use, and some are not practical.

A recent study showed that no matter what decision algorithm is used, all are affected by confounding variables that compromise the sensitivity and specificity of the instrument.[18] Confounding occurs when the estimate of a measure of association between drug exposure and health status is distorted by the effect of one or several other variables that are also risk factors for the outcome of interest.[19]

HARMONIZING DEFINITIONS

Part of the problem in studying and trying to prevent ADRs has been a bewildering array of differing definitions to describe ADRs. To overcome or substantially reduce this problem, a dedicated group

EXHIBIT 4.2. ADR Probability Scale

To assess the adverse drug reaction, please answer the following and give pertinent score

Question	Yes	No	Do not know	Score
1. Are there previous conclusive reports on this reaction?	+1	0	0	
2. Did the adverse event appear after the suspected drug was administered?	+2	−1	0	
3. Did the adverse reaction improve when the drug was discontinued or a specific antagonist was administered?	+1	0	0	
4. Did the adverse reaction reappear when the drug was readministered?	+2	−1	0	
5. Are there alternative causes (other than the drug) that could on their own have caused the reaction?	−1	+2	0	
6. Did the reaction reappear when a placebo was given?	−1	+1	0	
7. Was the drug detected in the blood (or other fluids) in concentrations known to be toxic?	+1	0	0	
8. Was the reaction more severe when the dose was increased, or less severe when the dose was decreased?	+1	0	0	
9. Did the patient have a similar reaction to the same or similar drugs in any previous exposure?	+1	0	0	
10. Was the adverse event confirmed by any objective evidence?	+1	0	0	

Source: From Naranjo CA, Busto U, Sellers EM, Sandor P, Ruiz I, Roberts EA, Janecek E, Domecq C, and Greenblatt DJ (1981). A method for estimating the probability of adverse drug reactions. *Clin Pharmacol Ther* 30(2): 239-245. Reprinted with permission.

of individuals convened by the Council for International Organizations of Medical Sciences (CIOMS) of the World Health Organization (WHO), has been working to harmonize adverse drug reaction terms. This effort started in 1966 with definitions of terms and minimum requirements for respiratory and skin disorders.[20] So far 13 reports have been published.

TREATMENT

The treatment choices for ADRs range from no treatment to heroic measures to save someone's life. Some ADRs do not need treatment, only the assurance that nothing negative is going to happen. Most other ADRs need symptomatic relief and dissipate after the drug is discontinued. A smaller group of ADRs need immediate medical attention, especially when there is bleeding, breathing difficulties, heart problems, or problems with the kidneys. The keys to minimizing the harmful affects of ADRs are early recognition and early treatment.

Pharmacogenomics: The Future of Managing Adverse Drug Reactions

The risk of experiencing an ADR is not evenly distributed throughout the population. Certain ethnic groups have a higher incidence of ADRs. For example, because many East Asians metabolize codeine differently than Caucasians, East Asians often require higher dosages for pain relief. Ashkenazi Jews are significantly more susceptible to a potentially life-threatening blood disorder that can be induced by the drug clozapine which is used to treat schizophrenia.[21]

The disparity in ADR risk is genetically linked, and many ADRs represent an interaction between environmental exposure and the host (genetic makeup). The study of this interaction is called "genetic epidemiology" (pharmacoepidemiology when a drug is the exposure).[22] Type B ADRs formerly considered "idiosyncratic" or "bizarre," because we could not explain them, are now seen as part of a different genetic population.

Decoding the human genome has fostered new disciplines such as pharmacogenetics and pharmacogenomics. *Pharmacogenetics* is the study of the impact of heritable traits on pharmacology and toxicology. *Pharmacogenomics* is the study of the interplay between genotype and drug efficacy. Genetic polymorphisms (a stable difference in DNA sequence at the same locus) have the potential to affect a drug's mechanism of action. For example, many drug-metabolizing enzymes (chiefly the cytochrome p-450 isoenzymes) exhibit polymorphic expressions that divide the human population into two groups: "poor" metabolizers and "extensive" metabolizers. "Poor metabolizers account for 3 to 7 percent of whites; the distribution of these polymorphisms can be very different in other ethnic groups."[23]

Different patients respond in different ways to the same medicine. We now have a better understanding of why.[24] Patients are starting to be tested for common polymorphisms and are being given "report cards." Doctors are given a report stating which drugs to avoid or to take in reduced dosages due to polymorphisms. However, this practice is in its infancy, and it will take time to see how practical this approach will be, and if the cost of the testing will be reduced.

SUMMARY

The extent of ADR morbidity and mortality and their companion costs have not been fully realized, until recently. Fatal ADRs may rank as one of the leading causes of death in the United States. In general, doctors and pharmacists need better tools to do a better job of discovering, documenting, assessing, identifying, and preventing ADRs. In the past, some ADRs have been considered unpreventable. However, due to genetic breakthroughs, patients with an increased likelihood of reacting to a drug may be identified early in life, and thus be able to avoid drugs that have a high likelihood of causing harm.

Chapter 5

Dangerous Allergic Drug Reactions

The previous chapter discussed adverse drug reactions (ADRs). This chapter will discuss a special ADR—the allergic drug reaction. These drug misadventures need to be discussed separately as they have unique mechanisms of action and need distinct procedures for detecting, documenting, treating, and preventing them.

DEFINITIONS

An *allergic drug reaction* is the adverse effect of medication that involves immunologic mechanisms. The term "hypersensitivity" implies an immunologic basis. Adverse effects not proven to be immune mediated (no drug-specific antibodies or T-lymphocytes), but resembling allergic reactions in their clinical presentation, are referred to as "allergiclike" or "pseudoallergic" reactions.[1]

TYPES OF ALLERGIC DRUG REACTIONS

There are several ways to classify allergic drug reactions. The most common schema is divided into five groups—Types I-V.[2]

Type I: Anaphylactic Reactions

In anaphylactic reactions the allergen binds to IgE on basophils or mast cells resulting in a release of inflammatory mediators, the typical onset is within 30 minutes, and drug reactions are revealed as urticaria, anaphylactic shock, angioedema, rhinitis, or bronchospasm.

Prescribed Medications and the Public Health
© 2006 by The Haworth Press, Inc. All rights reserved.
doi:10.1300/5688_05

Type II: Cytotoxic Reactions

In cytotoxic reactions the antibody reacts with a cell-bound antigen, activating complement and producing cell injury, the typical onset is 5 to 12 hours, and there may be decreased production of platelets (thrombocytopenia), a decreased production of new white blood cells (neutropenia), or dissolving red blood cells (hemolytic anemia).

Type III: Immune Complex Reactions

In immune complex reactions antigen-antibody complexes form and deposit on blood vessel walls or into basement membranes and activate complement, the typical onset is three to eight hours, and vaculitis, glomerulonephritis, or other basement membrane diseases may develop if the individual does not have normal mechanisms to clear the immune complexes from the body.

Type IV: Cell-Mediated Reactions
(Delayed Hypersensitivity)

In cell-mediated reactions the antigens cause activation of lymphocytes that release inflammatory mediators, the typical onset is 24 to 48 hours, and the result may be contact dermatitis.

Type V: Pseudoallergic Reactions

Some adverse drug reactions probably have an immunologic basis, but the mechanism is unknown. Examples are: drug fever, acute pulmonary infiltration, chronic pulmonary fibrosis, drug-induced asthma, pneumonitis, and skin reactions such as Stevens-Johnson Syndrome (SJS), and toxic epidermal necrolysis (TEN).

CASE EXAMPLES

The following are examples of each allergic reaction.

Anaphylactic Reaction

A 45-year-old man with low back pain collapses 15 minutes after an intramuscular injection of diclofenac. Twenty minutes after successful revival, he goes into a coma and never recovers.[3]

Cytotoxic Reaction

A four-year-old boy with recurrent otitis media (ear infection) starts taking trimethorpim 80 mg plus sulfamethoxazole 400 mg twice daily. On the ninth day of therapy, the boy is evaluated after a 24-hour history of multiple bruises and petechiae (small red dots or pimples). His platelet count is abnormally low. Discontinuing the trimethoprim and sulfamethoxazole and proper treatment returns the boy's platelet count to normal.[4]

Immune Complex Reaction

A 27-year-old woman receives minocycline hydrochloride for folliculitis, and develops a drug-induced vasculitis (polyarthralgia, intermittent low-grade fever, and light red reticulated erythemas with cutaneous nodules on her extremities).[5]

Cell-Mediated Reaction (Delayed Hypersensitivity)

A patient develops a maculopapular rash 48 hours after beginning oral therapy with flurbiprofen (an nonsteroidal anti-inflammatory drug like ibuprofen), and two days later develops angioedema and hypotension.[6]

Pseudoallergic Reaction

A cough syrup with codeine is prescribed for a two-year-old girl with symptoms of viral upper respiratory tract infection. She develops a painful red splotch on the back of her neck, and pains in her legs and hands. The following day, her entire body is covered with an erythematous, raised macular rash. Drug-induced erythema multiforme (a potentially lethal skin condition) is suspected. The cough syrup is discontinued and the rash goes away.[7]

RECOGNITION

Early recognition that an allergic drug reaction is taking place or has taken place is the key to prevention or successful treatment. However, recognizing an allergic drug reaction is not always easy. Some allergic drug reactions mimic other types of ADRs. Without direct immunologic evidence, the following criteria may be helpful in distinguishing allergic drug reactions:[8]

- Allergic drug reactions occur in a small percentage of patients.
- The clinical expression does not resemble any of the pharmacologic effects of the drug.

- Without previous exposure to the drug, no allergic expressions of the drug appeared when the drug was used for the first week of continuous therapy.
- The reaction resembles other known allergic reactions.
- The reaction reappears after small doses of the suspected drug are administered.
- There is blood or tissue eosinophilia (a rise in eosinophils).
- Drug-specific antibodies or T-lymphocytes react with the suspected drug.
- The manifestations of the reaction subside within several days when the drug is discontinued.

EPIDEMIOLOGY

Little epidemiological data exist on allergic drug reactions and "most of those available, including incidence, mortality and socioeconomic impact data, should be interpreted with caution."[9]

Prevalence

The incidence of allergic drug reactions in the public is unknown. This is because it is often difficult to discover if a drug reaction is immunologically mediated, and many reactions are not reported. In a sample of 340 adult patients in one hospital setting, 133 (39 percent) reported allergies to at least one drug.[10] In a study on the prevalence of drug allergies in 1,218 surgical patients, 15 percent reported being allergic to at least one drug.[11]

One study reports "ADRs occur in 10-20 percent of hospitalized patients, and up to one-third of these are of an allergic or pseudo-allergic nature."[9] Of the patients seen in an emergency room for a drug misadventure, about 21 percent had an allergic drug reaction.[12] "Allergic drug reactions are responsible for up to 5 percent of reactions to medications among hospitalized patients."[1] In a series of 11,526 consecutively monitored patients in one hospital, drug anaphylaxis was recorded in eight cases (0.6 in every 1,000 patients).[13] In a series of 1,520 published case reports of serious adverse drug events, 25 percent were allergic drug reactions.[14] Of these, 45 percent were type I reactions, 30 percent were type II reactions, 7 percent were type III reactions, 1 percent were type IV reactions, and 17 percent were type V reactions.

Patient Variables

Not much is known about the age distribution of drug-induced allergies. In a review of 447 published cases of fatal adverse drug events, "the frequency of allergic drug reactions increased with age."[15] Patients less than one year of age had 13 percent of the fatal allergic events, while 11 percent occurred in those over age 39.

Drug Variables

In a sample of 340 adult patients in one hospital, the most common drug allergies were to β-lactam (the penicillins) antibiotics, sulfa drugs, and opioid (morphine type) narcotics.[10] In general, the drug categories producing the most allergic drug reactions are: penicillins, radiocontrast media, insulins, nonsteroidal anti-inflammatory agents (such as ibuprofen), sulfa drugs, and dyes used to color tablets such as tartrazine (FD&C yellow dye no. 5).[1]

In a review of 1,520 published case reports of serious ADEs, the most common drugs causing allergic drug reactions were: heparin, dextran, sulfasalazine, carbamazepine, chlorhexidine, and cefazolin.[14] In one study of fatal ADEs, 26 percent of the fatal allergic drug reactions were thought to be caused by antimicrobial agents.[15]

Severity and Outcomes

Although most allergic drug reactions are mild, some are severe and at times fatal.[16] In surgical patients, the most severe reactions (16.4 percent of all allergic drug reactions) were associated with radiological contrast media (36.4 percent).[11] In this study, the skin was involved in 72.1 percent of all allergic drug reactions, the respiratory tract was involved in 6.9 percent, and the circulatory system was involved in 4.4 percent.

It is unknown how many people seek treatment for adverse drug reactions. However, most people having an allergic drug reaction do not incur much morbidity. In one study of published case reports of ADEs that were threats to life, 35 percent were allergic drug reactions, and anaphylaxis was the number one threat (11.9 percent).[17] How often people die of an allergic drug reaction is unknown. Of 447 published case reports on fatal ADEs, 19 percent were thought to have had an allergic basis.[15]

POOR PRACTICES

Poor practices contribute to allergic drug reactions. These poor practices include the way in which patient histories are taken, and the way a patient's history of previous allergic reactions is recorded in the patient's medical record. Standardized methods are needed. For example, most health care workers simply ask a patient, "Are you allergic to any medications?" The patient tries to think of previous reactions or what someone has told him or her about what drugs to avoid. This method seldom results in any concrete information. Next, the health care worker records whatever drugs the patient reports, and goes on to the next step in the medication process.

Taking the Patient's History of Medication Allergy

The first problem with this traditional method is that the patient usually thinks about only prescription drugs, and rarely reveals any problems with over-the-counter or nontraditional drugs such as herbal medications. Second, the patient's knowledge of what makes up allergic phenomena is often not correct. For example, gastrointestional upset is not an allergic event, but more accurately should be classified as "intolerance." In one study of patients claiming to be allergic to penicillin, 17.1 percent had "intolerance."[18] Thus, the drug for which they were intolerant might be safely used if dosed more carefully.

Documenting the Patient's Medication Allergy

The second problem is the manner in which drug allergies are recorded. The proper way is to list the drug, followed by what happens when the drug is consumed. For example, "penicillin—throws up." This gives more meaning to the potential problem. Contrast this with— "penicillin—stops breathing." Another question that is seldom asked is, "How do you know you have a medication allergy?" If the patient explains what happened when he or she took the medication, a much clearer picture is revealed. An even better question is, "Who said you are allergic to this medication?" The answer can be revealing. If the answer is "my grandmother," it reveals one fact, but quite another if the answer is "my allergist."

A study on wrong allergy documentation in pediatric patients took place in 2001.[19] In this study, 186 of 248 drug allergies identified in 1,591 patient records were challenged. Of these, 26 (14 percent), 103 (55 percent), and 57 (31 percent) were considered true, undetermined, and falsely reported drug allergies, respectively. Fifty-three (93 percent) of the falsely reported allergies were removed from patients' records with the consent of the attending doctors.

The value in finding and removing incorrect allergy information (i.e., adverse effects or intolerance) that is wrong information can increase the risk of using medications that are more toxic, less infective, or more costly.

In another study, 60 (45 percent) of 134 hospitalized patients reported 78 drug allergies.[20] However, "information from the interviews indicated the criteria for true allergy were met by only 36 (60 percent) of these patients and 39 drugs. Thus, the prevalence of allergy in the patients studied was 27 percent."

Another problem in documenting medication allergy information is that it is seldom done completely. The correct procedure in institutional settings is to document the allergy in five places: patients' medical records, their wristband, their chart cover, the nurse's medication administration record, and the pharmacy profile. In one study of 117 patients with a history of allergy to medication, the allergy was documented in 98.7 percent of patient charts and 96.7 percent of medication administration records. There was no mention of the other areas where the medication allergy should be recorded.[18] Symptoms of the allergic reaction were described in the patients' records only 34 percent of the time.

The quality of medication history taking and documentation in doctors' offices and in community pharmacies is unknown and needs to be explored.

Noticing an Allergic Drug Reaction

In general, nurses and patients need to do a better job of noticing when an allergic drug reaction is taking place. The early detection of an allergic drug reaction is much easier to treat than one that is in its full stages. Nursing students and practicing nurses need to be better educated on what to monitor, and patients need to be better educated by doctors, nurses, and pharmacists on what makes up an allergic reaction. However, this is seldom done because of lack of knowledge and not being aware of the patient's unspoken needs.

In a study assessing medication errors that involved drug allergies at a university hospital, most contributing factors were classified as "MD [the prescribing doctor] was unaware of the allergy."[10]

TREATMENT

Some allergic drug reactions can be resolved by simply discontinuing the drug. Mild reactions can be treated with antihistamines (such as dimenhydramine), orally or topically, or both. Progressive allergic drug reactions are usually treated using a corticosteroid (such as prednisone) in tapering doses. For anaphylaxis, prompt treatment is needed with antihistamines, sympathomimetic amines (such as epinephrine), and corticosteroid drugs, with provision of a satisfactory airway, when indicated. [21]

PREVENTION

Good Policies and Procedures

One of the main means of preventing allergic drug reactions is to have good policies and procedures in place and a more standardized approach to take and document allergy histories.[22] The procedure should spell out the proper approach including defining what is a "true allergy," what questions to ask, and how to discover the credibility of the information. Also, documenting what happens when the allergy takes place, where to document the allergy information, how to document the information, how to educate the patient, and how to monitor for reactions should be included.

Skin Testing

In allergic drug reactions the most serious concern is a systemic allergic reaction. Skin testing is used when there is a chance the person may be allergic—never when a true allergy exists. "Immediate-type skin tests are the most rapid and reliable method of proving the presence of IgE antibody."[23] This testing is reserved for evaluating drugs that are proteins such as chymopapain, streptokinase, and insulin.

A skin prick test is done by puncturing the skin with a sharp needle through an allergen solution.[23] "If negative at 20 minutes, this is followed by the intradermal test, which is accomplished by injecting 0.02 ml of solution, intradermally raising a small bleb. A positive test is defined as a 1 cm erythema and a negative saline control."

Good procedures are available for performing penicillin skin testing.[1]

Test Dosing

Test dosing is used in patients with a history suggestive of an allergic reaction. The drug in question is initiated at a dose below that which would cause a serious reaction, then with incremental doses until a full dose is safely established. The intent is to see if any allergic symptoms develop.

Desensitization

Converting a patient from a sensitive state to a normal state using incremental doses of a drug is called desensitization. The procedure implies the presence of a proven immunologic mechanism (sensitized IgE mast cells). "During desensitization, it is presumed the IgE antibody is gradually neutralized by reaction with increasing amounts of antigen or that IgE sensitized mast cells are degranulated without a systemic reaction or both."[23] Local reactions may happen, in which case the dose is reduced and progressive doses restarted when the dose is correct.

Pretreatment

A relatively new procedure is to pretreat the patient with an antihistamine or corticosteroid before a drug that is known to cause allergic reactions is administered. This procedure has worked well in patients about to receive radiocontrast media.

SUMMARY

Allergic drug reactions are ADRs that have an immunologic component. The number of adverse drug reactions is unknown so therefore it is unknown if the incidence rates are increasing, decreasing, or staying the same. The severity of allergic drug reactions ranges from discomfort to sudden death. Therefore, good practices are needed to minimize their incidence and outcomes. However, many changes are needed to make this minimization a reality.

Better practices include improvement in the history taking and recording of allergic drug information—how it is recorded and where it is recorded. Better policies and procedures are needed on how organized health care settings handle drug allergies, and all health care professionals need better training on handling allergic drug reactions. Finally, any patient receiving a drug known to cause allergic reactions should be educated on what to look for and how to seek help should an allergic reaction occur.

Chapter 6

Are Drug Interactions Really Dangerous?

Ideally, patients should not receive combinations of medication that cause harm, however, this is sometimes not the case. Medical journals often contain reports submitted by doctors and pharmacists summarizing the circumstances of a patient receiving a combination of drugs that caused the harm, and sometimes death. This chapter will discuss the problem of drug interactions.

DEFINITIONS

Not all combinations of drugs cause harm, but there are two types of combinations that have the potential to cause harm. The first type is when two or more drugs being used cause the same effect. For example, taking two drugs that depress the same area of the central nervous system can cause the respiratory system to slow down to the point where breathing is difficult. It is said that the effect is "additive" or "potentiated." This means the total effect is the added effects of each similar-acting drug being used. Such additive effects are classified under "adverse drug reactions."

The second potentially dangerous combination of drugs is when there is a "drug-drug interaction." The mechanism of this effect is different. One drug (the participant drug) interacts with a second drug (the object drug), and causes the second drug to either have more or less of an effect than if the drug was given by itself. Having less of an effect may mean being undertreated and possible treatment failure. Having more of an effect may mean harm. Most of the worry is on the side of possible harm.

CASE EXAMPLES

Harmful drug interactions rarely occur, but when they do they can be fatal. Following are some examples:

A patient suffering from depression was prescribed tranylcypromine. Eleven days later, the patient developed a cold and went to a second doctor who prescribed phenylproponolamine. The patient returned to the pharmacy where he had received the tranylcypromine. The pharmacy computer system detected a significant interaction between the two drugs, but the pharmacy technician overrode the system. The patient suffered a stroke and died of the interaction.[1]

A 47-year-old man was prescribed chlordiazepoxide and haloperidol as part of a supervised alcohol detoxification program. He also received 650 mg of acetaminophen twice a day for two days. On the third day, the patient experienced disorientation, hallucinations, low blood pressure, jaundice, and a tender liver. He progressively worsened and died on his twenty-eighth day in the hospital. His doctor suspected a drug interaction between the acetaminophen and alcohol.[2]

A 43-year-old man with schizophrenia was started on clozapine while he was receiving 1 mg of lorazepam three times a day. The dosage of clozapine was increased to 400 mg daily over two weeks. After 17 days of clozapine, the man became increasingly psychotic and received three doses of lorazepam 2 mg intravenously within nine hours. He went to bed and was found dead in his bed at 5 a.m. the next day.[3]

A 52-year-old woman, having a two-week history of loosely formed stools was prescribed 500 mg of metronidazole three times a day. The patient was already taking warfarin 5 mg daily for two and one-half years to prevent clotting of a heart valve. Shortly, the patient experienced multiple bruises on her body, headaches, fever, back pain, and diarrhea. Her blood-clotting time went from 21 to 27 seconds, to 75 seconds. Both drugs were stopped and the patient needed to be transfused with fresh frozen plasma and packed red blood cells.[4]

HOW DRUG INTERACTIONS HAPPEN

Drugs can interact in several ways. In general, one drug can act on a second drug to affect the second drug's absorption, distribution, excretion, or metabolism, either raising or lowering the blood or tissue levels of the second drug. The net effect may be: (1) *antagonism,* such as reduced blood pressure control by clonidine when a tricyclic antidepressant is added to a patient's drug regimen; (2) *synergism,* such as an increased anticoagulant effect when administering salicylates (like aspirin) and warfarin together; or (3) *idiosyncratic,* such as the rare but severe effects that can happen when meperidine and a monoamine oxidase inhibitor are used together.[5]

EPIDEMIOLOGY

Prevalence

How often do drug interactions occur?

Ambulatory

Some studies have tried to discover the prevalence of exposure to potentially harmful drug-drug interactions in the general population. One study in 2002 determined that one-third of the population in Denmark was exposed to concurrent use of two or more drugs, and among these, 15 percent were exposed to a drug carrying a risk of a drug interaction.[6]

Drug-drug interaction exposure studies have also been performed using pharmacy records. For example, a study performed in Sweden in 1999 showed that 13.6 percent of prescriptions dispensed by pharmacies included at least one potential drug interaction.[7] Potential interactions that might have serious clinical consequence were found in 1.4 percent of the prescriptions.

Using a drug claims database that included roughly 2.9 million patients with more than 30 million prescriptions dispensed in a 12-month period (September 2001 to August 2002), investigators found a low incidence (<1 percent) of potentially serious drug-drug interactions.[8] However the authors of this study caution that the incidence depends on the method of case finding.

Acute Care

A study to look into the frequency, nature, and side effects of drug-drug interactions in 1,000 geriatric (>70 years old) inpatients taking drugs at home during the two week period before hospital admission was undertaken.[9] A total of 538 patients were exposed to 1,087 drug-drug interactions.

Long-Term Care

In one exposure study using patient medication profiles, the prevalence of drug-drug interactions in geriatric patients in 132 nursing homes was 2.7 percent.[10] Two other exposure studies in nursing homes found exposure rates of 6.2 percent and 5.8 percent respectively.[11,12] How much harm occurred in these patients was not reported.

Harm

Although there are well-designed studies on drug-drug interaction exposure, there are few outcome studies on how often people are harmed from drug-drug interactions. In a review of nine studies of drug-drug interactions, 0 to 2.8 percent of hospital admissions were because of a drug-drug interaction.[13] In another study, the most frequent side effects of drug-drug interactions were neuropsychological impairment, arterial hypotension, and acute renal failure.[9]

A 2003 case control study looked at elderly patients hospitalized for drug toxicity.[14] Patients taking glyburide and co-trimoxazole were more likely to be admitted within seven days for hypoglycemia (low blood glucose levels) than those patients not taking this combination. Patients taking digoxin and clarithromycin were more likely to be admitted (within seven days) for digoxin toxicity than those patients not taking this combination. Patients taking ACE inhibitors and a potassium-sparing diuretic were more likely to be admitted (within seven days) for hyperkalemia (too much blood potassium) than those not taking this combination.

Only one controlled study (a matched-pair, case-control study) on drug interactions was found in the literature.[15] The researchers used a Medicaid claims database to discover the risk of hospitalization associated with drug-drug interactions. Patients were hospitalized and controls were not. Cases were matched with controls on Medicaid eligibility. Odds ratios for hospitalization in patients exposed to known drug interactions were compared with patients exposed to one of the interacting agents. Odds ratios were significantly raised for several interacting pairs of drugs versus the controls. However, like most drug interaction studies, this study was not designed to discover the incidences or the morbidity and mortality associated with drug-drug interactions.

Age of Patients

It is not known if drug-drug interactions are equally distributed among all age groups. However, one study in an inpatient population of pediatric patients with infectious diseases determined that these patients were prescribed potential drug interactions 3.5 percent of the time.[16] Another study discovered that drug interactions may increase with age.[6]

Geriatric patients may be exposed to the most drug interactions based on the number of medications they take. They also may be the most vulnerable to the effects of drug interactions because of decreased liver and kidney function.

Common Drugs

Studies in the general population suggest that the most common drug categories associated with drug-drug interactions are the cardio-vascular agents, nonsteroidal anti-inflammatory drugs (NSAIDs), oral antidiabetic agents, and anticoagulants.[6,8] Some of the most common serious drug-drug interactions are between potassium supplements and potassium-sparing diuretics, and between warfarin and NSAIDs.[8] Serious drug interactions can also occur between potassium-sparing diuretics and anticoagulants.[6]

In a review of case reports of clinically significant adverse drug events published over a 20-year period, 8 percent (of 1,520 reports) involved a drug-drug interaction.[17] The drugs most commonly involved in a drug-drug interaction were: methotrexate, cancer drugs, trimethoprim-sulfamethoxazole, levamisole, bleomycin, clozapine, filgastim, hydrochlorthiazide, hyralazine, lithium, trimethoprim, and warfarin.

In 2001, the M3 Project identified the top ten dangerous drug interactions in long-term care.[18] These interactions were: warfarin with NSAIDs, sulfa drugs, macrolides, quinolones, or phenytoin; ACE inhibitors with potassium supplements or spironolactone; digoxin with amiodarone or verapamil; and theophylline with quinolones.

Sometimes oral contraceptives can interact with other drugs or natural substances. A comprehensive review of these interactions is available.[19]

Concerns have been raised about drug interactions with natural products because these products are being used more often. Interactions between natural products and drugs are based on the same mechanisms as drug-drug interactions. Natural products reported to interact with drugs include: coenzyme Q_{10}, dong quai, ephedra, *Ginkgo biloba,* ginseng, glucosamine, sulfate, iprifavone, melatonin, and St. John's wort.[20]

COST

Only a few anecdotal reports exist on the added costs of drug-drug interactions. These adverse events usually result in visits to a doctor or the emergency room, the purchase of over-the-counter drugs or prescription-only medication, hospitalization, or extended hospitalization. Other costs include attorneys fees, and costs of verdicts and settlements from medical malpractice litigation.[21]

A case report of a patient experiencing two different drug interactions over a two-week period reported that "these drug interactions caused the patient significant morbidity and resulted in a hospitalization with total medical expenses of $17,213 which included charges from a 15-day hospitalization, emergency room visits, ambulance services, magnetic resonance imaging, electrocardiogram, laboratory tests, and consultations."[22]

A study of hospital admissions secondary to theophylline drug interactions reported a cost of $12,864 for two interactions—one involving cimetidine and theophylline, and another involving ciprofloxacin and theophylline.[23] The hospital stays were 16 days and 13 days, respectively.

Patients who have been harmed, or the relatives of patients who die of drug interactions, sometimes sue their health care providers. The basis for the suit is that their health care provider should have been aware that the prescribed combination of drugs would be harmful. Some patients harmed by drug interactions have received large legal settlements or judgments in the millions of dollars.[17]

PREVENTION

The drug interactions associated with the use of a new drug are not likely to be known when the FDA approves the drug. However, all known drug interactions are preventable. Drug-drug interactions become known as the drug is used in more and more people. Doctors and pharmacists send case reports on these events to medical journals for publication or report them to the FDA. Once the FDA has enough information to discover the drug-drug interaction commonly occurs, they require the manufacturer to revise its product labeling to include information about the drug-drug interaction. If the drug-drug interaction is significant, the FDA may take the added step of sending "Dear Doctor" and "Dear Pharmacist" letters to warn doctors and pharmacists of the interaction.

Pharmacists have a duty to not dispense drugs to patients already taking other medication that may cause harmful drug interactions that are known and foreseeable.[1] They do this by being vigilant and by employing drug interaction detection software.

DETECTING HARMFUL DRUG INTERACTIONS IS NOT SO EASY

The first problem in detecting drug interactions is that there are countless drugs on the market and countless combinations of drugs that can be taken. The second problem is lack of agreement on which drug-drug interactions are harmful. Why is this?

Reference texts are lacking.

Although there are many drug-interaction reference texts, the information in them is based on anecdotal case reports (sometimes only one report) of someone taking a drug combination and experiencing an adverse event.

The authors of these texts review case reports of drug interactions and try to discover a significance level based on various factors. However, the process is often more subjective than objective. Another problem is that some of the drug interactions in these texts are theoretical, based on the pharmacology or pharmacokinetics of the drugs being used together.

Various problems are associated with assessing and classifying potential drug interactions no matter how carefully it is done. There is no standard approach. Therefore, there is no agreement among existing compendia of drug interactions. In 2000, a study revealed disagreement among five drug compendiums on inclusion and severity ratings of drug-drug interactions.[24]

Researchers at the University of Arizona, working under a grant from the Centers for Disease Control and Prevention (CDC), performed a systematic review and identification of major drug interactions listed in four well-known tertiary drug-interaction references. A total of 406 major drug interactions were listed in all four compendia.[25]

The process for developing pharmacy software to detect major drug interactions, disturbingly, is similar to what is used to develop drug-interaction reference texts. In 1992, Jankel and Martin evaluated six computerized drug-interaction screening programs and found inconsistency and none of them ideal.[26]

Causality assessment needs improvement.

The lack of agreement between drug interaction compendia may exist based on the way case reports of drug interactions are assessed. Are objective criteria being used to assess each report? If so, how do these criteria vary from text to text? How is missing information handled in the assessment? An example of objective criteria for properly assessing drug interaction case reports is one used by Hansten and Horn.[26]

Drug interaction exposure studies tell us little.

Some of the drug interactions in reference documents have come from drug exposure studies. These types of studies use prescriptions or drug orders in pharmacy computer systems, or claims in insurance databases, to find out if drugs were prescribed for patients that had the potential to cause a drug-drug interaction. An example is the study by Bjerrum and colleagues.[6] In this study, 15 percent of the population studied was exposed to drugs carrying a risk of a drug interaction at all risk levels.

The problem with some studies (and there are many) is that they fail to report any harm results from these drug interactions. A hospital study in the United States estimated that only 9.5 percent of drug interactions are potentially clinically significant, but this figure has not been validated.[27]

What is needed are studies that compare the outcomes of using what is thought to be potentially dangerous drug-drug interactions with the outcomes of using only one drug in potentially dangerous combinations. The best way to do this is by designing a retrospective cohort (database) study.

Pharmacists are missing drug interactions.

Pharmacists must rely on pharmacy software to screen for potentially dangerous combinations of drugs. How well do pharmacists do this?

Several studies have shown that drug interaction detection in pharmacies is lacking. The most extensive and publicized study so far was performed by Georgetown University and reported in *U.S. News and World Report*.[28] In this study, three sets of prescriptions, representing moderate to serious drug interactions rated in drug-interaction texts, were "shopped" at 245 pharmacies in three major cities in the United States. Pharmacists dispensed 58 percent of the medicines without intervention.

How many of the interactions were detected by pharmacy software and why pharmacists missed these interactions are unknown. What is known is that drug-drug interaction software programs are suboptimal.

Drug-drug interaction software is lacking.

In 2001, Hazlet and colleagues tested nine different drug-drug interaction software programs in six fictitious patient profiles.[29] Software failed to detect drug-drug interactions one-third of the time. Chrischilles and colleagues recently concluded, "there is limited and inconclusive evidence whether pharmacy computer systems are effective in reducing harm to patients."[30]

In trying to explain what may have gone wrong in the study published in the *U.S. News and World Report,* one author surmised that: (1) the computer may have not been updated to include the drug interactions presented; (2) the computer program may not have enough roadblocks; or (3) pharmacists are being bombarded with too many insignificant drug interactions and have grown used to skipping by them.[31]

Too many meaningless drug interaction alerts.

A recent study showed that 10.3 percent of third-party claims in 41 pharmacies in Indiana resulted in an alert.[32] Of these, 14.7 percent were for drug interactions. These alerts were overridden 88.1 percent of the time because the pharmacist was aware of the problem (24.2 percent), the problem did not exist (33.6 percent), or the problem was not clinically significant (27.3 percent).

A 2002 study in the United Kingdom found that 22 percent of general practitioners admitted to frequently or very frequently overriding drug interaction alerts.[33] The most common reason for overriding a drug interaction alert was the view that the alerts were frequently irrelevant.

In a study, published in 2003, 3,481 consecutive alerts were generated at five adult primary care practices.[34] Doctors overrode 91.2 percent of drug allergy alerts and 89.4 percent of high-severity drug interaction alerts. There were few ADEs, suggesting the threshold for alerting was set too low.

In 1999, Dalton and colleagues showed that it is possible to decrease the number of false drug interaction alerts in a hospital-based system if the vendor of the system allows users to adjust alerts.[31] However, the number of alerts was still high. Housley and Kelly recently made some good suggestions on how pharmacy systems can be improved (Table 6.1) and what pharmacists can do (Exhibit 6.1) to detect drug interactions.[35]

Most pharmacy software systems allow only the pharmacist to bypass an alert. However, because of so many false alerts and the need to dispense so many prescriptions, some pharmacists give pharmacy technicians access to their identification number so that the pharmacy technicians can bypass the system when an alert goes off. This is a dangerous practice.

TABLE 6.1. How to Improve Drug-Interaction Detection Systems

Improvement Needed	Priority
The system should contain only drug interactions that are evidence based.	Major
The drug interactions that trigger an alert should be user (pharmacist) defined.	Major
The system should check for drug interactions only against medications the patient is currently taking.	Major
The system should include the management of the drug interactions.	Major
The system should be designed so that only the pharmacist can override a drug-interaction alert.	Major
The system should require an explanation for overriding a drug-interaction alert.	Major
The system should identify the source of the drug-interaction information.	Minor
The system should be updated at least monthly.	Minor

Source: Housley SC and Kelly WN. (2003). Drug-interaction monitoring: Good, bad, and ugly. *Drug Topics* 147:41-42. Reprinted with permission.

THE PHARMACIST'S DUTY TO WARN

Over the years, laws have been expanding to hold pharmacists responsible for warning about foreseeable problems with medications prescribed for patients. For example, in one case, a child was prescribed theophylline and erythromycin at the same time. The medication was dispensed resulting in seizures and permanent damage to the child. The doctor and pharmacist were both sued. The pharmacist tried using the defense that only the doctor was responsible. However, the court disagreed, ruling that the pharmacist had a responsibility to detect and act on drug interactions.[36] More and more courts are taking a similar position about the pharmacist's duty to warn about drug interactions.

EXHIBIT 6.1. Pharmacy Practices
That Promote Drug-Interaction Detection

Pharmacists need to:

- Know that studies show that community pharmacists are missing significant drug interactions
- Learn their pharmacy's policies and procedures for handling drug interactions
- Get out from behind the counter and ask patients which medications they are taking and update the patient's profile accordingly
- Take the time to screen thoroughly for drug interactions
- Recognize the drug interactions that can result in death
- Be less reliant on software systems to detect drug interactions
- Understand how to properly use the pharmacy software system
- Be aware of the limitations of the pharmacy software system
- Contact the prescribing physician when faced with a high severity alert

Pharmacy technicians need to:

- Enter 100% of the prescriptions into the system
- Know the pharmacy's policy and procedure on handling drug interactions
- Never override a drug-interaction alert without the pharmacist's permission

Source: Housley SC and Kelly WN. (2003). Drug-interaction monitoring: Good, bad, and ugly. *Drug Topics* 147:41-42. Reprinted with permission.

WHICH DRUG INTERACTIONS
ARE THE MOST HARMFUL?

Nearly 100,000 interactions between drugs have been reported in the medical or drug company literature.[37] However, most of these cause little harm. A good question is—what are the most dangerous drug interactions? This question is difficult to answer due to a lack of good outcome studies. Until these outcome studies are completed, other criteria can be used to identify the most harmful drug interactions.

One approach is to look in four of the most popular drug-interaction references to see which drug interactions were listed as the most dangerous in all four books. As shown in Table 6.2, there are only nine such interactions.[25] Some of the drugs in these drug interactions are rarely used, therefore, it may be worth expanding the list to the top 35 drug interactions of the highest severity found in three of the four drug interaction reference books. Another approach is to focus on those drug-interactions that can be fatal.[38,39] These are listed in Table 6.3.

Yet another approach is to assemble a group of experts in drug-drug interactions and use a Delphi process to reach a consensus on which drug interactions are the most clinically significant.[40] The results of this exercise are listed in Table 6.4.

Drug-Food Interactions

None of these tables include drug interactions between drugs and foods.[41] The most common drug-food interaction involves taking

TABLE 6.2. Drug Interactions Listed at the Highest Severity Level in Four Drug Interaction Compendia

Drug-Drug Interactions	Net Potential Effect
Anticoagulants and androgens	Bleeding
Anticoagulants and barbiturates	Bleeding[a]
HMG COA reductase inhibitors and macrolide antibiotics	Increased HMG-COA reductase
Meperidine and MAO inhibitors	Serotonin syndrome
Methotrexate and probenecid	Methotrexate toxicity
Potassium and potassium-sparing diuretics	High serum potassium levels
Sibutramine and MAO inhibitors	Serotonin syndrome
SSRI and MAO inhibitors	Serotonin syndrome
Thiopurines and allopurinol	Thiopurine toxicity

Source: Adapted from Abarca J, Malone DC, Armstrong EP, Grizzle AJ, Hansten PD, Van Bergen RC, Lipton RB. (2004). Concordance of major drug interaction classification among drug interaction compendia. *Am J Pharm Assoc* 44(2):136-141. Copyright American Pharmacists Association. Reprinted by permission of APhA.

[a]Upon discontinuation of the barbiturate

TABLE 6.3. Drug Interactions Associated with Fatal Outcomes

Drug Interaction	Net Potential Effect
Fluoxetine and phenelzine	Rapid heart rate
Digoxin and quindine	Digoxin toxicity
Sildenafil and isorbide mononitrate	Low blood pressure
Potassium chloride and spironolactone	High serum potassium levels
Clonidine and propranalol	High blood pressure
Warfarin and diflunisal	Gastrointestinal bleeding
Theophylline and ciprofloxacin	Theophylline toxicity
Pimozide and ketoconazole	Cardiac irregularities
Methotrexate and probenecid	Methotrexate toxicity
Bromocriptine and pseudoephedrine	Severe high blood pressure
Methotrexate and NSAIDs	Methotrexate toxicity
Phenytoin and dopamine	Dramatic low blood pressure

Source: Adapted from Burns SB and Kelly WN. (2002). 10 drug interactions every pharmacist should know. *Pharmacy Times* 68:46-48, and Howard T. (1997). Ten drug interactions every pharmacist should know. *Southern J Health-Syst Pharm* 2:13-16. Reprinted with permission.

certain drugs with grapefruit juice.[42] Grapefruit juice can either increase or decrease the effect of specific drugs taken at the same time. Therefore, grapefruit juice should be avoided when taking any of the drugs listed in Table 6.5. Health Canada has advised Canadians to never take drugs and drink grapefruit juice or eat grapefruit unless advised by a doctor to do otherwise.[43]

Drug-Herbal Drug Interactions

More and more Americans are using herbal medicines. Table 6.6 lists common herbal drugs that should not be taken with other drugs.[44]

TABLE 6.4. Drug-Drug Interactions of Clinical Importance

Object Drug	Participant Drug
Anticoagulants	Thyroid hormones
Benzodiazepines	Azole antifungals
Carbamazepine	Propoxyphene
Cyclosporine	Rifamycins
Dextromethorphan	MAO inhibitors
Digoxin	Clarithromycin
Ergot alkaloids	Macrolide antibiotics
Estrogen plus progestin products	Rifampin
Ganciclovir	Zidovudine
MAO inhibitors	Anorexiants
MAO inhibitors	Sympathomimetics
Meperidine	MAO inhibitors
Methoptrexate	Trimethoprim
Nitrates	Sildenafil
Pimozide	Macrolide antibiotics
SSRIs	MAO inhibitors
Theophyllines	Quinolones
Theophyllines	Fluvoamine
Thiopurines	Allopurinol
Warfarin	Sulfinpyrazone
Warfarin	NSAIDs
Warfarin	Cimetidine
Warfarin	Fibric acid derivatives
Warfarin	Barbiturates

Source: Adapted from Malone DC, Abarca J, Hansten PD, Grizzle AJ, Armstrong EP, Van Bergen RC, Duncan-Edgar BS, Solomon SL, Lipton RB. (2004). Identification of serious drug-drug interactions: Results of the partnership to prevent drug-drug interactions. *J Am Pharm Assoc* 44(2)142-151. Copyright American Pharmacists Association. Reprinted by permission of APhA.

TABLE 6.5. Drugs That Interact with Grapefruit or Grapefruit Juice

Drugs Affected by Grapefruit Juice	Net Effect
Calcium channel blockers	Flushing, headache, increased heart rate, decreased blood pressure
Felodipine (Plendil)	
Nifedipine (Procardia XL, Adalat CC)	
Nimodipine (Nimotop)	
Verapamil (Calan, Isoptin)	Decreased heart rate, constipation, decreased blood pressure
Nonsedating antihistamines	EKG abnormalities (prolongation of QT interval) and ventricular arrhythmias
Terfenadine (Seldane [currently off the market])	
Astemizole (Hismanol)	
Benzodiazepines	Increased sedation
Alprazolam (Xanax)	
Triazolam (Halcion)	
Midazolam	
Cholesterol-lowering drugs	Headache, gastrointestinal complaints, and muscle pain

Source: Adapted from National Emphysema Association http://emphysema foundation.org/GrapeJuice.aspx. Reprinted with permission.

TABLE 6.6. Drug-Herbal Interactions of Major Clinical Significance

Drug	Herbal Product
Warfarin	*Gingko biloba*
Aspirin	*Gingko biloba*
Sertraline	St. John's wort
Trazodone	*Gingko biloba*
Alprazolam	Kava
Cyclosporin	St. John's wort

Source: Adapted from Brazier NC and Levine MAH. (2002). Drug-herb interaction among commonly used conventional medicines: A compendium for health care professionals. *Am J Ther* 10(3):163-169. Reprinted with permission.

TREATMENT

The first step in treating someone experiencing a drug-drug interaction is to identify the offending drug, then to stop taking it. Usually, stopping the drug will result in improvement. If not, the most life-threatening symptoms are treated. Specific antidotes or agents that hasten the metabolism or elimination of the offending drug, if available, can be used.

PATIENT EDUCATION

Patients should be counseled when a drug they are taking may interact with another drug, especially if the interaction is known to cause harm. This advice should include any foods or herbal products to avoid. Pharmacists should list all active prescription drugs, over-the-counter drugs, and herbal products the patient takes routinely on the patient's medication profile.

SUMMARY

Drug interactions happen and can harm patients.[45] However, drug-interaction texts and detection software in pharmacy computer systems are lacking because of inadequate evidence-based information about which drug interactions cause harm.[46] Despite these limitations, and too many annoying drug-interaction alerts going off, the pharmacist has a duty to warn patients and doctors of foreseeable harm from drug interactions. Patients need to be counseled when they are taking a drug that potentially interacts with other drugs, foods (such as grapefruit or grapefruit juice), or herbal products.

Chapter 7

The Most Dangerous
Drug Misadventure

Probably the most dangerous drug misadventure is a medication error. It is also the one that is the least expected, the least reported, and the most preventable. The reasons for medication errors are complex—the etiology is interrelated between a breakdown in the medication-use system and human behavior. Fortunately, work is progressing to prevent medication errors, but the battle is challenging.

BACKGROUND

A 2002 American Society of Health-System Pharmacists (ASHP) survey revealed what patients were most concerned about regarding medication-related issues.[1] Three of the top concerns identified were: (1) being given two or more medicines that interact in a negative way (70 percent); (2) being given the wrong medicine (69 percent); and (3) potential harmful side effects from taking a medication (67 percent).

The problem of medication errors is not new. Most licensed health care professionals have known about the problem for years. Reports on the extent of injury from medical interventions and medications appeared as early as 1964.[2,3,4,5] In 1981, one investigator reported that 36 percent of the patients admitted to a medical unit of a university hospital suffered a medical injury and that 20 percent of these were serious or fatal.[3] More than half of the injuries were because of medication.

Until recently, the problem of medical and medication errors has been like an iceberg, mostly hidden from the public view. This was

Prescribed Medications and the Public Health
© 2006 by The Haworth Press, Inc. All rights reserved.
doi:10.1300/5688_07

not purposeful, but rather extended from the attitude of health care professionals that although these events were unfortunate, they were an inherent part of the health care process. The problem was accepted as a normal part of care and most people felt the problem could never be removed. Thoreau characterized this attitude as "a prevalent error that requires the most disinterested virtue to sustain it."[6] The irony is that in accepting medication errors as a part of the health care process, beneficence, the primary virtue of the healing arts, is neglected.

The problem of medical and medication errors was made public in 1999 when the Institute of Medicine (IOM), an arm of the U.S. Academy of Medical Sciences, issued its now famous report titled *To Err Is Human: Building a Safer Health System.*[7] This report not only caught the attention of health care professionals, but also the media and the public. The report stated "at least 44,000 people, and perhaps as many as 98,000 people, die in hospitals each year because of medical errors that could have been prevented, according to estimates from two major studies." It went on to estimate the total cost of this problem was between $17 and $29 billion a year in hospitals alone.

The data in the IOM report are only the tip of the medical misadventure iceberg—the morbidity, mortality, and cost of medical and medication mishaps in the ambulatory care environment was ignored. For example, a report in one journal stated, "nine out of ten pharmacists surveyed said they were aware of what they considered to be a medication error in their pharmacy in the past year."[8]

There are many causes of medication errors and most errors have more than one cause.[9] The increasing number of prescriptions being dispensed adds to the problem. One drug safety expert has provided insight on the cause of medical errors and some of these causes will be covered later in this chapter.[10]

What is a medication error? What are the various types? How often do they occur? What are the most common causes? What are the most common drugs involved? These are the questions addressed in this chapter.

DEFINITIONS

A *medication error* has been defined as "an unintended act (either of omission or commission) or as an act that does not achieve its intended outcome."[11] The National Coordinating Council for Medication

Error Reporting and Prevention (NCC MERP) defines a medication error as "any preventable event that may cause or lead to inappropriate medication use or patient harm while the medication is in control of the health care professional, patient, or consumer."[12] Medication errors are also adverse episodes associated with the use of medications that should be prevented through effective control systems.

ERROR CLASSIFICATION

The United States Pharmacopeia (USP) has the largest database of medication errors in the United States (MEDMARX) and receives anonymous medication error reports each year from over 500 hospitals. There are more than 1 million reports in the database. MEDMARX classifies medication errors in various ways. One classification is the stage in the medication-use process *when* the error occurred. For 2002, MEDMARX reported the following distribution: administering (33 percent), documenting (23 percent), dispensing (22 percent), prescribing (21 percent), and monitoring (1 percent).[13] Other error classifications by USP include *what* went wrong: omission (25.6 percent), improper dose or quantity (25.5 percent), prescribing error (18.5 percent), receiving an unauthorized drug (11.1 percent), receiving a drug at the wrong time (6.9 percent), extra dose (5 percent), wrong patient (4.7 percent), and miscellaneous (9.2 percent).

USP also classifies medication errors by their *cause*. In 2002, the leading causes of medication errors in hospitals that resulted in harm were: performance deficit (46.7 percent), a procedure or protocol not followed (29.4 percent), poor communication (17.7 percent), knowledge deficit (17.6 percent), inaccurate transcription or omission (11.2 percent), poor documentation (10.2 percent), and computer-entry error (8.2 percent).

Another way of classifying medication errors is to group the errors by contributing factors such as: distractions (29 percent), workload increases (15 percent), inexperienced staffing (12 percent), inadequate staffing (8 percent), shift change (8 percent), temporary staffing (5 percent), and cross coverage (4 percent).[14]

CASE EXAMPLES

In 1995, a health columnist for one of the largest newspapers in the country, was undergoing therapy for advanced breast cancer at an academic cancer center in the Northeastern United States.[15] The columnist's heart failed and she died after being given four times the maximum safe dosage of a toxic chemotherapeutic drug. "At least a dozen doctors, nurses, and pharmacists overlooked the error for four days while Lehman continued to receive an overdose of cyclophosphamide and a fourfold overdose of another drug meant to shield her from side effects."

Mike McClave mixed a couple of spoonfuls of prescription medicine he picked up at a pharmacy for his eight-year-old daughter with some 7-Up and gave it to her to relieve a raspy sore throat. The next morning Megan never woke up.[16]

In 1995, a children's hospital confirmed that its doctors accidentally gave powerful doses of a wrong drug to a six-year-old child suffering from seizures.[17] A representative for the hospital said, "It is our belief that there are no short-term adverse effects, and it is our belief there will be no long-term effects. Nevertheless, there was a series of errors which the hospital regrets deeply."

A baby girl was born on August 1, 1984.[18] A checkup at a well-baby clinic in 1985 revealed that she had Wilms' tumor—a cancerous, potentially lethal disease. She was in and out of doctors' offices and hospitals over the next few months. During this time, her parents noticed that medications which should have been given to her with food were given without food and conversely. In addition, several allergic reactions were narrowly avoided.

Back in the hospital, she started on a more potent cancer drug. The order read 10 mg. On the third day, she received 100 mg of the drug rather than 10 mg. "The doctor—and this happens every day and is probably happening right now—had meant to write 10 mg, and he thought he did, but when we looked at the documentation it sure looked like 100 mg to me," said her father. "The pharmacist missed it, the resident missed it, the fellow missed it, the on-call doctor missed it, and the nurse missed it, even though the first two doses had been 10 mg." She survived this overdose, but the story goes on.

One night, her mom woke up to find a nurse ready to put something into her daughter's IV line. She questioned the nurse. After the nurse succumbed to the pleas of a frantic mother, it was discovered the drug was for another patient.

The final error occurred later when a nurse came into her room at the end of the night shift to flush her IV line. The nurse, who had worked multiple nights in a row and was now on her second shift of the day, introduced air into the IV line. She had a cardiac arrest and died.

In summarizing what happened, her father said, "It was not as if the providers were not good people, that the doctors did not want to practice good medicine, that the nurses did not want to take care of the kids at that institution and do the very best they could do. These health care providers were all good people who needed better support and better systems."

EPIDEMIOLOGY

Medication Error Rates

Calculating medication error rates presents a dilemma. On one hand, calculating an error rate is an objective method to assess the extent of medication safety and is especially useful if the comparison is within the same facility and between two points in time. However, calculating medication error rates is fraught with complexity and confounding factors. Because of the latter, a comparison of medication error rates between different facilities is inappropriate.[19] Some of the problems associated in calculating and comparing medication error rates include differences in:

- defining medication errors,
- organizational culture,
- patient populations,
- detection methods, and
- denominators.

Large differences in medication error rates are based on the detection methods used. The observation method of studying medication errors yields higher rates than relying on incident reports of medication errors, which are notoriously underreported.[20] Including the criterion of administering medication at the wrong time will inflate medication error rates by almost 100 percent.

Despite the lack of standardized methods to document and calculate medication error rates, researchers have performed studies to discover medication error rates in various types of health care facilities and categories of patients. Some of these studies are listed in Table 7.1.

TABLE 7.1 Some Medication Error Rates by Health Care Site and Patient

Site	Year	Patients	Detection Method	Error Detection Rate	Harmful Error Rate
Emergency room[a]	2001	Emergency room	Incident Reports	1.95% of hospital errors	7.6% of errors in ER
Teaching hospital[b]	1990	Acute care	Prospective review of orders	3.13 errors/ 1,000 orders	1.81 errors/ 1,000 orders
Small hospitals[c]	1982	Acute care	Observation	12.2% of opportunities for error	–
Pediatric hospital[d]	2001	Pediatric	Prospec- tive/retro- spective review	57.1 errors/ 1,000 orders	1.94 errors/ 1,000 orders
Teaching hospital[e]	1994	Discharge	Discharge Rx review	5.8% of take-home prescrip- tions	–
Long-term care facilities[c]	1982	Long-term care	Observation	11.0% of opportunities for error	–
Home[f]	2001	Home health care	Criteria for inappropri- ate drug orders	17-19% of orders	–

[a]United States Pharmacopoeia (2003). Summary of information submitted to MEDMARX in the year 2002. November 18, 2003.

[b]Lesar TS, Briceland LL, Delcoure K, Parmalee JD, Masta-Fornic V, Pohl H. (1990). Medication prescribing errors in a teaching hospital. *JAMA* 263(17): 2329-2334.

[c]Barker KN, Mikeal RL, Pearson RE, Illig NA, Morse ML. (1982). Medication errors in nursing homes and small hospitals. *Am J Hosp Pharm* 39: 987-991.

[d]Kaushal R, Bates DW, Landrigan C. (2001). Medication errors and adverse drug event in pediatric inpatients. *JAMA* 285(16): 2114-2120.

[e]Schumock GT, Guenette AJ, Keys TV, Hutchinson RA. (1994). Prescribing errors for patients about to be discharged from a university hospital. *Am J Hosp Pharm* 51: 228, 2290.

[f] Meredith S., Feldman PH, Frey D, Hall K, Arnold K, Brown NJ, Ray WA. (2002). Possible medication erros in home healthcare patients. *J Am Geriatr Soc* 49: 719-724.

Hospital Errors

In a review of observation-based studies in hospitals, medication error rates ranged from 4.4 to 59.1 percent if wrong times were included, and from 0.4 to 24.7 percent if wrong times were excluded.[20] Medication error rates were consistently and significantly lower in hospitals using a unit-dose drug distribution system. A study of 36 hospitals and skilled nursing facilities in Atlanta and Denver revealed that 19 percent of the doses were in error, and of these, 7 percent were potentially harmful.[21] This was extrapolated to mean that hospitals make an average of 40 potentially harmful medication errors for 300 inpatients each day.

Some studies suggest that medication error rates may be highest in pediatric patients, patients in intensive care units (even when adjusted for the medication used), and in patients about to be discharged from the hospital.[22-24]

Emergency Room Errors

Medication errors occur in hospital emergency rooms.[25-26] Data for hospitals from MEDMARX show that about 2 percent of medication errors in a hospital happen in the hospital's emergency room, and that 7.6 percent of these errors resulted in harm.[13]

Medication Errors in Long-Term Care

Quality of care requirements under the Omnibus Budget Reconciliation Act (OBRA 90) specifies that long-term care (LTC) facilities must be free of any significant medication error rates of 5 percent or greater. A study of 12 LTC facilities in 2002 suggested the medication error rates (by the observation method) for these facilities ranged from 5.7 percent to 49.5 percent.[27]

Home Health Care Errors

A study to discover the frequency of possible medication errors in a population of older home health care patients using two different sets of criteria discovered that possible medication errors occurred 17 to 19 percent of the time.[28]

Medication Errors in Ambulatory Care

Medication errors also occur in the ambulatory environment. These will be discussed in Chapter 9.

Medication Error Types

The NCC MERP has a taxonomy for classifying medication errors. According to NCC MERP guidelines, information for each error should document: the event, the patient, the patient outcome, product information, the personnel involved, the error, the cause of the error, and contributing factors. The NCC MERP taxonomy document provides specific information to be collected in an organized and standardized format.[29]

Medication errors can be classified in different ways including during the processes of prescribing, documenting, dispensing, administration, compounding, or monitoring.

Prescribing Errors

Most medication errors occur at the prescribing stage. Rates vary by whom prescribed the medication. In one study, first-year postgraduate residents were found to have a higher error rate (4.25 /1,000 orders) than other prescriber classes. Obstetric/gynecology services (3.54 errors/1,000 orders) and surgery/anesthesia services (3.42 errors/1,000 orders) had a greater error rate than other services.[26] Although no medication error is acceptable, the rates for prescribing errors are relatively low because of pharmacist intervention. A study of 115 community pharmacies in Ohio discovered that pharmacists were often spotting problems in prescriptions.[30] Of the problems noted, most concerned inappropriate dose, regimen, or strength (25 percent); a drug interaction (31 percent); a problem in drug therapy monitoring (19 percent); or a prescription omission (16 percent). Despite the daily efforts of pharmacists, prescribing errors occasionally get through the system. For 2002, 21.3 percent of the medication errors reported to MEDMARX involved problems in prescribing.[13]

Documentation Errors

Errors in documentation involve recording inaccurate information or omitting relevant information. This can occur in the patient's record, the patient's pharmacy profile, or in nursing administration records. For 2002, 23 percent of the medication errors reported to MEDMARX involved errors in documentation.[13]

Dispensing Errors

Pharmacies dispense hundreds of thousands of prescriptions and drug orders every day. How many of these have errors? A recent study says 1.7 percent.[31] Of the errors discovered, 65 percent were judged clinically significant. The study was done in six cities and included chain-store pharmacies, independent community pharmacies, and health-system pharmacies (in hospitals or managed care organizations). This means about four errors a day happen in a pharmacy filling 250 prescriptions a day. About 3 billion prescriptions are filled every year in the United States; this means as many as 51.5 million dispensing errors may occur during a year, of which 3.3 million may be clinically significant. For hospitals during 2002, 21.6 percent of 162,337 medication errors reported to MEDMARX involved dispensing errors.

Compounding Errors

The art of measuring and mixing medicine or *compounding* was once the basis of the pharmacy profession. In the 1930s and 1940s, nearly 60 percent of medication was compounded. Medication compounding dwindled to about zero until the mid 1990s when some community pharmacists rediscovered the value of making customized medicinal products.

Compounding is the practice of pharmacy in which the product is made under a doctor's prescription and is produced one product at a time. Pharmacists follow standards of practice to help ensure that the product is made correctly. However, studies have shown that some products compounded by pharmacists may not be within safe limits. For example, an FDA undercover investigation in 2002 in 12 pharmacies reported that 10 of 29 compounded prescriptions failed testing, nine were subpotent, and one was contaminated.[32]

Fortunately, many of the products compounded by community pharmacists are for topical use and if made in error cause little danger. However, some compounding errors can be tragic. In 2001, a five-year-old child received a 1,000-fold overdose of clonidine because of a calculation error in which milligrams were substituted for micrograms.[33] Fortunately, the child survived.

Hospital pharmacists often compound sterile intravenous drug products for patients. An observational study on the accuracy of compounding in five hospitals was completed in 1997.[34] The range of error rates for the five hospitals was 6 to 10 percent with a mean of 9 percent. Two percent of the errors were considered clinically significant. Wrong dose or dose errors were the most common types of errors.

Administration Errors

Errors in administration occur when the nurse fails to give the medication correctly or, in the ambulatory environment, the patient does not take the medication correctly. The highest number of errors (33 percent) reported to MEDMARX in 2002 was for administration. However, it must be remembered that the nurse works near the end of the medication-use process and there is usually no double check on what they do or do not do. Some common administration errors are: giving the wrong drug or wrong dose to the right patient, giving the correct drug to the correct patient but in the wrong way or at the wrong time, or giving a drug to the wrong patient.

Monitoring Errors

Monitoring errors occur when drug therapy is not followed closely. For example, certain drugs need baseline laboratory values established before a drug is prescribed, and occasionally while the drug is being used.

In one study of 1,520 published adverse drug event reports, only 17 percent of the patients on drugs that should have been checked by blood-level monitoring were not monitored this way.[35] Monitoring errors represented 1.1 percent of the errors reported to the MEDMARX database in 2002.

PATIENTS

Medication errors are probably not evenly divided in the population. The distribution is determined by what drugs are prescribed or the dosage of the drugs administered, rather than any particular patient characteristic. However, patient risk factors contribute to outcome—harm or no harm.

Detecting harmful medication errors by age groups is difficult without adjusting for the drugs used by each age group. The youngest and oldest patients are more vulnerable to the effects of medication because of the maturity of key organs that metabolize and remove drugs from the body (the liver and kidneys, respectively). In addition, anyone with reduced liver or renal function is more susceptible to the harmful effects of drugs. Thus, monitoring these organ systems is critical when high-risk drugs are prescribed.

Some of the most dangerous drugs are those having a low therapeutic index—the minimum therapeutic dose is close to the minimum lethal dose. The FDA identifies a drug that has a narrow therapeutic index if small changes in the dosage level could cause toxic results.

The MEDMARX database contains medication errors reported from almost 500 hospitals in the United States. Table 7.2 lists the most common drugs involved in medication errors that caused 42.2 percent of the harm during 2002.

In one study, the most common drugs associated with errors in pediatric patients were anti-infective drugs (28 percent) and intravenous medication (54 percent). The most common error was dosing.[23] Errors with the use of cancer chemotherapeutic agents in pediatric patients has also been a problem, most notably in calculation errors and mix-ups between look-alike drugs such as vincristine and vinblastine.[36]

Another special population of patients are those who receive care at home. One study showed the drugs most inappropriately used in this population were: propoxyphene (an analgesic), chlordiazepoxide or diazepam (minor tranquilizers), disopyramide (heart drug), amitriptyline (antidepressant), and ticlopidine (platelet aggregation inhibitor).[28]

Getting a handle on which prescription and over-the-counter (OTC) drugs are most commonly associated with errors in the ambulatory environment has been difficult. This will be covered in Chapter 9.

TABLE 7.2. Some of the Most Dangerous Drugs Associated with Error

Narrow Therapeutic Drugs	Most Common Drugs Causing Harm to Hospital Patients
Aminophylline	Insulin (8.1%)
Carbamazepine	Morphine (5.5%)
Clonidine	Heparin (4.6%)
Isoproterenol	Potassium chloride (3.0%)
Lithium	Warfarin (3.0%)
Phénytoin	Hydromorphone (2.8%)
Procainamide	Fentanyl (2.2%)
Quinidine	Vancomycin (2.0%)
Theophylline	Enoxaparin (2.0%)
Valproic acid	Meperidine (1.9%)
Warfarin	Furosemide (1.7%)
	Diltiazem (1.5%)
	Metoprolol (1.3%)
	Dopamine (1.2%)
	Lorazepam (1.2%)

Source: Adapted with permission from Hicks RW, Cousins DD, and Williams RL. "Summary of information submitted to MEDMARX in the year 2002, the quest for quality," USP Center for the Advancement of Patient Safety, © 2003.

More work is needed to discover which drugs are associated with errors in various populations of patients.

Patient Outcomes from Medication Errors

The USP, through its MEDMARX medication reporting system, places each medication error into an outcome category (Figure 7.1). This is performed by using an algorithm (Figure 7.2). In 2002, only about half (49 percent) of the medication errors reported to MED-MARX reached the patient and 1.7 percent of these were harmful. Of those medication errors causing harm, 1 percent may have contributed to or resulted in permanent disability, 1.5 percent needed intervention to continue life, and 0.6 percent may have contributed to or

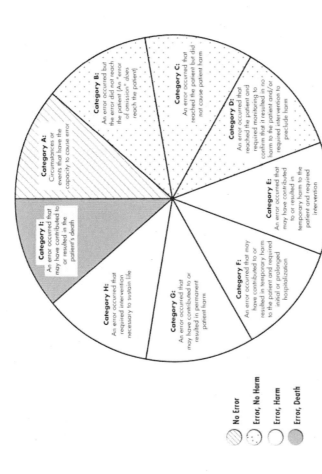

Definitions

Harm

Impairment of the physical, emotional, or psychological function or structure of the body and/or pain resulting therefrom.

Monitoring

To observe or record relevant physiological or psychological signs.

Intervention

May include change in therapy or active medical/surgical treatment.

Intervention Necessary to Sustain Life

Includes cardiovascular and respiratory support (e.g., CPR, defibrillation, intubation, etc.)

Category A:
Circumstances or events that have the capacity to cause error

Category B:
An error occurred but the error did not reach the patient (An "error of omission" does reach the patient)

Category C:
An error occurred that reached the patient but did not cause patient harm

Category D:
An error occurred that reached the patient and required monitoring to confirm that it resulted in no harm to the patient and/or required intervention to preclude harm

Category E:
An error occurred that may have contributed to or resulted in temporary harm to the patient and required intervention

Category F:
An error occurred that may have contributed to or resulted in temporary harm to the patient and required initial or prolonged hospitalization

Category G:
An error occurred that may have contributed to or resulted in permanent patient harm

Category H:
An error occurred that required intervention necessary to sustain life

Category I:
An error occurred that may have contributed to or resulted in the patient's death

No Error
Error, No Harm
Error, Harm
Error, Death

FIGURE 7.1. NCC MERP Index for Categorizing Medication Errors (*Source:* Copyright © 2001 by the National Coordinating Council for Medication Error Reporting and Prevention [NCC MERP]. All rights reserved. Reprinted with permission of the NCC MERP.)

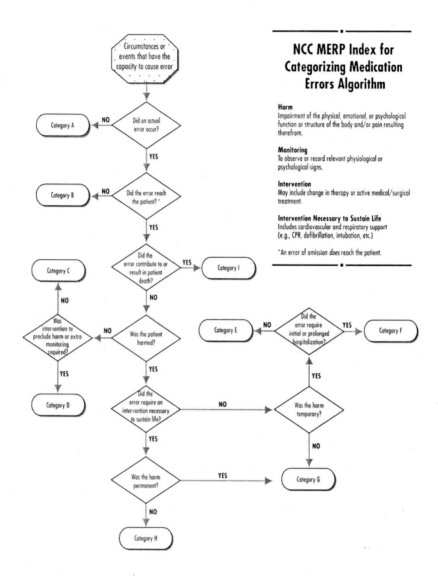

FIGURE 7.2. NCC MERP Index for Categorizing Medication Errors Algorithm (*Source:* Copyright © 2001 by the National Coordinating Council for Medication Error Reporting and Prevention [NCC MERP]. All rights reserved. Reprinted with permission of the NCC MERP.)

resulted in the patient's death.[13] Although the numbers of serious outcomes in MEDMARX are low, there may be reporting bias because of the negative nature of the data.

Medication Deaths

Studying the most serious medication errors may help in discovering clues as to how and why these events occur. Exactly how many people die each year in the United States from the legitimate use of medication is unknown and difficult to discover.[37]

Inappropriate extrapolations of how many people die as a result of their prescribed medication (as high as 140,000 yearly in the United States) have been calculated based on medication-related deaths of medical inpatients. However, these patients have more illnesses and take more medications than other categories of patients. The prevalence of medication-related deaths to hospitalized patients has ranged from 0 to 2.9 percent of admissions.[38] The possibility of death rises with the number of drugs prescribed, age, and the number of diseases being treated.[39]

In a 20-year review of published case reports, the drugs most commonly associated with a fatal medication error were: chlorpromazine (major tranquilizer), halothane (anesthestic), lidocaine (cardiac drug), meperidine (analgesic), and morphine (analgesic). MEDMARX reported 20 medication errors resulting in death in 2002 with 21 drugs involved once and two drugs involved twice—digoxin (heart) and dobutamine (heart).

In a study of fatal medication errors reported to the FDA's Adverse Events Reporting System (AERS) between 1993 and 1998, most patients were over 60 years old and in hospitals.[40] Most of the patients (46.7 percent) received central nervous system depressants, antineoplastic agents, or cardiovascular drugs. The most common error was improper dosing.

Life-Threats from Drug Errors

Sometimes people undergo a threat to life from a drug, but survive because of heroic measures. One study of this drug-related outcome discovered the most common drugs involved were: heparin (anticoagulant), methotrexate (cancer drug), vancomycin (antibiotic), phenytoin (seizures), and cyclosprorine (transplant).[41]

Permanent Disability from Medication Errors

Sometimes, people are permanently disabled from a medication error. They can lose their hearing or vision, have liver, kidney, or brain damage, or become quadriplegic or paraplegic. In a study of 227 published case reports of drug-induced permanent disability, the drugs most commonly involved were: doxorubicin (cancer drug), gentimicin (antibiotic), lithium (bipolar illness), neomycin (antibiotic), and oxytocin (labor-inducing agent).[42] About half of the patients received more than the usual dose and 29 percent were children less than ten years old.

COST

Although some studies estimate the cost of adverse drug events (ADEs) to a hospital ($3,244 to $5,857 a case), to a nursing home ($1.33 in health care resources for every $1 spent on drugs), and to society in general in the ambulatory setting ($76.6 billion a year), there is yet to be a well-designed study on what costs are associated with medication errors.[43,44,45,46]

WHAT IS THE PROBLEM?

So, why are these medication errors occurring? Many feel it is because the medication-use process is too complex. As shown in Figure 7.3, there are too many steps, too many things to remember, too many overlapping roles, too many gaps, and too many people involved in how medications are made, distributed, prescribed, dispensed, administered, managed, documented, and monitored. In a hospital, the procurement, preparation, and dispensing of drugs may include as many as 40 or 50 steps. The complexity and problems associated with the medication-use system was first documented in 1987 and the problem has gotten worse.[47]

Proof of the medication-use system being in disarray was shown in a computer field test performed by the Institute for Safe Medication

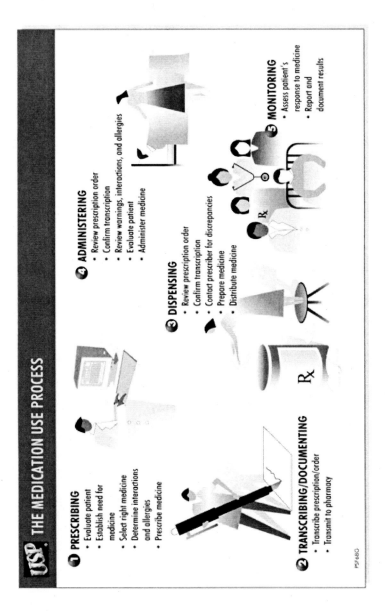

FIGURE 7.3. The Medication Use Process (*Source:* Reprinted with permission of the United States Pharmacopeial Convention, Inc., © 2003.)

Practices (ISMP) in over 300 hospitals in 1999.[48] Each hospital was provided with ten unsafe medication orders, each potentially lethal. Only four out of 307 (1.3 percent) pharmacy computer systems tested detected all ten unsafe orders. For each medication error, the detection for all hospitals tested ranged from a low of 12 percent to a high of 87 percent.

In addition, each of the hospitals taking part in the survey was asked ten questions about its pharmacy computer system. Answering "yes" to a question signaled a priority for safety. The range of "yes" answers was from a low of 13 percent to a high of 88 percent. The authors concluded: "pharmacy computer systems need serious improvement . . . it's frightening most of our nation's pharmacy computer systems may be incapable of detecting orders that exceed a set maximum dose."

COMMON TYPES OF MEDICATION ERRORS

The most reliable data on the most common types of medication errors come from the USP. In 2002, the most common types of medication errors that cause harm to patients in hospitals were: use of the wrong administration technique (6.2 percent), wrong route of administration (2.6 percent), a patient receiving an unauthorized drug (1.9 percent), using an improper dose or quantity of drug (1.9 percent), and providing an extra dose (1.9 percent).[13]

Errors with cancer chemotherapeutic medication and with the use of electronic infusion devices for drugs have been of major concern. Newer electronic infusion devices are starting to provide better safeguards. Why has this taken so long? A review of the ten most common lethal medication errors in hospital patients is provided.[49]

The extent and kinds of errors patients make in taking drugs or when they receive medication from a caretaker in their home is explored in Chapter 9.

SENTINEL EVENTS

The Joint Commission on Accreditation of Healthcare Organizations (JCAHO) requires health organizations to do more if the event is sentinel. A "sentinel event" is an adverse event that ends in death or is a "near miss event"—an event that could have ended in a tragic outcome. Also, the health care organization must perform a root cause analysis (RCA) of all sentinel events. On completion of the RCA, the health care organization must document what it will do differently to prevent a similar instance in the future. Guidelines on how to document sentinel events, how to perform RCA, and examples of sentinel events are available on JCAHO's Web site (http://www.jcaho.org). JCAHO also provides a guidance document on preventing medication errors for pharmacists.[50] Also available is a practical guide to medication safety and JCAHO compliance.[51]

MAJOR CAUSES OF MEDICATION ERROR

The causes of medication errors can be divided into two major problems—system problems and people problems. In 1995, Leape and colleagues performed an analysis to discover the proximal causes of adverse drug events such as medication errors.[52] They noted and identified sixteen underlying system failures, which they believed were to blame. System problems are easier to understand and correct than people problems.

System Problems

As previously discussed, the medication-use process is fraught with system problems. Some of these happen during the prescribing stage, some happen during the dispensing and administration stages, for example: handwriting, similar drug names, look-alike drugs, abbreviations, ambiguous and incomplete orders, misuse of decimals and zeros, look-alike labeling and packaging, verbal orders, not using a unit-dose system, miscalculating dose, and lack of patient education.

Handwriting

Many medication errors occur because:

1. the prescription was difficult to read,
2. the pharmacist thought he or she knew what the prescription said,

3. the pharmacist failed to double-check his or her interpretation with the prescriber, and
4. a medication different from what the doctor intended was dispensed.

Writing prescriptions by hand is an archaic practice that needs to be abandoned.

Similar Drug Names

Medication errors have occurred because many drug names look or sound alike. Confusion over the likeness of drug names (either written or spoken) accounts for roughly 15 percent of all reports to the USP Medication Errors Reporting System (MER). The USP publishes a list of more than 800 pairs of similar drug names. Some examples are: Iodine can sound like codeine, quinine can look like quinidine, and vinblastine can look like vincristine.

Look-Alike Drugs

The ISMP and FDA send out alerts when they notice errors because of look-alike drugs. For example, on October 9, 2003, the FDA advised health care professionals of the risk of dispensing errors between Keppra and Kaletra.

Adding to the drug-name confusion is that every drug has at least two names—a generic or common name, and usually a proprietary or trade name. Many names contribute to errors, and it has been argued that proprietary names for drugs should be eliminated.[53] However, major pharmaceutical companies love proprietary names. "Most companies hire consultants—at a cost of up to $200,000—whose creative departments brainstorm hundreds of names."[54] Unfortunately, many of the names eventually used for a drug sound or look like a drug already on the market. The problem of drug-name confusion is so bad that the Agency for Healthcare Quality and Research recently awarded $1.7 million to study the problem.[55]

Abbreviations

Many abbreviations are used in health care because they save time when writing prescriptions and orders, documenting what has taken place, and when communicating in writing. However, the use of abbreviations sometimes results in errors and patient harm. Several reasons exist for medical abbreviation errors.

First, there are so many abbreviations that it is difficult for health care workers to know what each one means. Here is an example:

> ....73 YO WDWNAAF BIBA admitted to CPETU c/o PND & DOE. TBNA in EDTU lask wk for CP relieved by NTG. Prev Adm for PTCA 1986, IATT 1997, & LARS 1999. ATSO Dr Jones[56]

The second reason is the same abbreviation may have more than one meaning. For example, does D/W mean dextrose and water or does it mean distilled water? Does MSO_4 mean morphine sulfate or magnesium sulfate?

The third reason is abbreviations often are confused with numbers that turn small doses into large doses. For example the abbreviation U for units has resulted in doses ten times normal. An order for 10U of insulin has been read as 100 units of insulin. The looping part of the handwritten letter F can wind up on the line below of an order that changes 100 mg into 1,000 mg. The use of the slash (/) has been interpreted as a 1. The abbreviation QD (every day) looks like and has been interpreted as QID (four times a day).

The fourth reason is that many health care organizations allow the use of any abbreviation, even those that people make up. Lists of acceptable abbreviations may be long, may have no definitions, have duplication, and probably will not show which definitions to never use.

The ISMP (http://www.ismp.org) publishes a list of error-prone abbreviations, symbols, and dose designations that can be used as the basis of creating a solid policy on the use of abbreviations.

Ambiguous and Incomplete Orders

Some medication orders are written with something missing, for example, "digoxin 1.5cc." One nurse may interpret this order as "1.5 cc of digoxin oral solution," while another nurse may interpret this to mean "1.5 cc of digoxin IV." Assumptions about what is missing on a prescription or drug order can be deadly. An order for cyclophosphamide (a cancer drug) written as "4 g/m^2 days 1-4" was interpreted to mean "4 g/m² each day for four days." This turned out to be lethal for a patient in Boston.

The Misuse of Decimals and Zeros

Using a trailing zero (that is 2.0) after a decimal point is a setup for a tenfold dosing error. In this case, misreading the decimal point, or if the decimal point is positioned on a line used to separate orders, would probably result in a patient receiving 20 mg rather than 2 mg. Not putting a zero before a decimal point (0.5 mg) is equally danger-ous. In this case, not seeing the decimal point (.5 mg) may also result in a patient receiving (5 mg)—a dose ten times what was ordered.

Errors also occur during the stages of dispensing and administra-tion.

Look-Alike Labeling and Packaging

Pharmaceutical companies like to standardize their packaging and labeling and make these distinctive so that users recognize their com-pany. This standardization has led to some major medication errors because packaging and labeling look so much alike.

An example of similar packaging and labeling is provided in Fig-ure 7.4. Little headway has been made in getting drug companies to understand that their labeling and packaging practices cause errors. A few companies have listened, but most have not.

Verbal Orders

Except for some narcotics and other controlled substances, it is le-gal for prescribers to give nurses and pharmacists verbal medication orders. Although convenient, this practice has led to some tragic medication errors. Seldane can sound like Feldene. A pharmacist or nurse unfamiliar with a person's accent can easily think they heard one thing when it was another. Most health care institutions have po-lices about verbal orders, but these are seldom enforced.

Not Using a Unit-Dose System

The unit-dose system is the safest system of drug distribution in or-ganized health care settings. In a unit-dose system, only a 24-hour

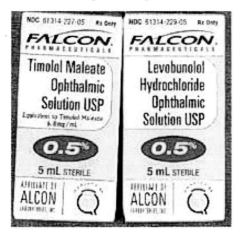

FIGURE 7.4. Photo of Timolol and Levobunolol—Similar Labeling/Packaging (*Source:* Reprinted from USP Quality Review No. 78, "Too Much Similarity," with permission of the United States Pharmacopeial Convention, Inc. Copyright 2004. All rights reserved.)

supply (or less) of medication is available on the patient care unit for a patient, and the medication is placed in the patient's own medication drawer. Each individual dose is labeled so it can be identified up to the point of administration. Despite the unit-dose method being evidenced based, some health care facilities still do not use this system.

Miscalculating Dose

Miscalculating a dose can lead to gross undertreatment or lethal overdose. At least three causes of dose miscalculations have been identified.

The first cause is that some pharmaceutical companies are not making their product available in unit-dose, ready-to-use packaging. Some companies say they are unaware of the need, while others say that it is too expensive.

The second cause is not using unit-dose-packaged, ready-to-give medication when it is available. Some hospitals claim it is too expensive, even though it is only pennies more a dose. This results in the pharmacist or nurse having to calculate and measure doses, increasing the opportunity for error.

The third cause is weak coursework in pharmaceutical calculations in the health profession schools, and not enough checking to evaluate who is weak in this area.

More contributing factors cause medication dispensing and administration errors. An excellent review, specific to pharmacy errors, has been written.[57] The American Society of Consultant Pharmacists (ASCP) also has a guide on common breakdown points in the medication-use process.[58]

Lack of Patient Education

Patients who are not informed or do not care to know about their medications are more vulnerable to medication errors than those patients who are informed. All health care providers, doctors, pharmacists, and nurses, have a duty to make sure patients understand their medications. Patients should be encouraged to ask questions and to become a partner in the medication-use process.

People Problems

System problems are much easier to understand and correct than people problems. The irony is that people problems cause most of the medication errors. Unfortunately, many people, even those working hard to reduce the problem of medication errors, sorely misunderstand this point.

In 1995, a study was conducted about the proximal cause of medication errors.[52] The most common causes were:

1. lack of knowledge about the drug,
2. lack of knowledge about the patient,
3. rules violations, and
4. slips in memory lapses.

In 1997, another study reported that over a one-year period, 2,103 prescribing errors were discovered in a large teaching hospital in the United States.[59] The most common groups of factors associated with these errors were:

1. those related to knowledge and applying knowledge on drug therapy (30 percent),

2. knowledge and use of knowledge on patient factors that affect drug therapy (29.2 percent),
3. use of calculations, decimal points, or unit and rate of expression factors (17.5 percent), and
4. nomenclature factors such as wrong drug name, dosage form, or abbreviations (13.4 percent).

Confirmation that people problems are the major cause of medication errors is shown in the 2002 MEDMARX report.[13] During 2002, the most common causes of the medication errors reported to MEDMARX were:

1. performance deficit (46.6 percent),
2. procedures or policies not followed (29.4 percent),
3. communication (17.7 percent), and
4. knowledge deficit (17.6 percent).

Slips versus Mistakes

Medication mishaps can also be classified as "slips" or "errors."[10] Slips are defined as attention-deficit errors. The person knew better, but because of inattention or distraction, he or she did something wrong. Almost everyone has made these errors. The major contributors to medication slips are: not reading labels, interruptions and distractions, and having too much to do.

Not reading labels. This happens all the time. An example is going to the supermarket and bringing home regular coffee when you thought you had bought decaffeinated coffee. Being familiar with what something looks like, rather than reading the label, contributes to these errors. This is why color-coding often does not help—people look for the color rather than read the label.

On October 9, 2003, the FDA sent a safety alert to health care professionals about accidental overdose and deaths from a high concentration morphine sulfate oral solution. In most of these cases, the morphine oral solution was ordered in milligrams (mg), but interpreted for milliliters (ml), resulting in twentyfold overdoses. The product was labeled correctly, thus the error was either because the person committing the error was unfamiliar with the product or did not read the label, or both.

Interruptions and distractions. In a 1999 study of interruptions and distractions in an ambulatory clinic pharmacy, the mean number of interruptions per hour was 2.99 (+/– 2.70) and the mean number of distractions per hour was 3.80 (+/– 3.17). The overall error rate was 3.23 percent while the error rate for prescriptions filled with one or more distractions was 6.55 percent.[60]

Between 1998 and 2002, nearly 35,000 medication error records were submitted to MEDMARX. Distractions were most often reported for errors that occurred during the drug administration (39.7 percent) and drug dispensing (27.8 percent) phases of the medication-use process, and least often during the prescribing phase (8.8 percent).[61]

Workload. The current shortages of nursing and pharmacy personnel started showing up in the mid-1990s and these have not subsided. In 1999, a study commissioned by the Massachusetts State Board of Pharmacy revealed that most pharmacists felt that hectic working conditions were a major reason in their making mistakes.[62] Dispensing the wrong drug or strength (two of the most dangerous medication errors) represented 88 percent of all errors.

Pharmacists have cited problems such as long hours (sometimes up to 14 hours a day), lack of rest breaks, distractions, and not enough help.[63] Harris Fleming, writing in the February 21, 2000, issue of *Drug Topics,* called the situation a "time bomb."[64] Robert L. Landschoot confirms Fleming's feeling.[65] Landschoot details the typical hectic day of the typical community pharmacist and says that most errors made by pharmacists are largely caused by workplace factors. The shortage of pharmacists will continue through 2010 while the number of prescriptions is expected to rise.[66]

"According to healthcare experts, the present nursing shortage is going to extend to 2020 with an estimated 400,000 RN vacancies."[67] How many more medication errors will be committed because of the shortage of nurses is unknown. Fewer nurses means less time to do tasks correctly.

In addition to the factors listed previously, performance lapses can also be based in workplace chitchat, poor working conditions, poor work flow, and uneven workload.[68]

Mistakes. Mistakes are made because of lack of knowledge. An example is prescribing two drugs that are known to interact. The prescriber should have known that the drugs interact. These types of errors, although just as bad as slips, cause just as much harm as slips, and are usually less forgiving. Knowledge of drugs and drug therapy is at the heart of being a professional health care provider. Not knowing something that most peers would know is negligence. When the proper application of the knowledge is called on, and there is lack of suitable action or no action at all, it is considered negligence.

Managing Human Behavior

Many medication safety experts emphatically state that medication errors are the result of system problems. Yet, "to err is human"—so why not also pay attention to the human? Managing behavior can reduce medical and medication errors.[69] Management must put into place a system that focuses on the solution rather than the problem, trains people well, pays attention to the details of behavior, and uses positive reinforcement for procedure compliance. This system of managing behavior has been shown to reduce dramatically errors in many types of settings and many different types of disciplines.

Focusing on the solution rather than the problem also involves moving beyond blaming individuals for making an error. A culture of blame pushes the discovery and reasons for medication errors underground. Blame does more harm than good. No health care practitioner wants to make an error, especially one that harms someone. Most health care practitioners take an oath to help, rather than to harm, patients. When a health care practitioner makes an error, he or she feels bad. If the error harms someone, they have a difficult time forgiving themselves. They are taught to be perfect, and thus punish themselves unmercifully.[68] Getting beyond blame for a medication error and making a culture of trust spurs the discovery, the documentation, the identification, and prevention of errors.[70]

SUMMARY

Medication errors are the most dangerous drug misadventure. Most medication errors occur because of a breakdown in the safety net setup. Knowledge deficits, lapses in human behavior, or willfully not following proper procedures are examples of the breakdown. Medication errors may be a way of life. However, if the entire medication-use process is reengineered, medication errors can be substantially reduced.[71]

Chapter 8

Are Vaccines Safe?

Most people understand that vaccines prevent debilitating diseases, but not everyone agrees that vaccines are safe. Some people believe vaccines cause problems, and the risks of immunizations outweigh the risks of getting the diseases that they prevent. Some vaccine devotees and groups believe the government withholds safety information or is not telling the truth about vaccines. What is the truth about the vaccines? How effective are they? How safe are they? What kinds of adverse effects are there? These questions will be discussed in this chapter.

BENEFITS VERSUS RISKS

No drug or vaccine has been developed that is 100 percent safe (no side effects) and there probably will never be one. This is because of the drug and vaccine ingredients and the biological and ethnic differences within the population. Even genetically engineered drugs and vaccines may have some adverse effects associated with their use based on added (and needed) ingredients other than the active drug. Therefore, the viability of a drug or vaccine depends on its benefit-to-risk ratio. Do the benefits of vaccines outweigh the risks?

The Benefits

Of all the therapeutic agents available, vaccines have the highest benefit-to-risk ratio to society and to individuals. Immunizations are responsible for preventing death and disability due to disease and are one of the most cost-effective and widely used health interventions.[1]

Prescribed Medications and the Public Health
© 2006 by The Haworth Press, Inc. All rights reserved.
doi:10.1300/5688_08

Table 8.1 displays the maximum and the recently reported morbidity from vaccine-preventable diseases in the United States.[2] The contrast is striking—almost a 99 percent decrease in morbidity from the earth's most lethal diseases. Naturally occurring smallpox has been wiped out globally, poliomyelitis is nearly wiped out, and there have been major decreases in the incidences, morbidity, and mortality of other vaccine-preventable diseases. Because of this, immunizations rank among the greatest public health accomplishments during the twentieth century in the United States.[3]

A recent example of the synergistic value of immunization is a report that pneumococcal vaccine given to children is starting to prevent illness in unvaccinated older children and adults.[4] The study credited the 25 percent overall decline in pneumococcal disease in those over five years old to "herd immunity," which occurs when enough people in a community are vaccinated to resist circulating bacteria.

TABLE 8.1. Comparison of Maximum and Current Reported Morbidity, Vaccine-Preventable Diseases and Vaccine Adverse Events, United States

Disease	Prevaccine Era[a]	2003[b]	% Change
Diptheria	175,885 (1921)	1	−99.99
Measles	503,282 (1941)	42	−99.99
Mumps	152,209 (1968)	197	−99.87
Pertussis	147,271 (1934)	8,483	−94.24
Polio (paralytic)	16,316 (1952)	0	−100.0
Rubella	47,745 (1969)	7	−99.99
Cogenital rubella syndrome	823 (1964-65)	0	−100.0
Tetanus	1,314 (1948)	14	−98.93
Haemophilus type b and unknown (<5 yrs)	20,000 (1984)	213	−98.84

Source: Adapted from the Centers for Disease Control and Prevention (1999). Achievements in public health, 1900-1999: Impact of vaccines universally recommended for children—United States, 1990-1998. *MMWR* 48:243-248.

[a]Year of maximum cases
[b]Provisional

The Risks

Ten million immunizations are administered to children (birth through five years old) yearly in the United States, and many millions are administered to adults. In 2003, 16,880 vaccine-adverse events were reported to the Centers for Disease Control and Prevention (CDC) and to the Food and Drug Administration (FDA) through the Vaccine Adverse Events Reporting System (VAERS). Table 8.2 displays commonly required or recommended immunizations administered versus the number of vaccine-adverse events reported to VAERS, 1991-2001.[5] Although most known side effects of vaccines are minor or self-limited, some vaccines administered in some people have been associated with rare but serious side effects.[6]

TABLE 8.2. Vaccine Adverse Events Reporting System (VAERS) Reports and Dose-Based Rates for Commonly Required or Recommended Vaccines—United States, 1991-2001

Vaccine	No. of VAERS Reports	Rate for Every 100,000 Doses Distributed
Diptheria-Tetanus	1,822	14.9
Diptheria-Tetanus-Accellular Pertussis	14,016	12.5
Influenza	15,652	3.1
Hepatitis B	32,559	11.8
Hepatitis A	2,734	8.6
Haemophilus b conjugate vaccines	22,145	18.1
Inactivated polio	7,920	13.1
Meningococcal	630	7.9
Measles-Mumps-Rubella	23,787	16.3
Pneumococcal 7-valent conjugate	3,688	12.8
Pneumococcal polyvalent	6,398	10.9
Tetanus-Diptheria	9,692	6.3
Varicella	15,180	50.0

Source: Centers for Disease Control and Prevention (2003). Surveillance for safety after immunization: Vaccine adverse event reporting system (VAERS)—United States, 1991-2001. *MMWR* 52:(SS-1):15.

EVALUATION OF RISK

The FDA approves vaccines and other immunizing agents as "generally safe and effective" and the CDC and FDA monitor the safety of vaccines once they are approved for use.

Prelicensure Evaluation

As with drugs, vaccines undergo extensive laboratory, animal, and human studies. Because of the experimental design process used, inferences on the causal relationship of an adverse event with a vaccine is straightforward and can detect common acute vaccine reactions such as fever and local reactions, or adverse events that would occur in most individuals.[7] However, the expense of such trials limits the number of individuals studied. Thus, such trials cannot provide data on rare adverse reactions (for example occurring less than 1 in 1,000 doses), reactions with delayed onset (for example 30 days or more after immunization), or reactions in small subpopulations (such as small ethnic groups or premature infants). Thus, it is essential to collect post-licensing data after the vaccine is approved for use.

Postlicensure Evaluation

The postlicensure evaluation of vaccines is a continuing process and involves several components.

Published Case Reports

One postmarketing surveillance process is the reporting (by health care practitioners) of unusual or new adverse vaccine events to a medical journal. Health care practitioners, vaccine manufacturers, and patients may also file paper or electronic reports (http://www.vaers. org) directly to VAERS.

VAERS

VAERS is a cooperative program for vaccine safety of the CDC and the FDA.[8] VAERS collects reports on adverse events following immunization (AEFI). Over 15,000 reports enter the VAERS system each year. An interdisciplinary group of medical and scientific researchers at the FDA and CDC constantly review and look for patterns and signals that may suggest a possible relationship between a vaccine and an adverse event that may need further study.

An example of the success of this process was a signal produced between rotavirus vaccine (approved for use in August 1998) and a gastrointestinal problem in children called intussusception in July of 1999. The incidence of this condition during prelicensure trials with the vaccine was 0.05 percent versus an incidence of 0.02 percent in infants receiving a placebo vaccine. The difference was not statistically significant. However, shortly after the recommendations for the use of rotavirus vaccine were published in March of 1999, the VAERS team noticed 15 reports of intussusception in infants administered rotavirus vaccine. These reports resulted in a more rigorous epidemiologic investigation that discovered a strong correlation between the use of the vaccine and the adverse event. This resulted in the manufacturer withdrawing the vaccine from the market.

VAERS has several strengths.[8] It provides: a reporting system for practitioners and the public, some important details about each adverse event, it can signal previously unreported events and unusual increases in known adverse events, it is used to form hypotheses on possible relationships between a vaccine and an adverse event and possible risk factors, and it is inexpensive to perform.

VAERS also has its limits.[8] The first limit is the underreporting of adverse vaccine events. It is unknown what part of all adverse vaccine events VAERS represents, but the part that is reported is thought to be representative. The second limit is lack of a comparison (control) group. This limits causality assessment. Another limit of VAERS is that the number of doses administered is unknown, thus removing an important denominator to discover the prevalence of adverse events. A fourth limit of VAERS is missing or ambiguous information in many of the reports. Lastly is confounding by drug or disease. The mere fact the vaccine was used may cause bias in the report.

Even with the limits, VAERS continues to be an invaluable tool to monitor vaccine-adverse events, to look for signals, and to hypothesize about relationships and risk factors.

The Vaccine Safety Data Link

As noted in Figure 8.1, four groups of patients are required to discover if there is causal relationship between a vaccine and an adverse event:

1. patients who receive the vaccine and have an adverse event (box a);
2. patients who receive the vaccine and do not have the adverse event (box b);
3. patients who do not receive the vaccine and do not have the adverse event (box c); and
4. patients who do not receive the vaccine, but do have the adverse event (box d).[9]

VAERS reports on vaccinated people with adverse events (box a). Nevertheless, VAERS reports can be used to form hypotheses that can be tested using more rigorous methods.

To test hypotheses about a relationship between a vaccine and an adverse event, the CDC uses a large-linked database (LLDB) called

Adverse Event

	Yes	No
Yes	a	b
No	c	d

(Vaccination)

FIGURE 8.1. Determining a Causal Relationship Between a Vaccine and an Adverse Event (*Source:* Iskander JK, Miller ER, Pless RP, and Chen RT. Centers for Disease Control and Prevention. Vaccine post marketing surveillance: The vaccine adverse event reporting system. Continuing Medication Education. http://www.phppo.cdc.gov/phtnonline.)

The Vaccine Safety Datalink (VSD). Through affiliation with multiple health maintenance organizations (HMOs) using the staff model, the VSD prospectively collects immunization histories, patient demographics, clinical and laboratory information, and medical outcomes.[10]

The VSD has conducted active surveillance on nearly 2 percent of the U.S. population in the birth- to six-years-old age group. Epidemiologic studies in the VSD collect all the information (Figure 8.1), and have the proper design and enough power to discover rare, causal relationships between a vaccine and an adverse event.

SEVERITY OF ADVERSE VACCINE EVENTS

Most adverse reactions to vaccines are mild and safe limiting. For example, the most common reactions reported to VAERS from 1991 through 2001 are shown in Table 8.3. Most reactions occur at the site of injection.

VAERS classifies reports as nonserious or serious. From 1991 through 2001, nonserious reports ranged from 84.2 percent (2001) to

TABLE 8.3. The Most Frequent Adverse Events Reported to VAERS 1991-2001

Adverse Event	No.	%
Fever	33,172	25.8
Injection-site hypersensitivity	20,359	15.8
Rash	14,112	11.0
Injection-site edema	13,960	11.0
Vasodilation	13,929	10.8
Injection-site pain	10,382	8.1
Infection	9,741	7.6
Agitation	9,443	7.3
Pruritis	8,908	6.9
Pain	8,755	6.8

Source: Centers for Disease Control and Prevention (2003). Surveillance for safety after immunization: Vaccine adverse event reporting system (VAERS)—United States, 1991-2001. *MMWR* 52:(SS-1):15.

87.1 percent (1996).[5] The range of serious reports during this time frame was 12.9 percent (1996) to 15.8 percent (2001). Serious reports are defined as: death (1.4 to 2.3 percent), life-threatening illness (1.4 to 2.8 percent), hospitalization (9.1 to 11.1 percent), prolonged hospitalization (0.3 to 3.8 percent), and permanent disability (1.4 to 4.0 percent).

Table 8.4 lists some adverse reactions by severity specific to some commonly administered vaccines.[11] Given the number of doses of vaccines administered each year, the low prevalence of severe reactions is remarkable. However, "there is a lower tolerance for reactions caused by products given to healthy people (for example, vaccines) compared with therapy for ill people (for example, cancer)."[12]

ASSESSING WHETHER A VACCINE IS THE CAUSE OF AN ADVERSE EVENT

Academic and government researchers, using the best scientific methods, continually seek to discover if there are causal relationships between various vaccines and reported adverse events. Large funds of money, both public and private, advance this work. Some causal relationships have been discovered. Sometimes accepted scientific and statistical methods show that the relationship is coincidental. It is difficult to explain to parents of a child that the vaccine was not the cause of their child's problem. Because of no other logical explanation, some parents believe the vaccine is the cause. After all (the thinking goes), the adverse event happened after immunization.

However, there is more to causality assessment than timing and calculating odds ratios and relative risks (the scientific method), and more than "It was the vaccine; I know it."

The formal process of assessing the causality of an adverse drug or vaccine event answers three questions: Can it? Did it? Will it?[13] When reviewing an individual case report, it is natural to answer yes to the questions "Can it?" and "did it?" However, in reality, a causal association may or may not exist.

Each adverse event report needs to be reviewed for the following questions: What was the previous experience with the vaccine? Is it biologically reasonable for the vaccine to cause this event? What is the mechanism? How susceptible was the person being vaccinated? Was the timing of the adverse event consistent? Were there any

TABLE 8.4. Adverse Reactions for Some Commonly Administered Vaccines

Vaccine	Severity (Prevalence)		
	Mild	Moderate	Severe
Diptheria, Tetanus, and Pertussis	Fever (up to 1 child in 4) Redness or swelling at injection site (up to 1 child in 4) Soreness or tenderness at injection site (up to 1 child in 4)	Seizure, jerking, or staring (about 1 child in 14,000) Crying for 3 hours or more (up to 1 child out of 1,000) Fever over 105F (About 1 child out of 16,000)	Serious allergic reaction (less than 1 child out of 1 million) Long-term seizures, coma, or lowered consciousness, or permanent brain damage (so rare it is hard to tell if they are caused by the vaccine)
Haemophilus influenzae, type B	Redness, warmth or swelling at injection site (up to 1 child in 4) Fever up 101F (up to 1 child in 20)		
Hepatitis B	Soreness at injection site (up to 1 child in 4) Mild to moderate fever (up to 1 child & adolescents out of 14, and 1 out of 100 adults)		

123

TABLE 8.4 *(continued)*

Vaccine	Severity (Prevalence)		
	Mild	Moderate	Severe
Inactivated polio	Soreness at injection site (about 1 person out of 4)		Life-threatening allergic reactions (rare)
	Redness or swelling at injection site (less than 1 person out of 50)		Guillain-Barré Syndrome (in 1976 swine flu vaccine)
	Muscle aches, joint pain, fever, chills (about 1 person out of 15 or less)		
Influenza	Soreness, redness, or swelling at injection site		Serious allergic reaction (less than 1 out of a million doses)
	Fever	Seizure, jerking, or staring (about 1 out of 3,000 cases)	
	Aches	Temporary pain and stiffness in joints (up to 1 out of 4)	
Measles, Mumps, and Rubella	Fever (up to 1 person in 6)	Temporary swelling of the lymph nodes	Deafness, long-term seizures, coma or lowered consciousness (so rare, experts cannot be sure they are caused by the vaccine)
	Mild rash (about 1 person out of 20)	Temporary inflammation of the parotid gland	
	Swelling of glands in the cheeks or neck (rare)		

Vaccine	Mild side effects	More severe side effects
Pneumococcal conjugate	Redness, tenderness, or swelling at injection site (up to 1 infant in 4) Fever over 100.4F (about 1 out of 3) Fever over 102.2F (about 1 in 50) Fussy, drowsy, or loss of appetite (some)	
Pneumococcal polysaccharide	Redness or pain at injection site (about 1 in 2) Fever, muscle aches, or more severe local reactions (less than 1% rare)	
Tetanus and diptheria	Soreness, redness, or swelling at injection site	Serious allergic reaction (rarely) Deep, aching pain and muscle wasting in upper arms (rarely)
Varicella	Soreness or swelling at injection site (about 1 child out of 5 and 1 out of 3 adolescents) Fever (1 person out of 10 or less) Mild rash (1 person out of 20 or less)	Seizures, jerking, or staring (less than 1 person out of 1,000) Pneumonia (very rare) Severe brain reactions, low blood count (so rare that experts cannot tell if they are caused by the vaccine)

Source: Centers for Disease Control and Prevention. Vaccine side effects http://www.cdc.gov/nip/vacsafe/concerns/side-effects.htm.

confirmatory laboratory findings? Are there other possible explanations? What happened after dechallenge? Was there a rechallenge? If so, what happened?

The question "Will it happen?" refers to the likelihood that an individual will experience the event or, for populations, the part of the population that will experience it (that is the attributable risk). A causal association between a vaccine and an adverse event can be established if there exists: (1) a unique laboratory diagnostic result, (2) a unique clinical syndrome, or (3) a properly designed epidemiologic study showing that vaccinated people are much more likely than unvaccinated people to experience the adverse event. In the latter case, the strength of association is most important.[14]

VACCINE INJURY COMPENSATION

In 1986, Congress passed the National Childhood Vaccine Injury Act. This act set up a program to compensate those individuals or families of individuals who may have been injured by childhood vaccines on a "no-fault" basis, based on a predetermined vaccine injury table. Accurate assessment of whether adverse events can be caused by specific vaccines is required to update the vaccine injury table to compensate justly to people injured by true reactions and to disallow false or unrelated claims.

As shown in Table 8.5, nine vaccine types are currently in the vaccine injury table. The vaccine injury compensation program meets its goals by compensating individuals, stabilizing the marketplace (supply and pricing), and reducing health care provider and manufacturer liability.[15]

EMOTION VERSUS SCIENCE

Disagreements on whether a vaccine can cause an adverse event should be determined using good scientific methods rather than emotion. However, there are some people who believe vaccinations cause many problems and are distrustful of the government, medical science, or both. This has sparked growth of some groups who are negative about vaccines. In a recent study of Web sites untrusting toward vaccines, researchers discovered that most of these sites "express a

TABLE 8.5. Vaccine Injury Compensation Table

Vaccine	Adverse Event	Time Interval
Tetanus toxoid-containing vaccine	Anaphylaxis or anaphylactic shock	0-4 hours
	Brachial neuritis	2-28 days
	Any acute complication or sequela (including death) of events	
Pertussis antigen-containing vaccines	Anaphylaxis or anaphylactic shock	0-4 hours
	Encephalopathy (or encephalitis)	0-72 hours
	Any acute complication or sequela (including death) of events	
Measles, mumps, and rubella vaccine	Anaphylaxis or anaphylactic shock	0-4 hours
	Encephalopathy (or encephalitis)	5-15 days
	Any acute complication or sequela (including death) of events	
Rubella virus-containing vaccines	Chronic arthritis	7-42 hours
	Any acute complication or sequela (including death) of event	
Measles virus-containing vaccines	Thrombocytopenic purpura	7-30 days
	Vaccine-strain measles viral infection in an immunodeficient recipient	0-6 months
	Any acute complication or sequela (including death) of events	

TABLE 8.5 *(continued)*

Vaccine	Adverse Event	Time Interval
Polio live virus-containing vaccines	Paralytic polio	
	in a nonimmunodeficient recipient	0-30 days
	in an immunodeficient recipient	0-6 months
	in a vaccine-associated community case	
	Vaccine-strain polio viral infection	
	in a nonimmunodeficient recipient	0-30 days
	in an immunodeficient recipient	0-6 months
	in a vaccine-associated community case	
	Any acute complication or sequela (including death) of events	
Polio inactivated-virus containing vaccines	Anaphylaxis or anaphylactic shock	0-4 hours
	Any acute complication or sequela (including death) of event	
Hepatitis B antigen-containing vaccines	Anaphylaxis or anaphylactic shock	0-4 hours
	Any acute complication or sequela (including death) of event	
Vaccines containing live, oral, rhesus-based rotavirus	Intussusception	0-30 days
	Any acute complication (including death) of event	

Source: U.S. Health Resources and Services Administration (HRSA). National Vaccine Injury Compensation Program. Vaccine Injury Table. http://www.hrsa.gov/osp/vicp/table.htm. Accessed February 23, 2004.

range of concerns related to vaccine safety and varying distrust in medicine."[16] Furthermore, "the sites rely heavily on emotional appeal to convey their message." This study was heavily criticized by the National Vaccine Information Center that runs (according to them) the oldest and largest safety advocacy Web site (no doubt one of the Web sites reviewed in the study).[17]

In addition to untrusting vaccine groups, it appears that some chiropractors, especially some in Canada, are warning patients about the dangers of vaccinating their children.[18] Why chiropractors, who usually do not have privileges to administer or manage immunizations, are doing this is unknown, but is worrisome to health officials. At one time, untrusting vaccines groups targeted pertussis whole-cell vaccines. In a 1998 study, four countries in which high coverage with diphtheria-tetanus-pertussis vaccines were maintained were compared with eight countries in which immunization was disrupted by groups concerned about the safety of vaccines.[19] Pertussis incidence was 10 to 100 times lower in the countries where high vaccine coverage was maintained versus those countries where immunization programs were compromised by groups concerned about the safety of vaccines.

CURRENT VACCINE SAFETY CONTROVERSIES

Controversies abound in vaccine safety. The Institute of Medicine (IOM) reviews and reports on these controversies routinely.

Autism and Vaccines

Perhaps the hottest current controversy in vaccine safety is whether there is an association between vaccines and a developmental delay and impaired social skills in infants called autism. Most of the evidence suggests that autism is mainly a genetic disorder and that some symptoms may appear immediately after birth but are too subtle to spot in the first year of life.[20] Since newborns and infants receive most of their immunizations during their first year of life, it is easy for a parent to blame vaccinations as a cause.

The IOM, in its review, decided that "the evidence favors rejection of a causal relationship at the population level between the MMR vaccine and autistic spectrum disorders.[21] Other researchers have stated that "the weight of the available epidemiological evidence does not support a causal association between MMR vaccine, or any other vaccine or vaccine constituent, and autism."[22]

Despite these findings, the parents of autistic children who feel that a vaccine caused autism in their child have launched a political battle with lawyers and members of Congress to try to overrule science and medicine.[23] A major U.S. financial study designed to be the definitive answer to this issue "will track 100,000 babies in Norway to identify biological and environmental factors that could combine to cause autism and other developmental disorders."[24]

Thiomerosal and Autism

Until recently, some vaccines contained thiomerosal (a mercury compound) as a preservative. Some parents of autistic children feel that this is the cause of autism. Their claim has scared many parents about immunizations.[25] However, the evidence shows that, except for one study, no others have linked thiomerosal with autism.

The IOM, in its review of this issue, stated "the evidence is inadequate to accept or reject a causal relationship between exposure to thimerosal from vaccines and the neurodevelopmental disorders of autism, ADHD, and speech or language delay."[26] This was before a medical journal published one study showing a relationship between thiomerosal and autism and later said they had made a mistake and regretted publishing the study.[27]

Hepatitis B Vaccine and Demyelinating Neurological Disorders

Concern has been raised that hepatitis B vaccine may cause demyelinating diseases such as multiple sclerosis and Guillain-Barré Syndrome in adults. Several epidemiologic studies have explored this possibility.

The IOM in its review stated, "evidence of possible biological mechanisms that could produce this effect was weak . . . epidemiological evidence favors rejection of a causal relationship between the hepatitis B vaccine and multiple sclerosis." Also, "the evidence was inadequate to accept or reject a causal relationship between the hepatitis B vaccine and other demyelinating diseases."[28]

Multiple Immunizations and Immune Dysfunction

As more vaccines have become available, it has become necessary to provide multiple immunizations at the same time. Some parents worry that this may harm or weaken their child's immune system. However, the IOM decided that "the evidence favors rejection of a causal relationship between multiple immunizations and increased risk of infections and for type I diabetes."[29] The IOM also concluded, "epidemiological evidence on risk for allergic disease, particularly asthma, was inadequate to accept or reject a causal relationship."

Immunization and Sudden Unexpected Death in Infancy

Sudden infant death syndrome (SIDS) is the most common cause of death during the postneonatal period. Thus, it is natural to ask the question "Do vaccines play a role?" The IOM, after carefully reviewing all the studies, concluded that "the evidence favors rejection of a causal relationship between some vaccines and SIDs"; and "the evidence is inadequate to reject a causal relationship between other vaccines and SIDs or SUDI (sudden unexpected death in infancy)."[30]

ETIOLOGY OF ADVERSE VACCINE EVENTS

The reasons recipients of vaccines may experience an adverse event are not always known. Is the problem due to something in the vaccine, because of the makeup of the recipient, or an interaction between the two? Clearly, the susceptibility to adverse vaccine events is variable, but why there is such variability is unclear. Unlike most drugs, vaccines do not need to be metabolized before they are excreted from the body. Therefore, a patient deficient in a certain enzyme responsible for metabolizing a drug will not be more vulnerable to the adverse effects of a vaccine. Something else is responsible.

Within all vaccines are three general categories of constituents: (1) the weakened disease antigen (either live or killed), (2) additives, and (3) low levels of leftover ingredients.

Weakened Disease Antigen

Some rare cases have occurred in which the recipient ends up getting the disease the vaccine was intended to prevent. This almost only happens when a live, attenuated (weakened) vaccine (such as oral polio vaccine) is used. In these cases, the patient's virus needs to be isolated and identified to distinguish it from a "wild-type" virus responsible for the natural disease. Oral (live) polio vaccine (OPV) was recently replaced with an inactivated form of polio for required vaccinations in the United States.

Vaccine Additives

Vaccines often contain preservatives (such as thiomerosal), adjuvants (such as aluminum salts) that heighten antibody response, buffers to adjust pH, and stabilizers such as gelatin and normal serum albumin. Some parents are concerned that some of these substances might harm their children.

A recent study reviewed data on thimerosal, aluminum, gelatin, human serum albumin, formaldehyde, and antibiotics.[31] The study stated that gelatin is contained in some vaccines in quantities enough to induce rare instances of severe, immediate-type hypersensitivity reactions. However, none of the other additives studied have been found to be harmful in humans or experimental animals.

Leftover Ingredients

Small quantities of reagents (such as formaldehyde) and leftover cell-culture ingredients (mostly animal proteins) may remain in the vaccine despite purification processes to remove them. One study reviewing the data on these constituents found that formaldehyde posed no problem.[31] The authors went on to state that egg proteins are contained in enough quantities in some vaccines to induce rare instances of severe, immediate-type hypersensitivity reactions.

Recent evidence suggests that leftover cell-culture ingredients in two canine vaccines induce antibodies, some of which are elevated in some immune diseases.[32] A similar finding has been found with some human vaccines.[33] However, there are several reasons this may occur, and more study is needed.

LESSONS LEARNED: CHANGES THAT ARE NEEDED

Despite the relative safety and intense postmarketing surveillance of vaccines, lessons are constantly being learned and changes are needed.[7]

Lessons Learned

The first lesson is that the probability of having an adverse event from a vaccine is higher than experiencing the disease. The danger in this is that some people may feel that the vaccinated public will "protect" them if they do not get vaccinated. History has shown that it does not take much of a drop in immunization coverage to spark a sudden rise in disease. Second, we now have at our disposal sophisticated tools to study potential adverse vaccine events. However, epidemiologic studies of rare associations are challenging, costly, and time-consuming. Third, there is a lower tolerance for reactions caused by products given to healthy people (for example vaccines) compared with therapy for ill people (for example cancer patients). This has caused a concern among a small, but vocal, number of people. Newly hypothesized vaccine safety concerns spread rapidly via the Internet and the mass media. Some of this can adversely affect the patient-doctor relationship, and may incite panic in some parents before the facts of such concern can be thoroughly researched by experts.

Recommendations

Part of the problem in vaccine safety is that it takes time before a potential problem with a vaccine is realized. It takes even more time to investigate thoroughly these potential problems using good scientific and epidemiologic techniques. Concerned parents get frustrated, as do investigators. Some of the problems are that vaccine safety resources are good, but not good enough, and these resources are fragmented. The vaccine safety infrastructure must be invested in and reorganized. Reorganization should separate vaccine approval, supply, and risk to minimize conflicts of interest.

One way to advance and improve the efficiency of vaccine safety surveillance and research is to assign these roles to an independent national vaccine safety board styled after the National Transportation

Safety Board (NTSB).[34] The NTSB is a small, nonregulatory, independent, and respected agency. NTSB's track history of improving the safety of air travel is unprecedented and some feel this success is because of its independent structure. Creating a national immunization safety board may do the same for vaccine safety.

SUMMARY

Based on the millions of doses administered each year and the low incidence of severe adverse events, vaccines are remarkably safe. However, this record of safety does not matter if a harmful adverse effect happens to you or someone you love. Because of this, the safety of vaccines is an issue that is here to stay. However, no matter how controversial the issue, there is no substitute for science in refuting the myth.[35] Therefore, emotion and politics should not be allowed to overrule good science.

Parents concerned about vaccine safety need to evaluate carefully information about vaccines and consider the source of the information. Various good resources on vaccine safety are available.[36,37,38]

Vaccine safety needs to become a higher priority, it needs to be reorganized, and the infrastructure improved. One way to advance and improve the efficiency of vaccine safety surveillance and research is to form an independent national vaccine safety board.

Chapter 9

Probing the Ambulatory Frontier

Although there is quantitative and qualitative data on drug misadventures in the acute care environment, and some data in the long-term care environment, there are little data on drug misadventures in the ambulatory setting. This chapter explores the drug misadventures patients experience when they are not in an organized health care setting and why data on ambulatory drug misadventures is rare.

AMBULATORY CARE

Ambulatory care is care provided to patients who can walk. In simple terms, it is when individuals still live at home and function reasonably well. However, there are other ambulatory care environments in which medication is routinely consumed, such as day care centers, prisons, schools, and independent living facilities.

Estimates show that there were 823,542,000 visits to doctors' offices in 2000.[1] This figure equates to three visits each year for every person in the United States. The ambulatory environment is where most of the medication (3 billion prescriptions a year plus over-the-counter medication) is consumed. Why data on drug misadventures in this environment are so meager is perplexing. Thus, the ambulatory environment is a frontier with a patient-safety mandate.[2]

The Accreditation Association for Ambulatory Health Care (AAAHC) states the following regarding the lack of data in the ambulatory environment. "There is lack of infrastructure—and associated inability to accurately and without much burden track, classify, and quantify ambulatory medical events—in ambulatory health care organizations that are not part of a health 'system' or 'network.'"[3] Health care organizations with an ambulatory component do not have the systems necessary to collect data on health outcomes.

EPIDEMIOLOGY

Some data are available on drug misadventures in the ambulatory environment.

Source of Medication

Ambulatory patients receive their medication from their doctor (in the form of samples), from a hospital pharmacy (when they are discharged from the hospital, or visit an ambulatory clinic in a hospital), or from a community pharmacy. They can also buy prescription medication, often illegally, over the Internet.

Patients also buy over-the-counter medication (OTC), herbal medicines, and nutriceuticals (without a prescription) from health food stores, community pharmacies, grocery stores, convenience stores, and the Internet. Also, patients sometimes share prescriptions and OTC medications.

Last, is the illegal market in drugs and abused substances that is readily available—from the street corner and the Internet. No matter the source, all medication has the potential to cause negative outcomes called drug misadventures.

Prevalence of Drug Misadventures

Only a few studies exist on the prevalence of drug misadventures in the ambulatory environment. Table 9.1 displays the result of a literature search on this subject.

Three prevalent studies suggest that from 19 to 28.5 percent of ambulatory patients said they experienced an ADE while taking medication, and 6 to 11 percent of these may have been preventable.[4,5,6] However, a more precise incidence study in older adults suggests that ADEs may be occurring at a rate of 50/1,000 person years which is a much lower rate.[7] The preventable ADEs in this study were 13.8/ 1,000 person years. Extrapolating the rate of ADEs from this study to

TABLE 9.1. The Prevalence of Drug Misadventures in the Ambulatory Environment

Patients	No.	Type	Drug Misadventure	
			All	Preventable
Recently discharged[a]	400	ADEs	19%	6%
Adult ambulatory[b]	661	ADEs	25%	11%
Older persons[c]	27,617	ADEs	50.1/1,000 person years	13.8/1,000 person years
Adult ambulatory[d]	1,026	ADRs	28.5%	not studied

Notes: ADE = adverse drug event—any injury from medical management (includes errors); ADR = adverse drug reaction—injury from a drug (does not include errors)

[a]Forster AJ, Murff HJ, Peterson JF, Gandhi TK, Bates DW. (2003). The incidence and severity of adverse events affecting patients after discharge from the hospital. *Ann Intern Med* 138:161-167.
[b]Gandhi TK, Weingart SN, Borus J, Seger AC, Peterson J, Burdick E., Seger DL, Shu K, Federico F, Leape LL, Bates DW. (2003). Adverse drug events in ambulatory care. *N Eng J Med* 348:1556-1564.
[c]Gurwitz JH, Field TS, Harrold LR, Rothschild J, Debellis K, Seger AC, Cadoret C, Fish LS, Garber L, Kelleher M, Bates DW. (2003). Incidence and preventability of adverse drug events among older persons in the ambulatory setting. *JAMA* 289(9):1107-1116.
[d]Hutchinson TA, Flegel KM, Kramer MS, Leduc DG, Kong HH. (1986). Frequency, severity, and risk factors for adverse drug reactions in adult out-patients: A prospective study. *J Chron Dis* 39(7):533-542.

the total Medicare population shows as many as 1.9 million ADEs may occur yearly.[8] The incidence for the entire population is unknown.

One study was reported of medication administration problems in 82 day care centers.[9] Two of the most common problems were missed doses (55.6 percent of centers reported this problem) and medication not available (48.8 percent of centers reported this problem). Eight centers (9.8 percent of all centers reporting) reported giving medication without authorization, and two centers (2.4 percent of all centers reporting) reported giving overdoses.

The extent of medication misadventuring in schools is unknown. In one study of 649 schools, 48.5 percent of school nurses said that medication errors had taken place, and the most common error was missed doses (79.7 percent).[10]

The literature search did not reveal any prevalent studies for drug misadventures in jails, prisons, summer camps, adult day care centers, group homes for the developmentally disabled, or independent living facilities.

Types of Errors

Problems with medication in the ambulatory setting occur during the prescribing, dispensing, compounding, and administration stages of drug use.

Prescribing Errors

In a study of 89 community pharmacies in five states, pharmacists intervened to resolve prescribing-related problems in 1.9 percent of new prescriptions.[11] The rate for prescribing problems was 20.69 for each 1,000 new prescriptions. Of these, 28.3 percent could have caused the patient harm.

The rate at which pharmacists resolved prescribing problems was negatively related to the number of prescriptions they dispensed in an hour. The most common error was omission (45.6 percent). The most dangerous errors were: wrong dose or regimen (20.8 percent), drug interactions (4.1 percent), allergy sensitivity (3.5 percent), duplicative therapy (2.5 percent), and wrong patient (1 percent).

In a study of inappropriate prescribing by doctors in elderly ambulatory patients, 3.7 percent of elderly patients in 2000, and 3.8 percent of elderly patients in 1995, were provided at least one drug that was considered inappropriate by an expert panel.[12]

Dispensing Errors

Patients buy their prescription medications from community pharmacies, outpatient pharmacies in hospitals, or mail-order pharmacies.

In a 1995 study, conducted with the support of ABC News' *Primetime,* an analysis of 100 prescription orders dispensed detected 24 dispensing errors, of which four were clinically significant.[13] None of the errors was for the wrong drug.

In a national observational study in 50 pharmacies, the overall dispensing accuracy rate was 98.3 percent.[14] Of the errors noted, 6.5 percent were judged to be clinically important. The authors of this study estimated that about four errors a day occur in a pharmacy dispensing 250 prescriptions a day. Generalizing these results means that "an estimated 51.5 million errors occur during the filling of 3 billion prescriptions each year."

The prevalence of drug misadventures in proprietary environments such as community and mail-order pharmacies is obscure. At least some medication error data exist from community pharmacies, but almost none from mail-order pharmacies. However, one description of a mail-order pharmacy error explains some of the issues.

In the late 1980s, the state of Idaho brought manslaughter charges against one mail-order pharmacy that dispensed warfarin (an anticoagulant) instead of predisone (a corticosteroid) and the patient died. Although the case was dropped, it offers important lessons.[15] The first is lack of patient counseling about the patient's medication by a pharmacist. This may lead to increased error rates.[16] Second, the medication error occurred because strict measures were not enforced to make sure a drug loaded into an automated dispensing device was correct. Third, speed was a factor. "One report indicated an average of 56 prescriptions being filled per hour" in one of the mail-order plants, with a high of 75. It was reported that a weekly bonus of 15 cents for each prescription filled beyond 53 prescriptions an hour was granted.

One study on the accuracy of dispensing in a high-volume outpatient hospital pharmacy found (using a double-check system on the final product) that errors occurred in 12.5 percent of the prescriptions dispensed.[17] Of these, 1.6 percent were potentially serious. The most common error was not placing an auxiliary label (30.1 percent of all errors) on the prescription container when needed. The most serious errors (wrong drug and wrong strength) represented 1.5 percent of all errors.

Compounding Errors

In the 1930s and 1940s, nearly 60 percent of all prescriptions were compounded—"made from scratch"—by pharmacists using various chemicals and medicaments. From 1950 to 1990, compounding medication by the pharmacist declined as pharmaceutical companies made almost all the medication dispensed by the pharmacist. However, during the 1990s, the benefit of custom making certain medication was rediscovered because: (1) the compounded preparation can be custom made for the patient, and (2) compounded products can avoid certain additives that may cause allergic reactions in a patient.

Today, about 1 percent of prescriptions (about 43,000) are compounded daily in the United States. This percentage is much higher in most other countries. The products compounded by pharmacists include: suspensions, topical creams and ointments, suppositories, eyedrops, lozenges, lip balms, throat sprays, sublingual troches, transdermal patches, slow-release capsules, and lollipops.

Compounding is considered the practice of pharmacy and there are standards of practice that need to be followed to help ensure safety. Weighing and measuring must be done carefully, and everything needs to be double checked, including all calculations.

A 2002 undercover investigation by the FDA in twelve pharmacies reported that 10 of 29 compounded prescriptions failed testing—nine were subpotent and one was contaminated.[18] The pros and cons of pharmacist compounding has recently been discussed.[19]

Self-Administration Errors

Most patients do not take their medications as prescribed. This causes 25,000 deaths yearly, and a loss of 20 million work days and $1.5 billion in earnings in the United States.[20] "It's also the cause of 10 percent of all hospital admissions among the elderly, 23 percent of all nursing home admissions, and $8.5 billion in excess hospitalization costs."

When doctors, pharmacists, and nurses provide information to patients about their medication, and stress how important it is to take the medication properly, patients are much more compliant and have better outcomes.

Not only do patients not take their medication as prescribed, but they also sometimes take it incorrectly. Thirty patients recently discharged from a hospital were studied to see what medication errors occurred.[21] Only 4 of 30 (13 percent) patients received all of their medications as prescribed. Errors of omission and extra-dose errors occurred in 25 percent of the patients. Also, 20 percent of the patients had resumed taking prescription drugs that had been prescribed for them before hospital admission. The percentage of patients using OTC drugs was 83 percent.

What is unclear is why patients have a difficult time taking their medication. One study discovered reasons such as the inability to understand directions, patients' attitudes toward taking drugs, and unclear directions as contributing to poor compliance and medication errors caused by the patient.[22]

Obtaining Drugs from the Internet

No studies were found on the extent of drug misadventures when patients buy their medication from the Internet or get them from other patients, but this is a source of concern.

Severity

Most drug misadventures experienced by ambulatory patients are mild, mostly causing worry or some discomfort. However, the most comprehensive study so far showed there may be as many as 180,000 people a year in the United States that experience a life-threatening or fatal ADE, and this is just in the Medicare population.[6]

One study discovered that 0.19 percent of outpatient department visits were because of adverse effects of medication.[23] About 4 percent of these patients had to be admitted to the hospital. The nature of injuries that ambulatory patients incur from medication was described in a recent study.[4] Three percent (3 percent) of the injuries were serious drug-induced laboratory abnormalities, 65 percent were symptoms, 30 percent were symptoms associated with a nonpermanent disability, and 3 percent were permanent disabilities.

The most common preventable ADE events in one large ambulatory study in older patients were: electrolyte and renal (26.6 percent), gastrointestinal tract (21.1 percent), hemorrhagic (15.9 percent), metabolic/endocrine (13.8 percent), and neuropsychiatric (8.6 percent).[6] In one study the most common ADEs were: faintness (14 percent), fatigue (9 percent), headache (9 percent), and nausea or vomiting (8 percent).[7] Note: some patients had more than one symptom.

Cost

In 1995, a group of academic researchers developed a model of drug-related morbidity and mortality in the ambulatory environment.[24] They estimated that in the United States the cost of drug-related morbidity and mortality in the ambulatory environment ranged from $30.1 to $136.8 billion yearly. This model was updated in 2001.[25] It was estimated the cost of drug-related problems in the ambulatory environment doubled.

Drugs

Differences exist between acute care and ambulatory environments in drugs causing the most morbidity and mortality. More injectable drugs are used in acute care than in ambulatory care, and more oral drugs are used in ambulatory care than in acute care. Table 9.2 shows the drug categories most commonly associated with ADEs in the ambulatory environment. The most common drug categories reported with ADEs in the ambulatory environment are: cardiovascular drugs, anti-infective drugs, and analgesics. Unfortunately, none of the studies reviewed listed the prevalence of individual drugs.

Prescribing in the elderly ambulatory population continues to be troublesome. A recent study suggested that in 1995 and 2000, at least one drug, which was considered inappropriate by the Beers expert panel, was prescribed at 7.8 percent of ambulatory care visits by elderly patients.[26] Also, at least one drug classified as never or rarely appropriate by the Zahn expert panel was prescribed at 3.7 percent and 3.8 percent of these visits in 1995 and 2000, respectively.

Ambulatory patients also take over-the-counter medication. A 2002 study showed that 59 percent of adults used nonprescription medicine in the past six months.[27] Consumers are more likely to read the label when taking an OTC that is new to them, but only one in ten read the label for possible adverse effects or use warnings.

This study also discovered that one-third of adults in the United States have taken more than the recommended dosage of a nonprescription medicine. Reasons given included: (1) the high dosage was believed to bring relief more quickly (69 percent), (2) the recommended dosage did not bring relief (64 percent), and (3) the OTC product contained the same ingredients as a previously taken prescription (38 percent).

TABLE 9.2. Drug Categories Most Commonly Associated with ADEs in the Ambulatory Environment

Patients	No. of Patients, Rxs, or Visits	Drug Category (%)
Outpatients >18[a]	661 pts	Oral corticosteroids (33)
		Nonnarcotic analgesics (32)
		Penicillins (21)
		SSRIs (20)
Outpatients >65[b]	30,397 pts	Cardiovascular drugs (26)
		Anti-infective agents (15)
		Diuretics (13)
		Nonnarcotic analgesics (12)
Internal medicine[c]	1,539 Rxs	Cardiovascular (5)
	1,026 pts	CNS (4)
		Electrolytes/diuretics (4)
		Anti-infective agents (3)
Outpatients attending clinic for ADE[d]	251,017 pt visits	Hormones (31)
		Antibiotics (21)
		Analgesics (11)
		Anti-infectives (11)

[a]Gandhi TK, Weingart SN, Borus J, Seger AC, Peterson J, Brudick E, Seger DL, Shu K, Federico F, Leape LL, Bates DW. (2003). Adverse drug events in ambulatory care. *N Engl J Med* 348:1556-1564.

[b]Gurwitz JH, Field TS, Harrold LR, Rothschild J, Debellis K, Seger AC, Cadoret C, Fish LS, Garber L, Kelleher M, Bates DW. (2003). Incidence and preventability of adverse drug events among older persons in the ambulatory setting. *JAMA* 289(9):1107-1116.

[c]Hutchinson TA, Flegel KM, Kramer MS, Leduc DG, Kong HH. (1986). Frequency, severity, and risk factors for adverse drug reactions in adult out-patients: A prospective study. *J Chron Dis* 39(7):533-542.

[d]Aparasu RR and Helgeland DL. (2000). Visits to hospital outpatient departments in the United States due to adverse effects of medications. *Hosp Pharm* 35(8):825-831.

MEDICATION RISKS
IN THE AMBULATORY ENVIRONMENT

Risk is always a factor in taking medication, however, risk factors may vary depending on where the medication is used—intensive care, acute care, home care, long-term care, or ambulatory care. Risk factors in the ambulatory environment include those associated with prescribing, dispensing, and patient use.

Prescribing Risks

No doctor wants to inappropriately prescribe medication, but unfortunately, prescribing problems occur much too often. One group of researchers described the seven all-to-often-deadly sins of prescribing:[28]

1. The "disease" for which the drug is prescribed is an adverse reaction to another drug, masquerading as a disease.
2. A drug is used to treat a problem that should first be treated with common sense lifestyle changes.
3. The medical problem is both self-limiting and unresponsive to treatments such as antibiotics or does not merit treatment with certain drugs.
4. Instead of using a "drug of choice"—the safest, most effective, and often least expensive treatment—the doctor prescribes a less preferable alternative.
5. Two drugs are prescribed that interact. Each may be safe and effective, but when used together can cause serious injury or death.
6. Two or more drugs in the same therapeutic class are used, the extra one(s) does not add to the effectiveness of the first, but clearly increases the risk to the patient.
7. Prescribing the correct drug, but the dose is dangerously high.

In addition to these seven deadly sins are other prescribing errors.

Using Doses That Cause or Heighten Side Effects

Recent evidence suggests that some of the starting doses of prescription medication recommended by the drug's manufacturer may be too high.[29] Indeed, a 1998 study published in *JAMA* showed "there are a large number of serious reactions even when the drugs are properly prescribed and administered."[30] Similar findings are found in studies of published adverse drug event reports.[31,32,33] In the *JAMA* study, 76.2 percent of the side effects were dose related, meaning the problem was not the drug itself, but how much was prescribed. Doctors need to dose newly used drugs by *starting low and going slow.*

Discounting the Side Effects Reported by Patients

Some doctors quickly discount side effects reported by patients. The thinking goes, "I am using the drug at the manufacturer's recommended guidelines—it must not be the drug." This overdependence on drug-company information leads to all sorts of prescribing problems including using one company's drug over another company's drug when the other company's drug is a far better choice.

Problem Use

A recent study on the problem use of drugs analyzed data from the National Household Survey on Drug Abuse.[34] The researchers found that nearly 1.3 million Americans aged 12 years and older, experience problem use of prescription drugs representing physiological dependence or heavy daily use. "Those at greatest risk include older adults, females, those in poor or fair health, and daily alcohol drinkers." Why does this happen? Why aren't doctors and pharmacists doing more to lessen this problem? What can be done about it?

Dispensing Risks

How often are patients exposed to risk in the dispensing process? A 2001 study asked this question of pharmacists in Texas and 34 percent said at least one patient a week is exposed to risk.[35] Pharmacists practicing in mail-order and/or chain-store pharmacies reported a higher risk than pharmacists working in independent community pharmacies and food store pharmacies.

A 2003 study of patient risk in Florida pharmacies discovered that in the three months before the survey, about half of the pharmacists wanted to report a significant patient-risk problem but felt helpless to do so.[36] Pharmacists in chain-store pharmacies were confronted with the most patient-risk problems, and pharmacists in independent community pharmacies the least.

Problems Patients Have in Using Medication

Patients have various problems in taking medication. Following are just a few:

Continuity of Care Problems

As patients move from one care environment (such as a hospital) to another (such as ambulatory), various issues commonly come into play. For example, the medication a patient receives as an outpatient may be different, or look different, than he or she received in the hospital. This may be all right, but seldom does anyone tell the patient this. Sometimes, refilled medication may look different, but be the same drug and strength of what was received and used previously. The change may be because of an insurance issue, but the patient is never told this. Or, it may be an error. Patients should always ask for explanations when the medication does not look exactly as before.

Administration Problems

Some patients put many of their medications into one bottle for convenience. This is asking for problems, as is taking medication in the middle of the night with the light off. Other safety issues are sharing prescription medication with friends and relatives when someone thinks they have the same health problem, and taking more or less of the medication than prescribed without checking with the doctor.

Tablet Splitting

Some patients, to save money, get twice the tablet strength than they need, then split tablets and use the half tablets as the dose. There are several potential dangers here. First, rarely can a tablet be split exactly in half. Second, studies have shown that some medications are not evenly spread in a tablet. Third, some tablets are made for controlled or sustained delivery that is destroyed by splitting the tablet. Sometimes, all the medication may be released at the same time, rather than over 8, 12, or 24 hours.

Poor Tablet Identification

As of yet, there is no standardized approach to placing imprint codes on oral prescription drugs and many OTC drugs have no identification. Health care professionals are often asked to identify tablets and capsules shown to them by patients and have a difficult time doing so.[37] The percentages of drugs able to be identified from seven electronic resources ranged from 24.8 to 86.4 percent. The poor identification was because the drug was not in the database, or the drug was not uniquely marked. The United States Pharmacopoeia (USP) is currently exploring the possibility of standardized identification for all oral dosage forms, but this is being resisted by most of the drug manufacturers as unneeded and too expensive.

Direct-to-Patient Advertising of Rx Drugs

Despite strong objections by many health care professionals, the FDA allows the advertising of prescription-only drugs directly to the public. Most of this advertising by drug manufacturers is on television or in magazines widely read by the public. This heavy advertising by the drug companies has paid off—sales of the advertised drugs have skyrocketed. Patients are putting heavy pressure on doctors to prescribe these drugs that often are more expensive than other drugs that may work just as well. Just as important, the advertising is often heavily weighted toward the benefits of the drug, with little or no time in the ads given to the drug's risks.

OTC Use

Many patients use OTC medication and usually do so on their own. Many feel because OTC drugs do not require a prescription, they are safe. However, this simply is not true. OTC drugs can and do cause harm.[38] All pharmacists receive extensive training in OTC products. However, few make themselves available to patients when the patient is wandering the aisles of pharmacies looking for something to relieve symptoms.

OTC products can multiply or interfere with the effects of prescription medication. Occasionally, OTC medication can interact and pose dangers with prescription medication.[39] A few other potential problems with OTCs include:[38]

- A missed self-diagnosis
- Inadequate treatment
- Side effects
- Overdoses
- Overuse
- Drug interactions
- Sensitivity
- Confusing names and labels
- Label limits

Patients should insist on talking with the pharmacist or talk to their doctor before using an OTC product.

SOME SOLUTIONS

The safety of using medication in the ambulatory environment can be improved in many ways.

Improving Communication Between Doctor and Pharmacists

Most of the prescription information flowing from the doctor to the pharmacist is in notoriously poor handwriting that leads to errors. In this age of computers, handwriting prescriptions and drug orders is archaic.[40] Prescription and drug orders should be sent to the pharmacist electronically. The Center for Information Technology Leadership states that computerized prescriber order entry (CPOE) in ambulatory care will: (1) avoid more than 2 million ADEs yearly (130,000 of which are life threatening), (2) save $44 billion, and (3) cut out more than $10 billion in rejected claims for an outpatient visit.[41]

More Patient Information for Community Pharmacists

Community pharmacists practice in a vacuum. The only information they receive about a patient is the patient's name. They receive nothing about the patient's diseases, condition, renal function, liver function, weight, or for what the medication is being used. The pharmacist can use this information to improve the drug's efficacy and safety—all of which is in the patient's best interest.

Better Communication Between Pharmacists and Patients

Many pharmacists claim that they are too busy to interact and talk with patients. Most pharmacists are busy, but not all the time. The truth is that many pharmacists don't like talking with patients. They prefer typing labels and counting and pouring medication—the functions of pharmacy technicians. Not only is this unfortunate, it also breaks federal (OBRA 90) and most state laws that state "the pharmacist must make an offer to counsel the patient about the patient's medication."

Shrewd lawyers from corporate pharmacy companies think they have developed a way around the law by having the pharmacy clerk hand a piece of paper to the patient and say "sign here." Most patients sign the piece of paper thinking they are signing that they are picking up the medication. What they are doing is signing away their right to be counseled by the pharmacist about their medication. Since there is not a personal offer by the pharmacist to counsel, the law is not being met. However, enforcement of the law is almost nonexistent.

Clinical Decision Support

Once e-prescribing is in place in the ambulatory environment, it needs to be supplemented by clinical decision support. Computer software should link the prescribing with the laboratory results of the patient, and provide warnings and stop signs when prescribing is not in the patient's best interest.[40]

Computerized Data to Identify ADEs

Computer software should be in place that constantly sifts through patient data to detect when an ambulatory patient may have already experienced an ADE.[42]

Better Identification of Patients at Risk

Medication risk is probably not evenly divided throughout the population. Therefore, certain patients are more likely to incur an ADE than other patients. We know some of the risks, but not all of them. For example, people at higher levels of risk are: the very young and the very old, patients with reduced liver function, patients on more than five drugs, patients in poor health, and patients on inherently toxic drugs. Indicators for selecting ambulatory patients who warrant increased monitoring have been published.[43]

Going Slower on Rx-to-OTC Switches

Drug companies make more money when their "prescription-only" products can be converted to OTC status, especially when the prescription product is about to come off its patent. The FDA requires assurance that the benefits of switching a "prescription-only" drug to OTC status outweighs the risks. The drug company wanting the switch has a difficult time proving the drug will be safe when switched and the FDA has a difficult time deciding to approve the switch. Also, it seems there are no data after the switch to OTC status to show the decision was a good one.

To solve this problem, "prescription-only" products, rather than being made an OTC product, should be made "pharmacist only" (no prescription needed, but it is only dispensed on the advice of a pharmacist) for two years until enough data are collected to prove the switch is safe. Only then can the drug become OTC. If not, it should remain pharmacist-only or go back to prescription-only status.

Standardized Imprint Codes on All Oral Drugs

All oral medication—prescription and OTC—should be required to have standardized imprint codes, and there should be an electronic database of these products updated daily by the FDA.

Improved Patient Education

Patients need to receive better education about their medication, both verbally and in writing. Presently, this education is inadequate and needs to be improved. There needs to be more recognition of this issue by health care providers, especially doctors, nurses, and pharmacists.[44] At the same time, patients need to take more of an active role in their own care and be more assertive in dealing with insensitive health care providers who rush from patient to patient.

Other Solutions

The National Coordinating Council for Medication Error Reporting and Prevention (NCC MERP) has issued five other recommendations to prevent or reduce medication errors in non-health care settings such as schools, day care centers, day camps, assisted living facilities, board and care homes, and correctional facilities:[45]

1. Develop written policies and procedures for personnel who administer medications.
2. Provide training to personnel who are responsible for medication management.
3. Ensure that controlled substances are stored properly to prevent theft and diversion.
4. Encourage personnel to report medication errors to the proper state and national medication-error reporting systems.
5. When a medication error occurs, evaluate possible causes to improve the facility's system for medication management and to prevent future errors.

An Improved Research Agenda

Information on drug misadventures in the ambulatory environment is severely lacking, as is the infrastructure to collect such data. Public health funds need to be specifically earmarked to fill this void to reduce the morbidity and mortality from ambulatory drug misadventures.

SUMMARY

Nearly four billion prescriptions will be dispensed in the United States in 2005, and this number is expected to grow dramatically as the population ages. With the rising number of prescriptions will come a rising number of drug misadventures and with these, more drug-related morbidity and mortality. The problem is already at the "orange" level of concern and approaching the "red" level.

Drug-related morbidity and mortality in the ambulatory environment represents the tip of an iceberg. What we know is just above the water. Much more efforts and resources are needed to see what is below the surface. Based on what we know already, drug misadventures in the ambulatory environment represent a significant threat to the health of the public and need to be addressed more forthrightly.

Chapter 10

The Liability for Drug Injury

This chapter reviews drug injury and liability for defective drug products or for malpractice and the role of expert testimony in litigation brought forth because of these problems. Since the author is not an attorney, a disclaimer is in order. This chapter is for educational purposes only, and should not be used to decide whether a case of drug injury has merit, nor used as prosecution or defense material in a legal action. In these cases, a qualified attorney should be consulted.

DRUG INJURY OUTCOMES

Most drug misadventures end with no injury.[1] Indeed, most problems with medication are expected and annoying side effects are usually mild to moderate and subside with time or on discontinuation of therapy. Sometimes, medical attention will be needed when an adverse reaction occurs from a medication. Occasionally, drugs cause severe and life-threatening reactions, and rarely, some drugs cause permanent disability or death.

These outcomes can happen because of:

1. the inherent toxicity of the drug,
2. a genetic susceptibility of the person taking the drug,
3. a drug product defect,
4. negligence by a health care provider, or
5. a combination of these factors.

The mechanism of drug injury includes type A adverse drug reactions (pharmacologic and dose related), type B adverse drug reactions

Prescribed Medications and the Public Health
© 2006 by The Haworth Press, Inc. All rights reserved.
doi:10.1300/5688_10

(bizarre—not pharmacological or dose related), a drug interaction, an allergic drug reaction, or a medication error.

The effects of drug injury can include: tissue and organ damage, pain and suffering, loss of organ function, lost time at work or school, inconvenience, expense, frustration, or the worse effect, loss of life. None of these unfortunate events can be erased, and sometimes life, as once known, cannot be restored. Because some of these injuries can happen without product defect or negligence, there is no remedy for the result—it is simply the drug and bad luck. However, if a product defect or negligence can be proven, or the defendant in the case wishes to settle, compensation is possible. However, for most people, financial compensation for a drug injury does not offer much emotional relief. They would much rather not have the drug injury or have their loved one back or back the way they were before the injury.

CASE EXAMPLES

The following drug misadventure cases resulted in successful litigation.

Prescribing

A 61-year-old female hospital patient was prescribed and received gentamicin (an antibiotic) during her hospital stay for a postoperative bone infection. An appropriate dose and duration for the drug was prescribed. However, the dose was doubled when the patient was transferred to a skilled nursing facility. She was maintained at that dose for two weeks, resulting in possible related hearing toxicity. The patient incurred permanent effects, including vertigo and oscillopsia. The defendant claimed that therapy with other drugs might have contributed to the loss of vestibular function. According to the report, the case was settled for $800,000.[2]

During the delivery of a second pregnancy at 40 weeks' gestation, a patient received misoprostol to ripen the cervix. The patient had delivered a baby four years earlier via a cesarean section (c-section). The dose was ordered and administered twice. The medication was being used "off-label" (not approved for this use by the FDA). It was noted the American Board of Obstetrics and Gynecology advised that this medication should not be used in a patient with a history of c-section, because of the potential risk of uterine rupture. The patient also received pitocin for six hours to speed delivery.

After nearly one to one-and-one-half hours of stage two delivery, the patient experienced a uterine rupture. It required 27 minutes to deliver a nine-pound baby boy by emergency c-section. The baby needed intensive care support and suffers from quadriplegic cerebral palsy. The defendant claimed the mother requested a vaginal delivery that carries a risk of uterine rupture after a c-section delivery. The case was settled with a $1 million payment and structured settlement for $6.258 million.[3]

Dispensing

A 76-year-old patient unintentionally was dispensed 200 mg doxepin for two days instead of the prescribed doxycylcine. The plaintiff claimed the medication error resulted in hospitalization for twelve days and eventual placement in a nursing home until the patient's death two months later. The plaintiff claimed the doxepin was responsible for the patient's decline in mental and physical functioning and death. The defendant claimed the death was a result of preexisting medical conditions. The jury awarded the plaintiff $400,000.[4]

An 87-year-old hospitalized patient with Addison's disease needed daily treatment with hydrocortisone for the previous 40 years. During the patient's hospital stay, his doctor ordered hydrocortisone. However, a pharmacist transcribed the drug order as hydrochlorothiazide. This was dispensed and administered for three days. The patient developed hypotension and heart failure, lost consciousness, and required transfer to the intensive care unit. The medication error was discovered there. The patient suffered anoxic brain damage which resulted in neurological deficits for the balance of his life. The patient eventually died of a cardiac-related illness three years later. The defendants admitted negligence by dispensing the wrong medication. The jury awarded $75,000 to the plaintiff.[5]

Compounding

An eight-year-old hospitalized patient with a urea cycle disorder received a preparation to remove ammonia from the blood. The product was prescribed correctly, but was unintentionally prepared at a lower concentration than was ordered by the doctor. The patient only received 25 percent of the prescribed dosage over a 19-hour period. This resulted in high blood levels of ammonia. It addition, hemodialysis was delayed. The report claimed the child suffered permanent brain injury because of the medication error. The case was settled for $2.5 million.[6]

Administration

A premature neonate was treated with dopamine for hypertension. The medication was to be administered as an intravenous infusion in the patient's foot. However, the medication was unintentionally administered into the patient's artery, rather than the vein. This resulted in vasoconstriction of the arteries from the foot to the spinal cord. The misadministration was not recognized for nearly 13 hours. This resulted in loss of leg function and eventually required below-the-knee amputation. It was also claimed that electrolyte imbalances went unrecognized for two days, resulting in paraplegia and bowel and bladder dysfunction. This resulted in a reported settlement of $4.5 million.[7]

A 68-year-old retired male patient experienced infiltration of doxorubicin during infusion into his hand. Following this, extravasation resulted in a disfiguring scar and carpal tunnel syndrome. This required skin graft surgery. The plaintiff claimed the infusion was misadministered, resulting in an infusion-related injury and permanent damage. The defendants noted that extravasation is an inherent risk when administering cancer chemotherapeutic agents. According to the report, a $612,500 settlement was reached.[8]

Monitoring

A patient was transferred to a nursing home to recuperate after developing endocarditis and was maintained on gentamicin therapy. While in the hospital, the patient was monitored for peak and trough gentamicin levels in the blood and followed for signs of gentamicin toxicity. A doctor verbally ordered gentamicin peak and trough levels on admission to the nursing home. However, there was no documentation that this monitoring took place and the patient experienced signs and symptoms of gentamicin toxicity, including confusion, and being incoherent. Laboratory measurements showed toxic ranges of the drug and permanent dysfunction. Despite starting dialysis because of the renal dysfunction, the patient's condition worsened and resulted in death. According to this report, the case was settled for $600,000.[9]

PREVENTABILITY

Some drug injury is clearly not preventable. For example, type B drug reactions—those reactions that are bizarre or idiosyncratic, have no basis in pharmacology, and are not dose related—are unforeseeable, and thus, not preventable. The adverse effects of the drug are not because of negligence or a product defect. On the other hand, many feel that all medication errors, all known drug interactions, known drug allergies, and type A adverse drug reactions are potentially foreseeable and preventable.

BLAME

Naturally we want to blame someone when a mishap occurs and to have the person punished, demand compensation, and receive assurance that the error will not occur again to someone else. However, blame is also harmful. "Blaming and punishing for errors that are made by well-intentioned people working in the health care system drives the problem of iatrogenic harm underground and alienates people who are best placed to prevent such problems from recurring."[10] Health care delivery is complex and often is the basis for error.

In October 1996, a medication error in Denver resulted in the tragic death of a newborn infant.[11] The error involved the intravenous administration of a large dose of penicillin G benzathine, a drug that should always be administered intramuscularly. Many were quick to blame the death solely on the nurses because nurses are supposed to know the potential dangers of the drugs they administer. The district attorney involved brought the case before a grand jury and the three nurses in the case were eventually indicted for criminally negligent homicide.

In preparation for trial, a systems analysis of the error, performed for the defense, revealed over 50 latent failures in the system that allowed the tragic error to occur. After being presented this evidence during the trial, the jury delivered a "not guilty" verdict. The jury sent an important message in this trial—we must go beyond blame and focus on the multiple, underlying system failures that result in error, so systems can be fixed to prevent the same errors from occurring again. However, it is also important to meet society's need to blame and gain retribution when suitable.[10]

REMEDIES

There are four administrative and legal remedies for drug injury:

1. direct discussion and negotiation between parties,
2. reporting the drug injury to an administrative board,
3. civil action by bringing suit for a product defect, or
4. civil action by bringing suit for medical malpractice.

Direct Discussion Between Parties

For those who experience minor drug injury, the most common recourse is to discuss the matter with the person the injured party thinks is responsible for the injury. Common objectives are to make sure those responsible know what happened so it does not happen again, and to gain an apology. Injured parties who do not think these objectives have been met may continue to one or more of the next steps.

Report the Injury to an Administrative Board

Patients who are injured by a drug and feel that the injury was because of negligence by a health care provider can report the event to the person's employer and to the health care provider's licensing board such as the state boards of medicine, osteopathy, pharmacy, dentistry, or nursing. Most state licensing boards record and investigate complaints, and take action against practitioners when the licensing board feels such action is warranted.

File a Lawsuit for a Drug Product Defect

Sometimes, a drug product, after it has been approved by the FDA and been on the market, is found to cause serious problems in patients and is removed from the market. In these cases, those injured have the alternative of suing the manufacturer of the drug product based on laws governing product defects. The product liability claim must prove the manufacturer is liable for the damages incurred because of design defects, faulty marketing claims, or manufacturing defects. This is no easy matter.[12]

Usually, those injured can join a class action suit already underway against the manufacturer of the drug product. An example of a class action lawsuit for a drug product defect is for the drug combination fen-phen. Fenfluramine, dexfenfluramine, and phentermine (Pondimin) were approved over 25 years ago for short-term use in the medical management of obesity. The use of the products together has never been approved in the United States. On the advice of the FDA, the manufacturers of these two agents withdrew the drugs from the market in fall 1997 because of abnormal echocardiograms signaling possible heart valve problems.

Some of the arguments used in drug product liability cases include: wrongful death, failure to adequately test the product, over-promotion, lack of fair balance between benefits and risks, a defect in the drug's performance versus others in its same pharmacological or chemical class, or the product was adulterated or contaminated.[10]

File a Lawsuit for Medical Malpractice

For patients seriously injured by a drug in which the injury is thought to be because of medical malpractice, an alternative is to sue the supposed party. However, the suit needs to be legitimate and if the action is based on negligence, the prosecution must satisfy the four elements of negligence:

1. a duty was owed to the patient,
2. the duty was breached by the defendant,
3. damage occurred (harm), and
4. the breach of duty (misconduct) was the direct cause of the damage.[13]

MEDICAL MALPRACTICE CLAIMS
FOR DRUG INJURY

Little information is available in the public domain on medical injuries, the number of claims filed, or the number of claims found negligent. A 1974 study in California found that in the 4.65 medical injuries for every 100 hospitalizations, 17 percent were because of negligence.[14] In 1985, one author estimated that about 1 in 10 patients injured through negligence file a claim for damages.[15] Whether these findings are still valid is unknown.

THE ROLE OF EXPERT TESTIMONY
IN DRUG INJURY CLAIMS

When a person experiences injury after taking a drug, it does not necessarily mean the drug caused the injury (see Chapter 4). It is easy to blame the drug when it could easily be something else. "Association" does not mean "causation." Often, it is difficult to decide causality. The adverse effect could be caused by another drug the patient is taking or by another substance to which the patient was exposed. Or, the patient may have experienced a new symptom of his or her disease, or developed a new health problem. Assessing the evidence of drug injury is the topic of the next chapter (Chapter 11).

Expert witnesses are often necessary in cases of alleged drug-induced injury. Common questions to be answered are: Can the ADE occur? Did the ADE occur? How did the ADE occur? Why did the ADE occur? The type of expert witnesses to retain in an alleged drug-induced injury case depends on which questions need answering.[16]

Can the ADE Occur?

The best people to discover whether cases of alleged drug-induced drug injury can occur include pharmacoepidemiologists and drug information specialists. Drug information specialists—pharmacists working in 140 drug information centers in the United States (many with the PharmD degree)—are best at locating previous cases of the ADE in question.

Pharmacoepidemiologists (many with MD, PhD, PharmD, or MPH degrees) may be better at interpreting the results of these literature searches, and are experts in assessing population-based risk for drug injury. They are excellent at reviewing, assessing, interpreting the risk evidence gathered, and deciding the likelihood that an adverse event can occur.

Did the ADE Occur?

Who are the best people to retain as expert witnesses for answering the question "Did the ADE occur?" The answer depends on what occurred. The best person to answer if the drug caused the ADR is the patient's attending doctor or a clinical pharmacologist. If the ADE is a medication error, the best person to serve is a specialist in medication safety (a doctor, a pharmacist, or a nurse). If the ADE in question is a drug interaction, there are several experts, most of whom are academic professors of pharmacy. If the ADE is an allergic drug reaction, a medical allergist is the best person to consult.

How Did the ADE Occur?

Pharmacologists can answer questions on a drug's action, its mechanisms of action, dosage, and dose response. There are two types of pharmacologists—basic science and clinical. Basic science pharmacologists are scientists who have a MS or PhD degree, while clinical pharmacologists confine their practice to humans and are usually doctors.

Questions about the absorption, distribution, metabolism, and excretion of a drug, or if calculations are needed to interpret drug levels (in serum, urine), are best directed to a clinical pharmacokinetist. This could be someone with a PhD, PharmD, or MD who specializes in this area.

Why Did the ADE Occur?

Once an expert witness shows causality, and other experts prove how the drug caused an adverse effect, it is natural to ask "Why did it occur?" and, most important, "Was it preventable?" In cases of medication error, it is helpful to seek an expert in medication safety or the opinion of a health professional with the same background as the person accused of committing the error.

CLAIMS, VERDICTS, AND SETTLEMENTS FOR DRUG INJURY

To say the process and outcomes of medical malpractice suits are interesting is an understatement. Many people feel that the process is broken and the outcomes are out of hand. An article in *Parade* magazine quotes one expert as saying "the system doesn't work. Only one-third who sue are injured, while most bad doctors are not identified."[17] That was said in 1993. The system today may be much worse.

Drug Injury Claims

A study in 1972 by the Insurance Company of North America (INA) revealed that 30 percent of the claims against its insured hospitals were based on providing drugs and treatment.[18] The Government

Accounting Office studied medical malpractice claims closed in 1984. They found that 7.8 percent of the claims were for medication or medication administration.[19] The Harvard Medical Practice Study in New York found that adverse events occurred in 3.7 percent of hospitalized patients. More than half of the adverse events were attributed to errors, including more than 25 percent because of negligent care.[20] Medication-related complications were the most common adverse event (19 percent).

The Physician Insurers Association of America (PIAA) completed a medication error study that was reported in 1993.[21] PIAA's study of 393 claims found 1,019 reported medication errors (2.6 for each claim). The most recent and most useful study analyzed a New England malpractice insurance company's claims records from January 1, 1990, to December 31, 1999.[22] It was discovered that ADEs represented 6.3 percent (129/2,040) of the total claims.

Causes of Drug Injury Claims

The PIAA study (1993) listed the top causes of drug therapy claims against doctors: incorrect or inappropriate dosage, medication inappropriate for the medical condition, and failure to monitor side effects.[22] The INA study (1972) listed the most common basis for drug-related claims as: allergic reactions (44.3 percent), overdose (17.5 percent), and receiving the wrong drug (9.3 percent).[18]

System deficiencies and performance errors were the most frequent cause of preventable ADEs in the study of claims from the New England malpractice insurance company study (2002).[22] These included: poor team communication (48 percent), inadequate handoffs of relevant information (23 percent), poor interdisciplinary communication (30 percent), and use of substitute or inexperienced professionals (23 percent).

Information from the Pharmacists Mutual Insurance Company indicates the most common causes of pharmacy liability claims are: wrong drug dispensed (49.3 percent), wrong strength dispensed (25.9 percent), intellectual errors (17.1 percent), and wrong directions (7.7 percent).[23]

In a study of ADE reports published in the medical literature over a 20-year period, the most common causes of lawsuits involving drug injury were: overdose (20 percent), poor or no monitoring of the drug (19 percent), and improper treatment (15 percent).[24]

Drugs Incriminated

In the INA study (1972), the most common drugs involved in a drug injury claim were: penicillin, other antibiotics, and adrenal steroids.[18] In the PIAA study (1993), the most common drug classes for drug injury claims were: antibiotics, glucocorticoids, and narcotics.[21] These drug classes represented 35 percent of the claims. In the New England malpractice insurance company study (2002), the most often involved medication classes were antibiotics, antidepressants, and antipsychotics.[22]

Outcomes of Drug Injury

In the INA report (1972), 19 percent of the drug injury claims were a threat to life or serious debilitation (7 percent death and 13 percent permanent disability).[18] In the PIAA study (1993), death occurred in 83 of 393 (21 percent) claims, and a medication error was involved in 70 of the 83 (84 percent) deaths.[21] In the New England malpractice insurance company study (2002), 31 percent of the preventable drug injury claims were life threatening and 16 percent were fatal.[22] The claims were nearly equally divided between the outpatient and inpatient settings.

Defendants

In a study of published ADE reports over a 20-year period, 13.1 percent of the reports mentioned a lawsuit.[24] The primary defendants in these lawsuits were: doctors (37 percent), hospitals (20 percent), pharmacists (6 percent), and other or unknown (36 percent). In the New England malpractice insurance company study, the primary defendants for preventable claims were: doctors (59 percent), nurses (15 percent), pharmacists (10 percent), and other or unknown (17 percent).[22] In the latter study, the primary defendant doctors practiced in primary care (27 percent), general and specialty surgery (24 percent), anesthesiology (18 percent), and other (16 percent).

Decisions

In one study, 33 percent of drug injury claims resulted in payment.[21] In the New England malpractice insurance company study, of the preventable claims for drug injury, 79 percent were decided in favor of the plaintiff.[22] Another study found that payments for drug injury claims were decided by jury verdict in 57 percent of the claims, and by settlements in 43 percent of the claims.[24]

Payments

In a 1993 study, indemnity payments for drug injury claims averaged $99,721 per claim.[21] In 2000, the average for a drug injury claim resulting from a medication error was $636,844, second only to childbirth claims ($2 million average).[25] In another study of drug injury cases from the mid-1970s to the mid-1990s, the mean drug injury claim involving death was $1.1 million; a drug injury claim involving permanent disability was $4.4 million; and a drug injury claim involving a threat to life was $1.2 million.[24]

Punitive Damages

In addition to rewards for malpractice resulting in drug injury, juries and courts can also assess punitive damage payments for gross negligence (willful, wanton, or reckless conduct). In an Alabama case, the Supreme Court affirmed a jury verdict against a pharmacy company, awarding $100,000 in compensatory damages and $150,000 for punitive damages. The basis of the punitive damages was that the pharmacy lacked institutional controls over how prescriptions were filled.[26]

In South Carolina, the Court of Appeals affirmed a lower court decision that awarded a patient $5 million in compensatory damages for a medication error, and punished the pharmacy with $11 million in punitive damages for allowing a pharmacist to work long hours despite his age, his personal difficulties, and his history of wrongly dispensing prescriptions.[27]

Costs

One study found the cost of defending preventable and nonpreventable inpatient and outpatient malpractice ADEs was about the same (mean $64,700 to $74,200), but costs were greater for defending preventable inpatient ADEs (mean $376,500).[22]

RISK MANAGEMENT

There are various ways to reduce the risk of drug injury and litigation for malpractice. Some risk management strategies involve improving the medication-use system, or helping doctors, nurses, and pharmacists to understand how and why they make errors.

Reducing System Problems

One study judged various methods to prevent drug injury claims.[22] The following methods could have prevented claims: computerized doctor order entry with decision support (38 percent decrease), on-site clinical pharmacists (64 percent decrease), general error proofing methods (88 percent decrease), improved standardization of processes (90 percent decrease), and use of built-in design redundancies (87 percent decrease).

Reducing Human Error

Every incident report, customer complaint, or other evidence of a medication-use problem must be classified and investigated to root out any problems. Some people make an occasional error while others continue to make the same mistake over and over. Reducing human error means making the environment a safe place to document errors without unfairly penalizing people.

Some sound risk management procedures for dispensing medication have been recommended by the Pharmacists Mutual Insurance Company:[28]

- *Triple-check—plus two:* The usual triple-check of the medication dispensed versus what is ordered is not enough. Nor is the triple-check of right patient, right drug, and right strength enough. In addition, the National Drug Code (NDC) number on the stock bottle should be checked against the NDC number in the computer.

- *Show and tell:* Counseling each patient about his or her medication should be the final check. This step has been shown to catch errors in dispensing and should be followed.
- *The two-second rule:* No prescription bottle containing medication should be allowed to remain unlabeled for more than two seconds.
- *A comfortable customer is willing to wait:* All pharmacists feel pressured during busy periods and there is a temptation to skip routine steps in the dispensing process. Such omissions have led to major errors.[29] In some pharmacies, a comfortable patient waiting area is all that is needed to relieve pressure and allow the pharmacist to make sure every step in the dispensing process is taken.
- *The basket system:* When more than one prescription is processed at one time, medications can easily get mixed up. Using a basket system keeps prescriptions separate and is a proven method to reduce error.
- *Special storage and handling:* High-risk, high-alert drugs such as digoxin, warfarin, phenytoin, and methotrexate deserve special storage and handling.
- *Echoing verbal orders:* Verbal orders raise the risk of making a mistake. To avoid problems with verbal orders, pharmacists (or anyone receiving the verbal order) should read back what they heard and ask, "Is that correct?"
- *Documenting patient counseling:* Six percent (6 percent) of claims against a pharmacist resulted from the pharmacist's failure to counsel the patient adequately or to prove that counseling took place.

Duty to Warn

Doctors have a duty to warn patients about the most likely problems that can occur with the medication they prescribe, especially when patients are to take the medication on their own. However, the pharmacist's duty to warn is less clear. At one time (before 1990), pharmacists could walk into any court and convince a judge or a jury that they had no duty to the patient—no duty to warn, no duty to counsel, no duty to question the appropriateness of a prescription. Since 1990, court decisions are slowly but methodically establishing that the pharmacist has a duty to warn (usually the patient's doctor), especially about potentially harmful drug interactions, when there is a clear error in a prescription or drug order, and when the prescribed medication has the potential to cause permanent damage or death.[30-38] The legal requirement for the pharmacist to offer counseling to patients about their medication has increased the pharmacist's duty to warn.

A case decided by the appellate court in Illinois and reported in 2001 imposed a "duty to warn" on a pharmacist, independent of a doctor.[39] In this case, a patient told the pharmacy staff of drug allergies to aspirin, acetaminophen, and ibuprofen and this information was entered in the pharmacy computer system. A prescription for ibuprofen was phoned into the pharmacy. When the prescription information was entered in the pharmacy's computer system, a warning flashed across the screen. However, this was ignored and the medication was dispensed. The patient experienced respiratory distress, was admitted to the emergency room, and was diagnosed as having anaphylactic shock.

Disclosure of Medication Errors

Controversy surrounds whether it is good practice to disclose to patients that a medical or medication error has taken place. Ethicists and professional organizations recommend that anyone committing a medical or medication error reveal this to the patient. Patients want to know about errors that affect them and would like an apology. However, many doctors are reluctant to disclose these errors for fear of lawsuits.[40] Yet, full disclosure of medical errors to patients and families at the New Mexico Veterans Affairs (VA) Health Care System did not increase malpractice claims.[41]

SUMMARY

Drug injury claims associated with malpractice claims are often severe, costly, and preventable. These claims can provide insight on why these events occurred, and some interventions have been identified that can potentially prevent drug injuries. However, in general, society lacks systematic and reliable mechanisms for improving drug use and prescribing practices drawn from successful and unsuccessful litigation. Deciding if injury from a drug can occur, did occur, and how it occurred is best left to expert witnesses that specialize in medication safety.

Chapter 11

Assessing the Evidence
of Drug Injury

Chapter 10 covered drug injury and litigation, and expert testimony in cases of drug injury where compensation is sought. This chapter explores the process of deciding if injury is possible from a particular drug, if the injury occurred, and how it might have occurred.

Deciding if a specific drug injury can occur involves biologic plausibility and evidence that others have been injured using the same drug under similar circumstances. If it can occur, the question then becomes—did it occur in this patient? This involves an assessment of patient risk factors and how the drug was used, with laboratory evidence and expert opinion. Finally, if the ADE is a medication error, it is important to discover how it happened.

FINDING SUPPORTING EVIDENCE
ON "CAN IT HAPPEN?"

The first question to be asked in drug injury is—can the drug cause this injury? Except in cases of bizarre or idiosyncratic (type A) adverse drug reactions (ADRs), there needs to be biologic plausibility. If the drug did cause the injury, what were the biologic and pharmacologic mechanisms? For type B ADRs, there is a pharmacologic basis or a dose-response curve, and the mechanism of action (and damage) is usually unknown. For allergic drug reactions, the basis is immnuologic. For drug-drug interactions, the interaction has a mechanism (how one drug affected the other) and a certain time course.

The second question in deciding whether a drug can cause a specific injury is—has the suspected drug been reported in other patients taking the suspect drug under similar circumstances? There are several ways to examine this. First, was the adverse effect noted in clinical trials before the drug was approved for use? Second, after the Food and Drug Administration (FDA) approved the drug for marketing, was the drug labeled for the adverse effect? Third, after FDA approval, have there been any similar cases reported to the FDA or published in the medical literature? Fourth, have there been any studies comparing the use of the drug versus not using the drug for the adverse effect being questioned?

Pre-FDA-Approval Studies

Before a potential new drug can be considered for approval, it must pass animal testing and three phases of human testing. *Phase I investigation* is completed in 20 to 30 healthy volunteers and mainly shows a dose response. *Phase II investigation* takes place in several hundred patients with the disease for which the drug is intended, and mainly shows short-term safety and effectiveness. In *phase III investigation,* the drug is studied in several hundred to several thousand patients— some who will receive the drug (study patients) and some who will not (control patients). Phase III investigations usually take place in multihospital settings. The groups are compared for drug efficacy and safety.

During these trials, side effects and ADRs are closely watched and documented. If the manufacturer seeks a new drug approval (NDA) for the drug, its drug safety information and recommended labeling is submitted to the FDA with the rest of the information. The FDA then assesses the drug's risks versus its benefits. If the benefits outweigh the drug's risks, it is approved for use.

Drug Labeling

The FDA decides how a drug will be labeled and what information will be required in the package insert. This is called "official labeling." Official labeling is available in the product's package insert, some of which may (but not always) be reproduced in the *Physicians' Desk Reference (PDR).* The FDA can require more labeling as more information becomes known about the drug. All official labeling is dated. Thus, what was required in the product's labeling when the drug first came on the market usually changes as time goes by. This latter point is important in legal work. What precautions were required when the drug was prescribed is what is important—not what is required now or when the drug came on the market.

Postmarketing Surveillance

Studies of a drug in only a few thousand patients during the pre-FDA-approval period cannot identify all the adverse effects associated with a new drug. Once the drug is approved for marketing, thousands of patients are suddenly exposed to the drug and new adverse effects are identified. These new ADRs become known in several ways.

Spontaneous Reporting to MedWatch

Spontaneous reporting is the first step in the postmarketing surveillance of ADRs. Doctors use their clinical judgment and experience to assess whether a drug may be causing an adverse effect. If the doctor concludes that a drug is associated with a particular adverse effect, he or she should report this case to the FDA's MedWatch program (http://www.fda.gov/medwatch/index.html). However, reporting is voluntary and many doctors do not take the time to report the adverse drug effect. Thus, it may be some time before the FDA has enough reports to cause concern and to take any necessary action.

The FDA is mostly interested in new and serious adverse drug effects (ADRs, drug interactions, allergic drug reactions, and even medication errors). The Centers for Disease Control and Prevention (CDC) and the FDA jointly sponsor a similar reporting system for vaccines called the Vaccine Adverse Events Reporting System (VAERS) where health care professionals and patients can document an ADR to a vaccine (http://www.vaers.hhs.org/). Access to information in these databases is through the freedom of information office (http://www.usdoj.gov/04foia/foiacontacts.htm).

The United States Pharmacopeia (USP) operates the only anonymous, national system for reporting medication errors in hospitals called MEDMARX. Work is advancing to expand MEDMARX's capability. In addition, the Institute for Safe Medication Practices (ISMP) captures and publishes medication safety cases and alerts for practitioners and consumers (http://www.ismp.org).

The FDA, CDC, and USP constantly review the incoming spontaneous adverse event reports to see if they detect a *signal*—a trend that may suggest a problem with the drug or vaccine. All signals are assessed scientifically and statistically to see if they are true or false. If something is of concern, the FDA publishes alerts for practitioners.

Published Case Reports

Another way of reporting a possible ADR is by publishing case reports in the medical and pharmaceutical literature. Sometimes a doctor will submit information to a medical journal about several patients who have taken the same drug and experienced the same ADR. This is a case series. Doctors write these case reports to alert other doctors that a drug may cause a certain adverse effect. They describe the patient, and the patient's disease state, the drug therapy involved, and the adverse effect. These can be helpful, however the quality of these reports have recently been questioned, chiefly because many reports have much missing information and few contain any formal causality assessment.[1]

Gathering evidence for "can a drug cause this injury?" is best carried out by a drug information pharmacist. These specially trained pharmacists work in one of 103 drug information centers in the United States.[2]

Although information from spontaneous reporting may be interesting, such reports are an unreliable measure of risk. They only "provide evidence of the relative awareness of specific toxic effects among reporters."[3]

EVIDENCE-BASED MEDICINE STUDIES

Signals from MedWatch or VAERs, or information from case reports or case series, are considered hypothesis-generating information, rather than cause-and-effect information. Thus, the information from these sources needs to be investigated using more rigorous study methods to establish an association between the drug or vaccine and an adverse event.

A study using simple rules of logic and science that can be applied to improve the clinical care of patients is called "evidence-based medicine" (EBM). "EBM de-emphasizes intuition, unsystematic clinical experience, and pathophysiologic rationale as sufficient grounds for decision making, and stresses the examination of evidence from clinical research."[4] Several types of EBM studies can discover a possible association between a drug and an adverse outcome.

Observational (Pharmacoepidemiologic) Studies

Observational or pharmacoepidemiologic studies can be used to discover the strength of an association. Pharmacoepidemiology is the study of the distribution and determinants of drug-related events in populations and the application of this study to efficacious drug treatment.[5] Pharmacoepidemiologic studies compare the records of many patients who received the drug with records of many patients who did not receive the drug, thus they are sometimes called "population-based" studies. There are three types of observational studies: cross-sectional, case control, and cohort.

Cross-sectional studies. A cross-sectional study is the simplest observational study and is done in present time (concurrently) to capture a snapshot, or *prevalence,* of an adverse effect at a certain point in time (see Figure 11.1).

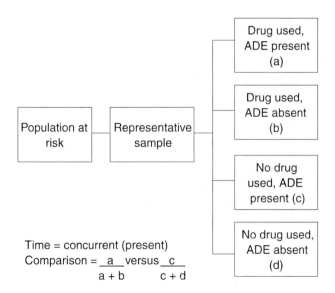

FIGURE 11.1. Design of a Cross-Sectional Study and Computation of Results

For example, 100 patients are selected on one day and the patients are divided into those who received and those who did not receive aspirin within the past 30 days. All patients are checked (endoscopically) to see if they have gastrointestinal (GI) bleeding. Bleeding rates are calculated and compared for those taking and for those not taking aspirin. Cross-sectional studies can be done quickly and are inexpensive. However, interpretations of these studies are limited, and thus used to generate hypotheses.

Case control studies. In case control studies, patients are selected by outcome (have or do not have the adverse effect of interest). Thus, these are usually *retrospective* studies (looking back) to see whether a person received the drug of interest (see Figure 11.2).

Case control studies discover the odds or odds ratio (OR) of a person receiving a drug when they have the adverse effect of interest versus someone who does not experience the adverse effect of interest. For example, if 100 patients are selected and divided into two groups—those with and those without GI bleeding—you can look back to see which patients received aspirin during the past 30 days and calculate an OR.

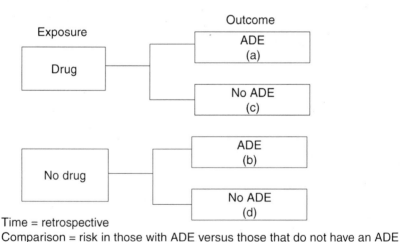

Time = retrospective
Comparison = risk in those with ADE versus those that do not have an ADE
Odds Ratio (OR) = $\dfrac{a \times d}{b \times c}$

FIGURE 11.2. Design of a Case Control Study and Computation of an Odds Ratio (OR)

Case control studies are convenient to use when the adverse effect is rare. The studies are relatively inexpensive and can be done quickly. However, they cannot be used to calculate an incidence rate (the number of new cases with time) for the adverse effect.

Cohort studies. Cohort studies are sometimes called "longitudinal" or "follow-up" studies. Patients are selected based on exposure (received or did not receive the drug), then followed prospectively (forward in time) to see if they develop the adverse effect of interest (see Figure 11.3). Cohort studies can discover the true *incidence* of an adverse effect (the rate for so many people for so many years). They also discover the relative risk (RR) of a person experiencing a particular adverse effect when they have taken a drug versus someone who has not taken the drug.

For example, 100 patients with no GI bleeding are divided into those taking aspirin and those who are not taking aspirin. The patients are followed for three months to see who has developed GI bleeding and a RR is calculated.

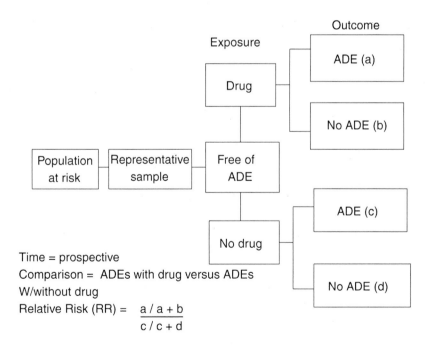

Time = prospective
Comparison = ADEs with drug versus ADEs W/without drug
Relative Risk (RR) = $\dfrac{a\,/\,a + b}{c\,/\,c + d}$

FIGURE 11.3. Design of a Cohort Study and Computation of Relative Risk (RR)

Randomized Clinical Trials (RCTs)

Observational or epidemiologic studies are used when you cannot randomly assign patients to the study or control groups. In observational studies, the investigator has little to no control over the study and control groups. The investigator studies the data he or she has available after patients have already been selected.

In a randomized clinical trial (RCT), the study is a pure experiment controlled by an investigator. The investigator draws potential patients from a population of similar individuals and randomizes them into a study sample and a control sample (see Figure 11.4). This increases the chance the groups are comparable except for the exposure (drug versus no drug, drug versus placebo, or drug A versus drug B).

The investigator in an RCT is also able to control the size of the groups to make sure there is enough statistical power to show a significant difference between groups (if one exists). The patients and investigator can also be blinded (not sure if the drug or a placebo was given) and the studies are *prospective* (move forward in time). These

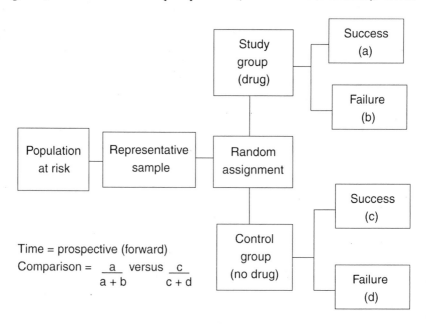

FIGURE 11.4. Design of a Randomized Clinical Trial (RCT) and Computation of Results

added conditions increases control over the study, thus RCTs are often termed *randomized controlled studies.*

Calculations

All studies use a 2×2 (two columns by two rows) contingency table (see Figure 11.5) to calculate RRs, ORs, or to compare proportions. The table is always laid out the same. Quadrant A contains the number of people exposed to the drug who experienced the adverse effect of interest. Quadrant B contains the number of people exposed to the drug who did not experience the adverse effect of interest. Quadrant C contains the number of people not exposed to the drug who experienced the adverse effect of interest. Quadrant D is for the number of people not exposed to the drug who did not experience the adverse effect of interest.

The formula for calculating a OR is shown in Figure 11.2. Figure 11.3 contains the formula for calculating a RR. ORs and RRs are *point estimates* of risk (like 1.5) and are computed with *confidence intervals*. For example OR = 2.4 (1.8, 3.1). The most common confidence interval is the CI^{95}, that means there is 95 percent confidence the *actual risk estimate* lies between 1.8 and 3.1.

For cross-sectional studies (Figure 11.1) and RCTs (Figure 11.4), proportions are compared. The comparison is between the proportion (percent) of patients who receive the drug and experience the adverse

	Present (AE)	Absent (AE)
Present (R)	A	B
Absent (R)	C	D

R = exposure to drug
AE = adverse effect

FIGURE 11.5. The 2 × 2 Contingency Table Used to Calculate the Results of Research Studies on Drugs

effect, and the proportion of patients who did not receive the drug and experienced the adverse effect (during the same time period).

Interpretation

What does an OR or RR of 1.5 mean? Let's say we are trying to discover the risk of GI bleeding when taking nonsteroidal anti-inflammatory drugs (NSAIDs) such as ibuprofen. When interpreting point estimates, the statement starts with how the study started. For example, in a case control study, an OR of 1.5 would be interpreted—people with GI bleeding are 50 percent more likely to be taking NSAIDs than those people who do not have GI bleeding. In a cohort study, a RR of 1.5 would be interpreted—people on NSAIDs are 50 percent more likely to have GI bleeding than people who are not taking NSAIDs.

An OR or RR of 1.0 means there is no difference between groups. ORs and RRs less than one (<1) are interpreted as a protective effect of the exposure (drug). However, because of limits inherent in observational studies, most pharmcoepidemiologists do not feel point estimates are significant unless both confidence limits are great than 1. The following point estimate would not be considered significant: OR = 1.6 (0.8, 2.0); while a point estimate of OR = 1.6 (1.1, 2.0) would be significant. When the adverse effect is rare, the OR and RR are about the same.

The proportion of people experiencing the adverse effect from the drug in an RCT (let's say 8 percent), can be divided by the proportion of people experiencing the adverse effect and are not taking the drug or taking the placebo (let's say 2 percent). This provides a ratio (8:2 or 4:1) that can be interpreted—those taking the drug may be four times more likely to experience the adverse effect than those not taking the drug. However, there is danger in doing this. Typically, RCTs use relatively small numbers of patients that decreases the precision of this estimate.

Systematic Reviews

A *systematic review* is a process of using statistical methods to combine the results of different studies. A *frequent application* is pooling results from several RCTs, none powerful enough to show statistically significant differences, but in total, capable of doing so. Systematic reviews are also used when the results of trials are conflicting to see the net effect.

The most common systematic review today is the meta-analysis. A meta-analysis statistically synthesizes the data from separate but similar, i.e., comparable studies, leading to a quantitative summary of the pooled results. Meta-analyses can be powerful tools to assess combinations of RCTs and observational studies.

Study Limitations

Every study has limitations. For example, cross-sectional studies can only provide a prevalence rate at one point in time. In case control studies, the study and control groups are not randomized, thus the results are susceptible to unmeasured confounders, and thus there may be threats to internal validity (the results are solely based on the hypothesized effect being measured). Therefore, the strength of the inference drawn from the results may be limited. Also, a true incidence rate of the adverse effect cannot be calculated.

Although a true incidence rate for an adverse drug effect can be calculated, cohort studies possess most of the same limitations as case control studies, including the bias *confounding by indication*. For example, if a cohort study shows that people taking nonsteroidal anti-inflammatory agents have a higher incidence (relative risk) of having upper gastrointestinal (GI) bleeding than those patients who do not take NSAIDs, it could be because the GI bleed is not because of the NSAIDs. There may be something different about the patients that needed the NSAIDs. Thus, the strength of the inference from a cohort study is always less than that of a rigorously conducted RCT.

The RCT is the "gold standard" for studies. The RCT is a true experiment in which patients are assigned, by a mechanism similar to flipping a coin, to either the putative causal agent or some alternative experience (either another agent or no agent at all). The strength of the RCT is based on the confidence that study and control groups are comparable. However, the limitations of the RCT are that they are time-consuming and expensive to conduct. Thus, if the study and control groups are not large enough, this can limit the study's power and thus the strength of the inference.

Study Quality

In general, the hierarchy of studies (from the most desirable to least desirable) are RCTs > cohort studies > case control studies > cross-sectional studies. Where to place systematic analyses on this scale is highly debated. There are concerns on how systematic reviews are completed.[6,7] Assessing the quality of each study in the meta-analysis is of primary importance and this needs to be done using strict criteria.[8]

A well-done meta-analysis may be weighted between a RCT and a cohort study, but a poor one would fall below a case control study. Each study needs to be conducted using quality methods. For example, guidelines for good epidemiology practices for drug, device, and vaccine research need to be followed.[9]

Most studies contain flaws in methodology, or bias—deviations from the truth. Major flaws should be detected by peer review before a manuscript is accepted for publication. Minor flaws and biases should be identified by the author and discussed as a limitation in the discussion section of the manuscript.

In July 2002, the Women's Health Initiative (WHI) stopped a large randomized trial assessing the risks and benefits of estrogen plus progestin in healthy postmenopausal women.[10] The study was stopped after 5.2 years of follow up because the overall health risks of taking the medication exceeded the benefits of taking the medication. Specifically, there was an increased risk for cardiovascular disease and invasive breast cancer.

The result of the WHI study has caused concern in the health care community. The results are the opposite of what was believed before this, most of which was based on observational studies. These differing results may have been the result of an inherent limitation in observational studies—confounding by indication.

Rating the Quality of Individual Studies

Trying to discover if a specific drug can cause a specific adverse effect needs to be done carefully. Besides assessing the relative merits of each study, each individual study needs assessment. An EBM approach to deciding if the results of a study on harm are valid would include answering the following questions:[11]

- Are the results of the study valid?
  - —Were there clearly identified comparison groups that were similar for the important determinants of outcome, other than the one of interest?
  - —Were the outcomes and exposures measured in the same way in the groups being compared?
  - —Was the follow-up sufficiently correct?
  - —Is the temporal relationship correct (did the drug exposure come before the outcome)?
  - —Is there a dose-response gradient (did the severity of the outcome increase with more dosage?)
- What are the results?
  - —How strong is the association between exposure and outcome?
  - —How precise is the estimate of the risk?

Grading the Strength of the Evidence

Scales and checklists are available to use in grading the strength of the evidence. In general, the number of RCTs, the quality of each RCT, and the strength of the association between the drug exposure and the adverse outcome is what is most important. Well-designed cohort, case control, and systematic reviews can also help in discovering if there is a true association between a drug and an adverse effect.

DID THE DRUG CAUSE THE ADVERSE EVENT?

If it is determined the drug or vaccine in question can cause the adverse effect in question, the next step is to discover if it happened in this patient. The first step in discovering this is to document that the patient received the drug before the adverse event occurred. If the answer is yes, then it is time to discover causality.

When a person suffers an adverse event after taking a medication, it does not mean the drug caused the adverse event. It is easy to blame the drug when it could easily have been something else. "Association" does not mean "causation."

It is often difficult to discover causality. The adverse effect could be caused by another drug the patient was taking or by another substance to which the person was exposed. Or, the patient may be experiencing a new symptom of his or her disease or has developed a new health problem. For example, someone starts taking a medication in the evening. The next day, the person has a rash over his or her shoulders, back, and chest. Did the medicine cause this? In this case it was not the medicine, but a dye in a shampoo the patient used in the morning.

Causality Assessment

Sir Austin Hill was one of the first to delineate out what needs to be considered when determining causation.[12] Today, the Naranjo method (see Table 4.2) is the easiest and most reliable method for estimating the probability that a drug caused an adverse reaction.[13]

Hansten and Horn have developed a modified Naranjo probability scale (Table 11.1) for assessing the likelihood of a drug-drug interaction.[14]

Each question needs to be answered when using the Naranjo or Hansten probability scales. Mark zero for those statements where no information is available. Once each statement is graded, the scores are added, and the total score is compared to the scale of definite, probable, possible, or doubtful. These algorithms work for all ADEs except for errors.

Laboratory Confirmation

Laboratory findings or objective evidence help confirm the drug as the possible cause. Levels of the drug in various bodily fluids (e.g., serum, salvia, hair, tears, or urine) are critical, if available. With a live viral vaccine, was a wild-type virus isolated and identified in the body versus the weakened virus used in the vaccine?

Patient and Drug Risk Factors

Was the patient more vulnerable to the negative effects of the exposure in question? Factors such as age, gender, severity of illness, ethnicity, renal or liver compromise, and weight might need consideration when determining if a specific drug cause harmed to a patient.

TABLE 11.1. A Drug Interaction Probability Scale

	Yes	No	Unsure or N.A.	Score
1. Are there previous credible reports of this interaction in humans (i.e., rating "possible" or higher on this algorithm)?	+1	0	0	
2. Is the observed interaction consistent with the known interactive properties of the precipitant drug (the one causing the interaction)?	+1	−1	0	
3. Is the observed interaction consistent with the known interactive properties of the object drug (the drug affected by the interaction)?	+1	−1	0	
4. Is the event consistent with the known or reasonable time course of the interaction (onset and/or offset)?	+1	−1	0	
5. Did the interaction remit upon dechallenge of the precipitant drug with no change in the object drug? If no dechallenge, use NA.	+1	−2	0	
6. Did the interaction reappear when the precipitant drug was readministered in the presence of continued use of object drug?	+2	−1	0	
7. Are there alternative reasonable causes for the event?[a]	−1	+1	0	
8. Was the object drug detected in the blood or other fluids in concentrations consistent with the proposed interaction?	+1	0	0	
9. Was the drug interaction confirmed by any objective evidence consistent with the effects on the object drug (other than drug concentrations from question 8)?	+1	0	0	
10. Was the reaction greater when the precipitant drug dose was increased or less when the precipitant drug dose was decreased?	+1	−1	0	

Source: Published with permission by P. Hansten & J. Horn. H & H Publications.

Note: Highly probable >8; Probable = 5-8; Possible = 2-4; Doubtful = <2

[a]Consider the patient's diseases and clinical condition, other drugs, lack of compliance, risk factors for the object drug toxicity (e.g., age, inappropriate doses of object drug). A "no" answer presumes that enough information was presented so that one would expect any alternative causes to be mentioned. When in doubt, use unsure.

Also, the dose, route, and duration of the drug may also be important. The risk for and prediction of ADEs will be covered in more detail in Chapter 14.

Medication Errors

Many patients do not connect problems they are suddenly having to their medication or consider that there may have been an error in prescribing, dispensing, or administration. However, pharmacists, and especially medication safety experts, can rapidly discover if an error has occurred by using policies, procedures, standards of practice, and laws, rules, and regulations. It is usually harder to discover *how* the error happened, than *if* it happened.

HOW DID IT OCCUR?

Except for medication errors, if the ADE can occur and did occur, discovering how it occurred is academic. If there are enough cases and studies of the ADE in question, there should be enough information on the drug's possible mechanisms for the harm in question.

With medication error, how the error occurred is of supreme importance. Where in the medication-use system was there a breakdown? How many breakdowns were there? Were their any rule violations? Was a duty not fulfilled? Did the duty violation result in direct harm? Someone who knows about medication safety should investigate these questions carefully. How medication errors should be detected, documented, investigated, and reported are covered in Chapters 12 and 13.

GAPS BETWEEN WHAT IS KNOWN AND PRACTICE

A lag exists between what is known scientifically (evidence) and what is done in clinical practice. For example, a well-designed RCT may show an association between the use of a drug and a serious adverse effect. If the study is published in a medical journal, it may be some time before it is noticed by the FDA or the manufacturer. A patient's doctor may never see it. In the latter case, the doctor may be a surgeon who mainly reads surgery journals. He or she never sees the article because it was published in an internal medicine journal.

It would be wonderful if all doctors kept up with all the medical literature, but this is impossible. However, there are too many medical journals, too many articles, and many constraints on doctors' time. Therefore, a doctor will not know everything about drugs they prescribe, and it may be a long time before they learn something current about the drugs.

Does this mean doctors should not be held accountable for prescribing a drug that causes harm? What should they know? This problem is handled in the legal system by asking the question "What is the standard of practice?" What do other doctors with similar credentials and practices know? Would they prescribe the drug under similar circumstances?

SUMMARY

When a patient is injured and a drug or vaccine is suspected as causing the injury, the adverse event needs to be investigated using sound investigative methods; emotion should not rule. There could be other reasons the adverse event occurred. The questions to be answered are: Can it happen? Did it happen? When an error has occurred, another question needs to be asked: Why did it happen? The best person to answer these questions is a medication safety expert, or a team of health professionals well versed in medication safety. The ADE needs to be properly documented, assessed, and reported. If the ADE is preventable, procedures and training should be put in place to help prevent the adverse event from occurring again.

Chapter 12

Detecting and Documenting Adverse Drug Events

Knowing when an adverse drug event has occurred, and knowing sooner is better than knowing later. This chapter will discuss detecting and documenting ADEs and retrospective and concurrent ways of detecting them.

The sooner an adverse drug event (ADE) is detected, the sooner the offending drug can be discontinued (which may limit the injury), and the patient can receive treatment for the ADE, if needed. When an ADE has occurred it should be documented in the patient's record and an incident report filled out. The patient should be made aware of the ADE and precautions should be made to prevent the ADE from occurring again in the patient.

In general, two ways to detect that an ADE has occurred are through clinical recognition and through manual and automatic systems. In the past, these two modes of recognition occurred retrospectively (after the ADE took place). Today, newer systems are being investigated to discover if an ADE is starting to take place (concurrently) or to predict (prospectively) when an ADE will occur.

Once detected, ADEs should be documented through an incident reporting system, and in the patient's medical record. This documentation records what happened and satisfies accreditation standards. Accurate and timely documentation is good risk management practice.

RETROSPECTIVE METHODS OF DETECTING ADEs

Until recently, ADEs were detected retrospectively—after they occurred. This has been done in several ways.

Prescribed Medications and the Public Health
© 2006 by The Haworth Press, Inc. All rights reserved.
doi:10.1300/5688_12

Clinical Recognition

It is not always easy to recognize that an adverse effect may be the result of a drug. Patients often do not think that a drug they are taking may be causing the adverse effect they are experiencing. Many doctors and nurses also have a low level of suspicion. Sometimes it is easier to attribute the adverse effect to an extension of the underlying disease or to other nondrug causes.

Doctors are unfamiliar with the possible adverse effects of a medication when it first comes on the market, but most doctors closely monitor a new drug for any adverse effects. They check any effects against the product labeling to see if this adverse effect was also seen in the preapproval trials of the drug.

Doctors routinely prescribe the same drugs and become familiar with how well they work and with their limitations, including common adverse effects. They are encouraged to report any new, unexpected, or serious adverse effects to the FDA's MedWatch program.

The role of a drug in an adverse effect is only one aspect of the classic medical diagnostic process which includes a differential and an etiologic diagnosis.[1] This is based on evidence for or against a temporal relationship—the timing of the drug and the event—and on ruling out other nondrug causes for the event.

Precise temporal data must be investigated to make a proper diagnosis of a drug-induced event. Data to be collected include:

1. the exact time the suspect drug was first administered,
2. the time when other doses were given,
3. if other drugs were given (and if so when),
4. the time the first symptoms of the adverse event occurred,
5. when drugs were discontinued, and
6. what effect this had on the adverse event.

Chronology is of utmost importance when trying to link a drug to an adverse event. The drug must have been given before the adverse event began. More than likely, the drug may have contributed to the adverse event if it appeared within minutes or hours of taking the drug, versus days and weeks.[1]

If the suspect drug was continued and the adverse effect disappeared, than more than likely, the drug was not the cause of the adverse event. There is likelihood the drug was associated with the adverse effect if, on the drug's discontinuation, the adverse effect quickly resolved. An even stronger clue that the drug was the culprit is when the adverse effect returns on reuse of the drug.

The Naranjo probability scale can be used for discovering whether a drug caused an adverse drug reaction (ADR).[2] Drug interaction probability scales can also be used.[3] These scales are discussed in Chapter 11.

Incident Reports

A Joint Commission on Accreditation of Healthcare Organizations (JCHAO) standard states that all ADEs should be documented using the organization's incident reporting system. Thus, some ADEs are documented, but most are not. Organizations typically report only 1 of every 20 ADEs.[4] This problem is illustrated in Figure 12.1. Various

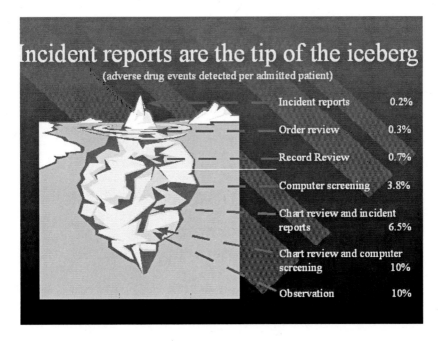

FIGURE 12.1. Source of ADE Incident Reports (*Source:* Reprinted with permission of ISMP.)

reasons contribute to this including: lack of time, the task is low priority, the feeling that nothing will be done, and fearing that if reported, the reporting may come back to haunt the reporter.

Discharge Summaries

A manual review of patients' hospital discharge summaries to find ADEs is fruitful, but time-consuming. A more cost-effective method is scanning these records using computer software programmed to recognize key words that may suggest an ADE.[5]

Chart Reviews

ADEs should be documented in the patient's chart. However, this is not always the case, especially when the ADE is an error. Most doctors hesitate to do this for medical and/or legal reasons. However, most doctors document ADRs when they think the adverse effect was associated with the use of a drug. Performing studies of ADEs by doing chart reviews is time-consuming and expensive. However, chart reviews are needed to validate other means of discovering ADEs that may be more productive and cost effective.

When looking for ADEs in medical records, most people use a standardized form and check the discharge summary, the progress notes, the medication orders, and the laboratory tests for confirmation or signals of an ADE.[6] Events to look for include: change in mental status, abnormal lab values, a sudden change in the patient's condition, a new rash or diarrhea, and orders for antidotes.

Medical Record Coding

Another way of detecting ADEs is through medical records coding. Medical records personnel use the International Classification of Diseases (ICD-10) to code diagnoses, procedures, and some outcomes (such as ADEs). Unfortunately, this is usually not done consistently.

CONCURRENT METHODS OF DETECTING ADVERSE DRUG EVENTS

Observing Medication Errors

Few health care professionals look for medication errors unless they are doing a study. Perhaps they should, as medication errors occur much too often. Observation is the most accurate and valid method of discovering the incidence of medication errors.[7,8] For example, one study using the observation method showed the number of errors discovered was 1,422 times the number identified by incident reports.[9] There are three requirements for observational studies: the event must be visible, predictable, and of limited duration.

Computer Alerts

The newest method to detect that an ADE has just occurred is by constant computer monitoring. When a signal is detected, a computer alert is sent to doctors, pharmacists, and nurses. The alert indicates a potential ADE.

To detect adverse drug events, an infrastructure is needed that contains an event monitor. "An *event monitor* is a program that checks all of a system's applications and looks for evidence of particular events. The applications run and produce new data."[10] The parts of the event monitor include a rule editor, enunciators to rout information to the correct individuals, and a coverage list to let co-workers know which clinician is responsible for a given patient at a given time.

The *rule editor* is at the heart of the system. Composing the rules engine is of supreme importance.[11] Examples of some rules and triggers for electronically checking for ADEs are shown in Table 12.1. The rules and triggers lie chiefly in four areas: laboratory data, drug levels, drug orders, and diagnoses. The key is to use enough rules and triggers to detect or prevent potential or serious ADEs, yet not activate so many alarms that practitioners ignore the warnings. The rules need continuous improvement to minimize false positive alarms.

TABLE 12.1. Some Typical Triggers Used in Electronic Adverse Drug Event Monitoring

Laboratory Data (Serum)	Drug Levels	Drug Orders	Diagnoses
Alkaline phosphatase >350	Amikacin peak >25	Digibind	Angioedema
ALT or AST >150	Carbamazepine >12	Diphenhydramine	Aplastic anemia
Bilirubin >10	Digoxin >2	Diphenoxylate/Atropine	GI bleeding
BUN >50	Gentamicin peak >10	Flumazenil	Hepatotoxicity
Creatinine clearance <50	Lidocaine >5	Kaolin/pectin	Hypoglycemia
Eosiniphil % >6	Phenytoin >20	Loperamide	Ototoxicity
Glucose <50	Theophylline peak >10	Naloxone	Rash
INR >6	Tobramycin peak >10	Phytonadione	Renal failure
Platelets <50,000	Valproate >120	Protamine sulfate	Seizures

More and more hospitals are testing these electronic systems to detect and alert personnel of a potential adverse drug effect or potential medication error.[12-14] However, it will be some time before these systems are perfected and commonly used.

COMPARING THE VARIOUS WAYS TO DETECT ADVERSE DRUG EVENTS

Work is ongoing to discover the best way to detect ADEs. Incident reporting and chart reviews are the traditional methods of detecting ADEs. Some work has been done on scanning discharge summaries and looking at medical record coding. The observation method has been confined to studies of medication errors. Using computer alerts to detect ADEs is in its early stages. Table 12.2 displays some studies on ADE detection and their success rates.

The compelling question remains: Which system best detects ADEs? Three measurements are important in comparing methods: sensitivity, specificity, and predictive value. *Sensitivity* is the proportion of true ADEs detected or true positives. *Specificity* is the proportion of ADEs detected that are not true ADEs or false positives (see Table 12.3).

TABLE 12.2. Some Studies on Detecting ADEs

Year	Setting	Event	Total	Detection					
				IR	DS	CR	MRC	OBS	CA
1991[a]	Hospital	ADEs	731	92					631
1996[b]	Hospital	ADRs	824	621			203		
1998[c]	Hospital	ADEs	696	23		398			275
1998[d]	Hospital	ADEs	596						1,116*
2000[e]	Hospital	ADRs	46	17					34
2001[f]	Hospital	ADEs	42	1		5	6		30
2002[g]	Hospital	ADRs	2,571	2,571					
2003[h]	Hospital	ADRs	109	109		109			109
2003[i]	Hospital	ADRs	157	157		126			
2003[j]	Hospital	AMEs	131		251*				
1990[k]	Hospital	PME	420						696*
1997[l]	Hospital	PME	2,859						2,859
2003[m]	Ambulatory	ADEs	1,523	173	749**				437
2002[n]	Hospitals	Errors	142	0		12		128	
1995[o]	Hospital	Errors	530			530			
2001[p]	Hospital	Errors	616			616			
2002[n]	LTC	Errors	239	0		7		185	
1987[q]	LTC	Errors	1,802			1,608		194	

Notes: ADE = adverse drug event; ADR = adverse drug reaction; AME = adverse medical event; PME = potential medication error; IR = incident reporting; DS = discharge summaries; CR = chart review; MRC = medical record coding; OBS = observation; CA = computer alerts.

[a] Classen DC, Pestotnik SL, Evans RD, and Burke JP. (1991). Computerized surveillance of adverse drug events in hospital patients. *JAMA* 266:2847-2878.

[b] Seeger JD, Schumock GT, and Kong SX. (1996). Estimating the rate of adverse drug reactions with capture-recapture analysis. *Am J Health-Syst Pharm* 53:178-181.

[c] Jha AK, Kuperman GJ, Teich JM, Leape L, Shea B, Rittenberg E, Burdick E, Seger DL, Vander Vliet M, Bates DW. (1998). Identifying adverse drug events: Development of a computer-based monitor and comparison with chart review and stimulated voluntary report. *J Am Informatics Assoc* 5(3):305-314.

[d] Raschke RA, Gollihare B, Wunderlich TA, Guidry JR, Leibowitz AI, Peirce JC, Lemelson L, Heisler MA, Susong C. (1998). A computer alert system to prevent injury from adverse drug events: Development and evaluation in a community teaching hospital. *JAMA* 280(15):1317-1320.

[e] Egger T, Dormann H, Runge U, Neubert A, Criegee-Rieck M, Gassmann KG, Brune K. (2003). Identification of adverse drug reactions in geriatric inpatients using computerized drug database. *Drugs and Aging* 20(10):769-776.

[f] Senst BL, Achusim LE, Genest RP, Cosentino LA, Ford CC, LIttle JA, Raybon SJ, Bates DW. (2001). Practical approach to determining costs and frequency of adverse drug events in a health care network. *Am J Health-Syst Pharm* 58:1126-1132.

[g] Winterstein AG, Hatton RC, Gonzalez-Rothi R, and Segal R. (2002). Identifying clinically significant preventable adverse drug events through a hospital's database of adverse drug reaction reports. *Am J Health-Syst Pharm* 59(18):1742-1749.

TABLE 12.2 *(continued)*

[h] Dormann H, Criegee-Rieck M, Neubert A, Egger T, Levy M, Hahn EG, Brune K. (2002). Implementation of a computer monitoring system for detection of adverse drug reactions by laboratory signals. Presented at the 18th International Conference on Pharmacoepidemiology. August 20, Edinburgh, Scotland.
[i] Troutman WG and Doherty KM. (2003). Comparison of voluntary adverse drug reaction reports and corresponding medical records. *Am J Health-Syst Pharm* 60:572-575.
[j] Murff HJ, Forster AJ, Peterson JF, Fiskio JM, Heiman HL, Bates DW. (2003). Electronically screening discharge summaries for adverse medical events. *J Am Med Informatics Assoc* 10:339-350.
[k] Pestotnik SL, Evans RS, Burke JP, Gardner RM, Classen DC. (1990). Therapeutic antibiotic monitoring: Surveillance using a computerized expert system. *Am J Med* 88(1):43-48.
[l] McMullin ST, Reichley RM, Kahn MG, Dunagan WC, Bailey TC. (1997). Automated system for identifying potential dosage problems at a large university hospital. *Am J Health-Syst Pharm* 54:445-549.
[m] Gurwitz JH, Field TS, Harrold LR, Rothschild J, Debellis K, Seger AC, Cadoret C, Fish LS, Garber L, Kelleher M, Bates DW. (2003). Incidence and preventability of adverse drug events among older persons in the ambulatory setting. *JAMA* 289(9):1107-1116.
[n] Flynn EA, Barker KN, Pepper GA, Bates DW, Mikeal RL. (2002). Comparison of methods for detecting medication errors in 36 hospitals and skilled-nursing facilities. *Am J Health-Syst Pharm* 59:436-446.
[o] Bates DW, Boyle DL, Vander Vliet MB, Schneider J, Leape L. (1995). Relationship between medication errors and adverse drug events. *J Gen Intern Med* 274:29-34.
[p] Kaushal R, Bates DW, Landrigan C, McKenna KJ, Clapp MD, Federico F, Goldmann DA. (2001). Medication errors and adverse drug events in pediatric patients. *JAMA* 285:2114-2120.
[q] Shannon RC and DeMuth JE. (1987). Comparison of medication-error detection methods in the long-term care facility. *The Consultant Pharmacist* 2:148-151.
*Number of times the alert system fired
**Free-text electronic searching

TABLE 12.3. Sensitivity and Specificity of ADE Detection

Screening Results	True Status		Total
	ADE	Non ADE	
Positive	A	B	a + b
Negative	C	D	c + d
Total	a + c	b + d	a + b + c + d

a = ADEs detected by the screening method (true positives); b = Non-ADEs detected as positive by the screening methods (false positives); c = ADEs not detected by the screening method (false negatives); d = Non-ADEs detected as negative by the screening methods (true negatives)

$$\text{Sensitivity} = \frac{a}{a+c}; \text{Specificity} = \frac{b}{b+d}; \text{Predictive value} = \frac{a}{a+b}$$

Source: Figure: "Sensitivity and Specificity of ADE Detection, p. 166," from *A Dictionary of Epidemiology, Third Edition* by John M. Last, edited for the Intl. Epidemiological Assn. By, copyright—1995 by Oxford University Press, Inc. Used by permission of Oxford University Press, Inc.

Predictive value is the probability that a person with an ADE is a true positive.

Source

Using calculations to discover the sensitivity, specificity, and predictive value of the various methods of detecting ADEs is essential. However, many studies have not determined these values even though the data were available. One problem in this arena is how to discover accurately the true number of ADEs since this is what (the method of interest) is used to compare against. Traditionally, the standard to measure against has been chart review. However, some newer methods can find more true ADEs than by chart review, and there is little overlap between the two. Thus, using more than one method will find more ADEs than either method alone.

Some studies comparing more than one method of detecting ADEs use the total number of ADEs discovered for all methods as the denominator, and the number found by a single method to discover the sensitivity. This is probably the best method. Table 12.4 reports the sensitivity, specificity, and predictive value for studies reporting these values. Sometimes, the values were calculated by using the previous method. Please keep in mind the limitations of discovering these values as stated previously.

Some information about detecting ADEs is becoming clear. First, electronically screening for potential ADEs using computer alerts (see Table 12.1) or by searching discharge summaries yield many "hits." Using these methods is efficient and may become the method of choice for detecting ADEs if the search terms can be refined to reduce the number of false positives. Second, no single method will be able to find all ADEs. For example, in one study, among 281 severe ADEs, computer monitoring detected 139 (49 percent).[15] Both methods detected 67 (12 percent). To show the power of computer monitoring, incident reporting detected only three ADEs.

In one study, computerized monitoring was more effective than chart review for finding events associated with laboratory test results and specific medications.[16] Chart review was better for detecting symptom-related ADEs, such as altered mental status. A comprehensive review of using information technology to screen for ADEs is available.[10]

TABLE 12.4. The Sensitivity, Specificity, and Predictive Values for Various Methods of Detecting ADEs

Method	Sensitivity (%)	Specificity (%)	Predictive Value (%)
Incident Reporting	4[a], 11[b], 13[c], 37[d], 75[e]	98[d]	
Discharge Summaries	11[b], 69[f]	48	
Chart Review	2[g], 49[b], 65[a], 89[h]		
Medical Record Coding	14[g], 25[e]		
Observation*	11[h], 90[i]		
Computer Alerts	2[b], 46[a], 60[j], 71[g], 74[d], 86[c], 100[l]	75[d]	53[k]

[a]Jha AK, Kuperman GJ, Teich JM, Leape L, Shea B, Rittenberg E, Burdick E, Seger DL, Vander Vliet M, Bates DW. (1998). Identifying adverse drug events: Development of a computer-based monitor and comparison with chart review and stimulated voluntary report. *J Am Informatics Assoc* 5(3):305-314.

[b]Gurwitz JH, Field TS, Harrold LR, Rothschild J, Debellis K, Seger AC, Cadoret C, Fish LS, Garber L, Kelleher M, Bates DW. (2003). Incidence and preventability of adverse drug events among older persons in the ambulatory setting. *JAMA* 289(9):1107-1116.

[c]Classen DC, Pestotnik SL, Evans RD, and Burke JP. (1991). Computerized surveillance of adverse drug events in hospital patients. *JAMA* 266:2847-2878.

[d]Egger T, Dormann H, Ahne G, Runge U, Neubert A, Criegee-Rieck M, Gassmann KG, Brune K. (2003). Identification of adverse drug reactions in geriatric inpatients using computerized drug database. *Drugs and Aging* 20(10):769-776.

[e]Seeger JD, Schumock GT, and Kong SX. (1996). Estimating the rate of adverse drug reactions with capture-recapture analysis. *Am J Health-Syst Pharm* 53:178-181.

[f] Murff HJ, Forster AJ, Peterson JF, Fiskio JM, Heiman HL, Bates DW. (2003). Electronically screening discharge summaries for adverse medical events. *J Am Med Informatics Assoc* 10:339-350.

[g]Senst BL, Achusim LE, Genest RP, Cosentino LA, Ford CC, Little JA, Raybon SJ, Bates DW. (2001). Practical approach to determining costs and frequency of adverse drug events in a health care network. *Am J Health-Syst Pharm* 58:1126-1132.

[h]Shannon RC and DeMuth JE. (1987). Comparison of medication-error detection methods in the long-term care facility. *The Consultant Pharmacist* 2:148-151.

[i] Flynn EA, Barker KN, Pepper GA, Bates DW, Mikeal RL. (2002). Comparison of methods for detecting medication errors in 36 hospitals and skilled-nursing facilities. *Am J Health-Syst Pharm* 59:436-446.

[j] Pestotnik SL, Evans RS, Burke JP, Gardner RM, Classen DC. (1990). Therapeutic antibiotic monitoring: Surveillance using a computerized expert system. *Am J Med* 88(1):43-48.

kRaschke RA, Gollihare B, Wunderlich TA, Guidry JR, Leibowitz AI, Peirce JC, Lemelson L, Heisler MA, Susong C. (1998). A computer alert system to prevent injury from adverse drug events: Development and evaluation in a community teaching hospital. *JAMA* 280(15):1317-1320.

l Criegee-Rieck M, Neubert A, Dormann H, Egger T, Geise A, Hahn EG, Bruen K. (2002). *Implementation of a computer monitoring system for detection of adverse drug reactions by laboratory signals.* Presented at the 18th International Conference on Pharmacoepidemiology. August 20, Edinburgh, Scotland.

* for medication errors

INNOVATIVE METHODS OF DETECTING ADVERSE DRUG EVENTS

Some unique methods of ADE detection are being investigated. One method is comparing medical record reviews with information from quality assurance records and risk management and litigation records.[17] This study determined that medical record reviews discovered most ADEs and negligent care.

Another innovative method of detecting ADEs is having patients self-monitor for ADEs. One group has studied the benefits and limitations of using patients to monitor the effects of their medication, and found more benefits than limitations.[18] No other postmarketing surveillance method exists that can gain early, reliable, and accurate reports of ADEs in outpatients.

Another study compared the rates of potential ADEs identified from self-reports from elderly outpatients and self-reports combined with chart reviews for elderly inpatients.[19] Overall, 141 patients reported an ADE. Self-reports accounted for 44 percent of the potential ADEs. Of the self-reported potential ADEs, 56 percent were also detected by chart review.

Based on the successful results of patient self-reporting, some community pharmacists in some European countries have started to monitor patients for ADEs.[20,21] Using community pharmacists to detect ADRs in new drugs is a way to speed reporting of ADRs not seen in preapproval studies. Randomly assigned pharmacies could be part of a reporting network that monitors all patients taking a new drug during for the first six months after approval.

Pharmacists could collect some baseline data and the patient's treatment goal at first dispensing. Then, during the first refill of the medication, the pharmacist would ask the patient how the drug was performing (a check on efficacy) and if there are any adverse effects (a check on safety). Any ADR not seen during preapproval trials would be reported to the patient's doctor and the FDA. Although pharmacists will need incentives for doing this monitoring, the benefit would be faster detection of ADRs.

Another simple innovation for documenting ADEs was developed at Cook County Hospital in Chicago.[22] A box is used on computerized discharge summary forms and doctors check if the patient experienced an ADE. This improves reporting ADEs.

DOCUMENTING ADVERSE DRUG EVENTS

Documentation of ADEs is severely lacking. For example, an analysis of medication-related incidents at 33 not-for-profit community hospitals found that most of these organizations grossly underdocumented these incidents.[23] In this eight-month study, 28 hospitals reported recording fewer than three total incidents a month, and 26 hospitals recorded two or fewer medication errors a month. Unfortunately, this pattern of underreporting ADEs is the norm.

This study also found that the quality of the documentation was lacking. Critical elements of the incidents were often missing or illegible. Only 60 percent of the incident reports recorded notification of the patient's doctor after the ADE occurred.

Document What?

All ADEs (adverse drug reactions, drug interactions, allergic drug reactions, and medication errors) need to be documented.

Why Document?

ADEs should be documented for at least four reasons. First, an ADE is part of a patient's medical history, thus there is a duty to the patient to make sure the ADE is properly documented. Second, to meet the JCAHO standards, ADEs need to be documented. Third, documenting ADEs is good risk management. Good documentation provides clear understanding of what happened. Fourth, the FDA and CDC encourage documenting and reporting serious ADEs.

When Should ADEs Be Documented?

ADEs should be documented when they are discovered.

Who Should Document the ADE?

Usually the person who discovers the ADE does the documenting, however, each health care location should have its own policy on this.

Where Should the ADE Be Documented?

All ADEs need to be documented using an incident reporting system that uses a standardized form. Most doctors document ADRs, allergic drug reactions, and drug interactions in the patient's record, but some hesitate or refuse to document medication errors for medical and/or legal reasons. Most risk managers would like to have something in the patient's record.

How Should ADEs Be Documented?

Documentation of ADEs must thoroughly represent complete and accurate findings.

ADRs

Most people would agree that ADRs should be documented using terms such as "the patient may have experienced an adverse reaction to _____ (drug)."

Drug Interactions

The same reporting format is also good for drug interactions. An article covering what is needed in community pharmacies has been written.[24]

Allergic Drug Reactions

Some hospitals document allergic drug reactions poorly. Rather than documenting that the patient experienced an allergic drug reaction to a drug, the documentation should describe how much drug was given, over what period of time, and what happened to the patient. This is important for the patient's future welfare.

Medication Errors

The JCAHO requires documentation of medication errors. Some hospitals use the same incident report form to document medication errors, and this seldom provides enough information. Customized incident reports for medication errors should be created. Some hospitals use a detailed medication error report that assigns a severity ranking of the error to reflect the patient's outcome through a point system.[25] This procedure is helpful in assessing the error, however, the method has been criticized as most systems do not consider the patient's prior health status before the error.[26]

Little is known about detecting and documenting medication errors in community pharmacies. The reasons for this may include:

1. Community pharmacies are privately or corporately owned.
2. Only a few states require documenting medication errors.
3. There are no professional standards to meet.
4. They do not want anyone to know what errors are occurring as it is bad for business.

A recent study however, documented potentially significant patient risk problems in pharmacies in one state.[27] Using a scale of 4 for always, 3 for usually, 2 for rarely, and 1 for never, 164 pharmacists were asked how often their pharmacy documented medication errors. The results were: chain stores 3.0, hospitals 3.2, independent pharmacies 2.5, food store pharmacies 3.1, and other pharmacies 3.2.

One article provides a strong appeal and explanation of why community pharmacists should carefully document medication errors, especially those that reach the patient.[28] This article includes a sample medication error reporting form for community pharmacies. It also outlines the innovative and well-designed quality assurance system that the state of Florida has set up to document medication errors in community pharmacies.

Documenting in incident reports the specifics of what happened is of supreme importance. This should include the time of day, where it happened, information about the drug (what was received versus what should have been received), and information about the patient. It is probably best (for medical malpractice reasons) to document in the patient's record what was received, and not mention anything about it being an error. In this way the facts are documented without incrimination.

Policies and Procedures

Every organized health care setting should have a policy and procedure on detecting, documenting, investigating, assessing, and reporting ADEs. However, some preliminary data indicate that this may not be the case, especially in independent community pharmacies.

SUMMARY

ADEs are grossly underdetected, and therefore, undocumented in most health care settings. This occurs despite JCAHO requirements, policies and procedures in most health care settings, and strong urgings from the FDA and CDC. The quantity and severity of ADEs from the drugs dispensed from community pharmacies is unknown. Yet patients often encounter ADEs from the drug they receive from these pharmacies. ADEs need to be detected and documented to protect patients from experiencing similar events in the future, to meet quality assurance standards, to practice good risk management, and to help future patients taking this medication.

Chapter 13

Investigating, Assessing, and Reporting Adverse Drug Events

Once ADEs are detected and documented, they need to be investigated, assessed, and reported. The purpose of investigating ADEs is to make sure all the facts about the ADE are collected. Once this step is completed, the ADE needs to be assessed for root causes, then measured, identified, and implemented to help prevent the ADE from occurring again. Reporting ADEs informs others and furthers research on why they occur and how they may be prevented.

INVESTIGATING ADVERSE DRUG EVENTS

Institutional Settings

All ADEs in institutional settings should be documented, investigated, and followed up. Someone other than the person documenting the ADE should investigate the ADE as this improves objectivity. A second person may spot something new about the ADE or something important that is missing in the documentation. This person is usually a risk manager, a medication safety officer, or a pharmacy or nurse manager. Although an incident report is the basic record for documenting an ADE, supplemental records can be used for further documentation.

Good ADE investigation is like peeling back the layers of an onion. Ask questions of those involved or those who saw the ADE. Asking those involved why they did or did not do something may be important in understanding why something happened. The investigator needs to know the policies and the proper procedures to discover

Prescribed Medications and the Public Health
© 2006 by The Haworth Press, Inc. All rights reserved.
doi:10.1300/5688_13

whether there were any rules violations. The patient's record needs to be checked to see what was ordered, what was dispensed, and what was administered. Knowing the environmental conditions (such as workload, staffing, and system status) when the ADE occurred may be important.

Ambulatory Care Settings

Institutions should collect and stratify their ADEs by patient care settings, i.e., critical care, acute care, and ambulatory care. In ambulatory care, added information may be needed to document what happened. For instance, was the patient transferring from one level of care to another?

Ambulatory patients provided medication by a community or outpatient pharmacist rarely have their ADEs documented or formally investigated by the pharmacy.[1] Reasons for this may be that community pharmacists are not required to investigate ADEs in their patients. Also, many community pharmacists are too busy to notice, ask, or investigate any ADEs. They are not reimbursed to do much beyond provide the medication.

Many pharmacists will not do more than dispense the medication until they get reimbursed to do so. Payers will not pay pharmacists until there is a proven need and pharmacists show the value of reporting ADEs. Having the pharmacist ask each patient how his or her medication is working, and if there are any problems is logical and easy to do, yet it is rarely done. This procedure makes the best use of the pharmacist's education. Unfortunately, what is in the best interest of patients is not seen by many pharmacy managers (many of whom are not pharmacists) as being in the best interest of pharmacy corporations.

An ADE will be documented only if a patient returns to his or her doctor or goes to an emergency room. Thus, only a tiny proportion of ADEs from community pharmacies are reported to the FDA's Med-Watch program.

ASSESSING ADVERSE DRUG EVENTS

Because assessing ADRs is discussed in Chapter 11, this chapter will assess medication errors. All medication errors deserve assessment for: (1) severity, (2) cause, (3) preventability, and if preventable,

(4) measures that need to be reinforced or put into place to prevent the error from occurring again. However, the extent of assessment is determined by organizational policy.

Institutional Settings

The Joint Commission on Accreditation of Healthcare Organizations (JCAHO) accredits most health care institutions. According to a JCAHO standard, health care organizations must collect data to monitor performing processes that involve risks or may result in a sentinel event. Furthermore, undesirable patterns or trends in performance and sentinel events must be intensely analyzed. This includes significant adverse drug reactions and significant medication errors. The organization must also identify changes that will lead to improved performance and reduce the risk of sentinel events.

Sentinel Events

JCAHO has a standard regarding sentinel events. A *sentinel event* is defined by JCAHO as:

> An unexpected event involving death or serious physical or psychological injury, or the risk thereof. Serious injury specifically includes the loss of limb or function. The phrase, "or the risk thereof" includes any process variation for which a recurrence would carry a significant change of a serious outcome. Such events are "sentinel" because they signal the need for immediate investigation or response.[2]

Between 1995 and 2003, medication errors represented about 13.5 percent (range 7-24 percent) of all sentinel events reviewed by JCAHO.[2]

JCAHO states what should be reported, i.e., an event that resulted in an unanticipated death or major permanent loss of function not related to the patient's disease process.

Root-Cause Analysis

JCAHO standards call for a root-cause analysis of all sentinel events. A root-cause analysis (RCA) according to JCAHO is:

> A process for identifying the basic or causal factors that underlie variation in performance, including the occurrence or possible occurrence of a sentinel event. A RCA focuses primarily on systems and processes, rather than individuals. It identifies system vulnerability and potential improvements or systems that reduce the likelihood of a similar event in the future.

RCA is a retrospective, multidisciplinary process that looks back over the course of a patient's care to see why it went wrong. As shown in Figure 13.1, the most common root causes of sentinel medication errors reviewed by the JCAHO were: communication, orientation and training, and standardization.[3]

From 1995 to 1998, certain medication error trends emerged through JCAHO's sentinel event system. These included problems with insulin, opiates and narcotics, injectable potassium chloride or

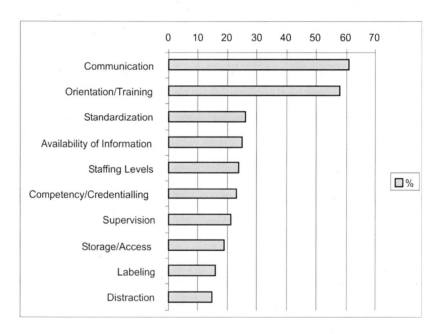

FIGURE 13.1. Root Causes of Medication Errors (1995-2003) (*Source:* JCAHO. Sentinel events: http://www.jcaho.org/accredited+organizations/ambulatory+ care/sentinel+events/rc+of+medication+errors.htm. Copyright Joint Commission on Accreditation of Healthcare Organizations, 2004. Reprinted with permission.)

phosphate concentrate, intravenous anticoagulants, and sodium chloride above 0.9 percent. Later, JCAHO issued alerts about infusion pumps, look-alike and sound-alike drugs, and potentially dangerous abbreviations.

Performing RCA is not easy; it takes time, patience, and teamwork. To be most effective, it also means focusing on the system rather than on individuals and avoiding turf battles. Donnelly and Alteri give an interesting and descriptive narrative of a fictitious RCA written as a one-act play that provides insight and a practical look at how RCAs are done.[4]

Several tools are available for RCAs. One is a list of system breakdown points in the medication-use system.[5] Major breakdown points can occur before the order reaches the pharmacy, while the order is in the pharmacy, or after the order leaves the pharmacy. Another useful tool in performing RCAs is a standardized taxonomy for medication errors.[6]

One technique that may yield fruitful results is assessing the RCA of many medication errors in many different settings to see what trends emerge. One study suggests that the same root causes will appear across time and technology.[7]

Ambulatory Care Settings

Medication errors that occur in ambulatory care settings within an institution should be assessed in the same manner that medication errors are assessed in the inpatient setting. The big question is—how do community pharmacists assess medication errors? Unfortunately, no one knows. The data are hidden from public view. No pharmacist wants to make errors and no pharmacy owner wants his or her error rate to be known. However, one study reveals that medication errors in community pharmacies are usually assessed for severity, but rarely is RCA completed.[1]

Severity

Many organizations assess medication for the severity of the outcome. A good system for doing this was developed by the National Coordinating Council for Medication Error Reporting and Prevention (NCC MERP). This is the basis for USP's MEDMARX medication error reporting system.[8] The system uses nine severity categories from A (no error) to I (death). USP recently validated the interrater reliability of these categories.

Some hospitals have developed their own severity ratings for medication errors. Many ratings are based on changes in the level of care after the error occurred or the increase in stay for the patient.[9,10] Some have tied the severity of the error to levels of discipline for those associated with the error.[11] However, others have been critical of this approach as most medication errors happen because of various system flaws and that correcting the system is more important than blaming and disciplining practitioners.[12]

Action Plans

The product of RCA is an action plan that may include a change in policy, education, or a system change the organization intends to implement to reduce the risk of similar events occurring in the future. Such action plans are needed to make the health care environment safer. These plans are required by JCAHO and the state of Florida for medication errors documented by pharmacies.

REPORTING ADVERSE DRUG EVENTS

Serious ADEs should always be reported, but most cases are not documented, let alone reported. Underreporting is a serious problem. It limits assessment of problems with medication and breakdowns in the medication-use system, and where people are committing rules violations.

The most prominent excuses for not reporting ADEs are: too busy, it takes too long, do not want to get into trouble, and do not want to get someone else in trouble. Historically, doctors have not liked reporting ADEs because of the possible stigma that could potentially come back to them in the form of a malpractice suit.[13] Not documenting and reporting ADEs means that others will probably be harmed by the same mechanism in the future. All health care providers should be held accountable for documenting and reporting all ADEs. Unfortunately, this responsibility is not stamped into the minds of all health care graduates.

Principles

NCC MERP has published general principles for patient-safety reporting systems. To be effective, they must be: nonpunitive, provide proper confidentiality and legal protections, and facilitate learning about errors and their solutions.[14] There needs to be recognition that medication errors are a reflection of system problems, not individual competency. The only way errors should be linked to performance is to reward for increased reporting. There also needs to be legal protection for reporting, for without it, errors will continue to be buried.

Internal Reporting

The first place to report a serious ADE is internally. Except for community pharmacies, there are usually policy and procedure guidelines to follow. In most community pharmacies, there is either no policy, or the policy is ignored.[1,15] Internal incident reports on ADEs document what happened, serve as good tracking documents, and can help protect the institution from overreaching litigation. These incident reports, once investigated and assessed, need to be reviewed by management, and in a hospital, nursing home, or managed care facility, by a pharmacy and therapeutics committee.

Voluntary Reporting

Reporting ADEs voluntarily outside the health care institution is sometimes called "spontaneous reporting," and is encouraged. Because of recent privacy legislation, specifically the Health Insurance Portability and Accountability Act (HIPAA), any personal identifiers are to be removed before reporting. Various organizations exist to which one can voluntarily report ADEs.

FDA MedWatch Program

MedWatch is the FDA's postmarketing surveillance program for reporting ADRs. The program is voluntary for practitioners, but mandatory for pharmaceutical companies who must report any ADR report they receive. Reports may be filed using a form (Figure 13.2) or on the Internet (https://www.accessdata.fda.gov/scripts/medwatch/).

U.S. Department of Health and Human Services

MEDWATCH

The FDA Safety Information and Adverse Event Reporting Program

For VOLUNTARY reporting of adverse events, product problems and product use errors

Page ___ of ___

Form Approved: OMB No. 0910-0291, Expires: 10/31/08
See OMB statement on reverse.

FDA USE ONLY

Triage unit sequence #

A. PATIENT INFORMATION

1. Patient Identifier ______ In confidence
2. Age at Time of Event, or Date of Birth:
3. Sex ☐ Female ☐ Male
4. Weight ______ lb or ______ kg

B. ADVERSE EVENT, PRODUCT PROBLEM OR ERROR

Check all that apply:

1. ☐ Adverse Event ☐ Product Problem (e.g., defects/malfunctions)
☐ Product Use Error ☐ Problem with Different Manufacturer of Same Medicine

2. Outcomes Attributed to Adverse Event (Check all that apply)
☐ Death: ______ (mm/dd/yyyy) ☐ Disability or Permanent Damage
☐ Life-threatening ☐ Congenital Anomaly/Birth Defect
☐ Hospitalization - initial or prolonged ☐ Other Serious (Important Medical Events)
☐ Required Intervention to Prevent Permanent Impairment/Damage (Devices)

3. Date of Event (mm/dd/yyyy)
4. Date of this Report (mm/dd/yyyy)

5. Describe Event, Problem or Product Use Error

6. Relevant Tests/Laboratory Data, Including Dates

7. Other Relevant History, Including Preexisting Medical Conditions (e.g., allergies, race, pregnancy, smoking and alcohol use, liver/kidney problems, etc.)

C. PRODUCT AVAILABILITY

Product Available for Evaluation? (Do not send product to FDA)
☐ Yes ☐ No ☐ Returned to Manufacturer on: ______ (mm/dd/yyyy)

D. SUSPECT PRODUCT(S)

1. Name, Strength, Manufacturer (from product label)
#1
#2

2. Dose or Amount / Frequency / Route
#1
#2

3. Dates of Use (If unknown, give duration) from/to (or best estimate)
#1
#2

4. Diagnosis or Reason for Use (Indication)
#1
#2

5. Event Abated After Use Stopped or Dose Reduced?
#1 ☐ Yes ☐ No ☐ Doesn't Apply
#2 ☐ Yes ☐ No ☐ Doesn't Apply

6. Lot #
#1
#2

7. Expiration Date
#1
#2

8. Event Reappeared After Reintroduction?
#1 ☐ Yes ☐ No ☐ Doesn't Apply
#2 ☐ Yes ☐ No ☐ Doesn't Apply

9. NDC # or Unique ID

E. SUSPECT MEDICAL DEVICE

1. Brand Name
2. Common Device Name
3. Manufacturer Name, City and State
4. Model # / Lot # / Catalog # / Expiration Date (mm/dd/yyyy) / Serial # / Other #
5. Operator of Device
☐ Health Professional
☐ Lay User/Patient
☐ Other:
6. If Implanted, Give Date (mm/dd/yyyy)
7. If Explanted, Give Date (mm/dd/yyyy)
8. Is this a Single-use Device that was Reprocessed and Reused on a Patient?
☐ Yes ☐ No
9. If Yes to Item No. 8, Enter Name and Address of Reprocessor

F. OTHER (CONCOMITANT) MEDICAL PRODUCTS

Product names and therapy dates (exclude treatment of event)

G. REPORTER ***(See confidentiality section on back)***

1. Name and Address
Phone # / E-mail
2. Health Professional? ☐ Yes ☐ No
3. Occupation
4. Also Reported to:
☐ Manufacturer
☐ User Facility
☐ Distributor/Importer
5. If you do NOT want your identity disclosed to the manufacturer, place an "X" in this box: ☐

PLEASE TYPE OR USE BLACK INK

FORM FDA 3500 (10/05) Submission of a report does not constitute an admission that medical personnel or the product caused or contributed to the event.

FIGURE 13.2. MedWatch Registry Form

The FDA is only interested in unusual, unexpected, or serious events. Figure 13.3 shows the number of postmarketing adverse drug events reported to the FDA from 1995 to 2002.[16] The FDA continually mines the MedWatch database for potential ADR signals that may suggest a serious trend.

VAERS

The Vaccine Adverse Events Reporting System (VAERS) is a national vaccine safety surveillance program cosponsored by the Centers for Disease Control and Prevention (CDC) and the FDA. VAERS collects and analyzes information from reports of adverse events following immunization. Anyone may submit a report by using a form (Figure 13.4) or by accessing the Web site (https://secure.vaers.org/VaersDataEntryintro.htm).

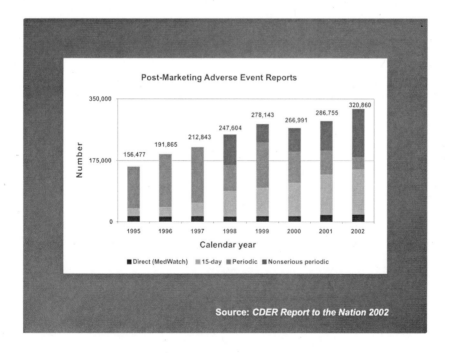

FIGURE 13.3. ADE Reports Submitted to FDA, 1995-2002

WEBSITE: www.vaers.org   E-MAIL: info@vaers.org   FAX: 1-877-721-0366

VACCINE ADVERSE EVENT REPORTING SYSTEM
24 Hour Toll-Free Information 1-800-822-7967
P.O. Box 1100, Rockville, MD 20849-1100
PATIENT IDENTITY KEPT CONFIDENTIAL

VAERS

For CDC/FDA Use Only

VAERS Number _____

Date Received _____

Patient Name:

Last   First   M.I.

Address

City   State   Zip

Telephone no. (____) ____

Vaccine administered by (Name):

Responsible
Physician _____
Facility Name/Address

City   State   Zip

Telephone no. (____) ____

Form completed by (Name):

Relation   ☐ Vaccine Provider ☐ Patient/Parent
to Patient ☐ Manufacturer ☐ Other
Address (if different from patient or provider)

City   State   Zip

Telephone no. (____) ____

| 1. State | 2. County where administered | 3. Date of birth /mm /dd /yy | 4. Patient age | 5. Sex ☐ M ☐ F | 6. Date form completed /mm /dd /yy |

7. Describe adverse events(s) (symptoms, signs, time course) and treatment, if any

8. Check all appropriate:
☐ Patient died   (date __ /mm __ /dd __ /yy)
☐ Life threatening illness
☐ Required emergency room/doctor visit
☐ Required hospitalization (_____ days)
☐ Resulted in prolongation of hospitalization
☐ Resulted in permanent disability
☐ None of the above

9. Patient recovered   ☐ YES ☐ NO ☐ UNKNOWN

10. Date of vaccination /mm /dd /yy Time ____ AM PM

11. Adverse event onset /mm /dd /yy Time ____ AM PM

12. Relevant diagnostic tests/laboratory data

13. Enter all vaccines given on date listed in no. 10

Vaccine (type)	Manufacturer	Lot number	Route/Site	No. Previous Doses
a.				
b.				
c.				
d.				

14. Any other vaccinations within 4 weeks prior to the date listed in no. 10

Vaccine (type)	Manufacturer	Lot number	Route/Site	No. Previous doses	Date given
a.					
b.					

15. Vaccinated at:
☐ Private doctor's office/hospital   ☐ Military clinic/hospital
☐ Public health clinic/hospital   ☐ Other/unknown

16. Vaccine purchased with:
☐ Private funds   ☐ Military funds
☐ Public funds   ☐ Other/unknown

17. Other medications

18. Illness at time of vaccination (specify)

19. Pre-existing physician-diagnosed allergies, birth defects, medical conditions (specify)

20. Have you reported this adverse event previously?
☐ No   ☐ To health department
☐ To doctor   ☐ To manufacturer

Only for children 5 and under

22. Birth weight ____ lb. ____ oz.

23. No. of brothers and sisters

21. Adverse event following prior vaccination (check all applicable, specify)

	Adverse Event	Onset Age	Type Vaccine	Dose no. in series
☐ In patient				
☐ In brother or sister				

Only for reports submitted by manufacturer/immunization project

24. Mfr./imm. proj. report no.

25. Date received by mfr./imm.proj.

26. 15 day report?   ☐ Yes ☐ No

27. Report type   ☐ Initial ☐ Follow-Up

Health care providers and manufacturers are required by law (42 USC 300aa-25) to report reactions to vaccines listed in the Table of Reportable Events Following Immunization. Reports for reactions to other vaccines are voluntary except when required as a condition of immunization grant awards.

Form VAERS-1(FDA)

FIGURE 13.4. VAERS Reporting Form

Since 1990, VAERS has received over 10,000 reports per year, most of which are mild side effects such as fever. These reports are also mined for signals that may suggest a serious trend.

MER

The USP manages two reporting systems for medication errors—one open and one closed. The open system, started in 1991, is called the Medication Errors Reporting (MER) Program and is presented in cooperation with the Institute for Safe Medication Practices (ISMP). MERs is a spontaneous, voluntary, practitioner-based reporting program that allows health care professionals to confidentially (and, if requested, anonymously) report medication errors.[17] Practitioners may report by using a form (Figure 13.5), telephoning (800-23-ERROR), or by using the Web site (http://www.usp.org/patientSafety/mer/).

MEDMARX

The second medication error reporting system operated by USP is called MEDMARX and is available to hospitals on a subscription basis. MEDMARX is a comprehensive, Internet-accessible, anonymous medication error reporting program and quality improvement tool. The program facilitates productive and efficient documentation, tracking, trending, and prevention of medication errors.

MEDMARX allows subscribing facilities to access and share information (http://www.usp.patientsafety/medmarx/). More than 1 million medication error records are in the database submitted by more than 800 participating facilities. The database is mined by USP to spot reporting trends, publish safety alerts, develop education and training programs, and to develop standards. A recent example of a trend discovered by MEDMARX mining had to do with medication errors in hospital emergency departments.[18]

State Reporting Programs

Some states mandate reporting systems for medical errors. For example, it is required to report any medication-related fatalities in North Carolina to the North Carolina Board of Pharmacy.

MEDI-CATION ERRORS

REPORTING PROGRAM

USP MEDICATION ERRORS REPORTING PROGRAM
Presented in cooperation with the Institute for Safe Medication Practices
USP is an FDA MEDWATCH partner
Reporters should not provide any individually identifiable health information, including names of practitioners, names of patients, names of healthcare facilities, or dates of birth (age is acceptable).

Date and time of event:

Please describe the error. Include description/sequence of events, type of staff involved, and work environment (e.g., code situation, change of shift, short staffing, no 24-hr. pharmacy, floor stock). If more space is needed, please attach a separate page.

Did the error reach the patient?　　☐ Yes　☐ No
Was the incorrect medication, dose, or dosage form administered to or taken by the patient?　　☐ Yes　☐ No
Circle the appropriate Error Outcome Category (select one—see back for details):　A　B　C　D　E　F　G　H　I

Describe the direct result of the error on the patient (e.g., death, type of harm, additional patient monitoring).
Indicate the possible error cause(s) and contributing factor(s) (e.g., abbreviation, similar names, distractions, etc.).

Indicate the location of the error (e.g., hospital, outpatient or community pharmacy, clinic, nursing home, patient's home, etc.).
What type of staff or healthcare practitioner made the initial error?
Indicate if other practitioner(s) were also involved in the error (type of staff perpetuating error).
What type of staff or healthcare practitioner discovered the error or recognized the potential for error?
How was the error (or potential for error) discovered/intercepted?
If available, provide patient age, gender, diagnosis. Do not provide any patient identifiers.

Please complete the following for the product(s) involved. (If more space is needed for additional products, please attach a separate page.)

	Product #1	Product #2
Brand/Product Name (If Applicable)		
Generic Name		
Manufacturer		
Labeler		
Dosage Form		
Strength/Concentration		
Type and Size of Container		

Reports are most useful when relevant materials such as product label, copy of prescription/order, etc., can be reviewed. Can these materials be provided?　☐ Yes　☐ No　　Please specify:

Suggest any recommendations to prevent recurrence of this error, or describe policies or procedures you instituted or plan to institute to prevent future similar errors.

Name and Title/Profession	Telephone Number (　　)	Fax Number (　　)
Facility/Address and Zip		E-mail

Address/Zip (where correspondence should be sent)

Your name, contact information, and a copy of this report are routinely shared with the Institute for Safe Medication Practices (ISMP). Copies of reports will be sent to third parties such as the manufacturer/labeler, and to the Food and Drug Administration (FDA). You have the option of including your name on these copies.

In addition to releasing my name and contact information to ISMP, USP may release my identity to these third parties as follows (check boxes that apply):
☐ The manufacturer and/or labeler as listed above　☐ FDA　☐ Other persons requesting a copy of this report　☐ Anonymous to all third parties

Signature	Date

Return to:
USP CAPS
12601 Twinbrook Parkway
Rockville, MD 20852-1790

Submit via the Web at www.usp.org/mer
Call Toll Free: 800-23-ERROR (800-233-7767)
or FAX: 301-816-8532

Date Received by USP	File Access Number

FIGURE 13.5. USP Medication Error Reporting Form (*Source:* Reprinted with permission of the United States Pharmacopeial Convention, Inc., 2003-2003. All Rights Reserved.)

Case Reports

Doctors and pharmacists sometimes send case reports of serious ADEs to medical and pharmacy journals. This provides a "heads up" for fellow practitioners. Publishing ADE cases is a valuable way of reporting ADEs. However, a recent study questioned the quality of some of these reports as lacking because of missing information and no formal causality assessment of the ADE reported.[19]

OTHER REPORTING METHODS

Several other methods of reporting potential ADEs are worth mentioning.

Point-of-Care Reporting

Several hospitals have implemented systems that involve targeting the dispensing of antidotes (such as naloxone, vitamin K, and protamine) from automated dispensing machines (such as Pyxis) located on patient care units. The unit functions like an automated teller machine (ATM) at banks. Anytime one of these drugs is dispensed, a screen pops up asking "Removing for an Adverse Reaction?" If the nurse selects "yes," there is a same-day warning of this information to the pharmacy's system.

Three methods of detecting and reporting ADEs were compared in a large community hospital: manual occurrence reporting (MOR), ICD-9 chart reviews (ICD-9 coding), and Pyxis antidote transactions (PAT).[20] Over a six-month period 1,528 ADEs were identified. Of these, 1,191 (78 percent) were identified by PAT, 318 (21 percent) by ICD-9, and 19 (1 percent) by MOR. PAT identified 19 percent of the ICD-9 cases, and ICD-9 identified 5 percent of the Pyxis cases. The 1,191 PATs for ADEs represented 12.3 percent of all Pyxis transactions. The beauty of this system is its automatic capture and reporting feature. It allows nurses to easily produce a report while providing patient care.

ADE Capture on Discharge Summary

Another simple, but effective method of capturing ADE data and automatically reporting them internally is to use a check box on computerized discharge summary forms. Doctors can check the box if the patient experienced an ADE during hospitalization.[21]

COMPARING MEDICATION ERROR RATES

Some researchers want to compare medication error reporting rates between different facilities, however, there is no value in doing this.[22] The dangers in comparing error rates include differences in culture, defining a medication error, patient populations, types of reporting systems, and what is used as a denominator.

DEFICIENCIES IN REPORTING
ADVERSE DRUG EVENTS

Despite internal and external reporting systems for ADEs, many deficiencies exist. The first problem is vast underreporting of ADRs and medication errors. ADE detection, documentation, assessment, and reporting are low priorities within the health care setting. Yet thousands of people continue to be harmed. Compare this to the airline industry where lately, there have been few accidents and deaths, and yet safety is still the priority in this industry.

Second, when ADEs are reported, the data trickle in slowly and no real trend can be noted. A new drug may be on the market for over a year before there is enough data to substantiate an inherent problem with the drug and that it needs to be removed from the market. Meanwhile, many people are harmed, and some may die.

Third, incidence and severity of ADEs in the ambulatory setting can be compared to an iceberg—one that is almost submerged below the waterline. ADEs in this environment just do not get reported. Is this because no good reporting mechanisms are in place? Reporting probably does not happen because the owners of community pharmacies do not wish this information to be known. Corporate owners would rather use pharmacists for their technical skills rather than their clinical expertise.

Fourth, there is no national requirement to report all ADEs associated with a fatal outcome. Those who condemn this requirement as an affront to their professional freedom need to look into the eyes and listen to a parent whose child died of a medication error. We need data on what contributes to fatal medication errors versus error-free cases to know for sure what is causing these mishaps and what can be done about them. Satisfactory legal protection can be built into this reporting requirement. Such a requirement may dramatically drop the death rate from ADEs.

SUMMARY

All ADEs need to be investigated, and all serious or unusual ones need to be assessed by having RCA performed. An action plan should be written and recommendations implemented to help prevent the ADE from occurring again. All serious and unusual ADEs should be reported to a national reporting database.

However, ADEs are underreported, especially in the ambulatory environment. Because of this, trends cannot be identified quickly and many patients are harmed before drugs causing ADEs can be removed from the market.

The detection, documentation, assessment, and reporting of ADEs need to be a much higher priority, and better systems need support to reduce the preventable morbidity and mortality from medication.

Chapter 14

Can Serious Adverse Drug Events Be Predicted?

Fortunately, medication-induced deaths are rare, considering the thousands of drugs administered each year, but even one death is too many. Too many people experience threats to their lives, incur permanent disability, or die of events related to prescribed medication. These serious adverse drug events (ADEs) are disturbing and worthy of investigation.

An example is two people the same age and gender receive the same drug, in the same dose, and follow the same dosage schedule for the same condition. One person is treated successfully while the other one experiences an adverse effect from the medication and dies.

This raises the question—is the risk of experiencing a serious adverse effect from medication evenly divided throughout the population? If the answer is yes, then no further investigation is needed. However, if the answer is no, can the patients at high risk for harm be identified before they are prescribed medication?

WHAT CAUSES ADVERSE DRUG EFFECTS?

Adverse drug effects are caused by certain host factors, exposure factors, or environmental factors. *Host factors* are those variables within an individual that increase the person's chance of experiencing an ADE. These may include such variables as age, gender, renal and liver function, and genetic predisposition. *Exposure factors* include the drug, its dosage, how it is administered, and other drugs that may be administered at the same time. Figure 14.1 shows the sources of

Prescribed Medications and the Public Health
© 2006 by The Haworth Press, Inc. All rights reserved.
doi:10.1300/5688_14

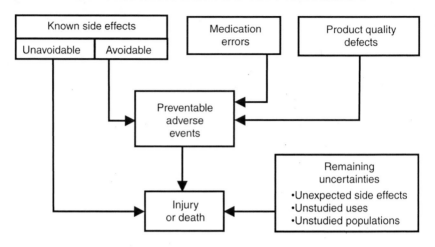

FIGURE 14.1. Sources of Risk from Drug Products

risk from drug products, some of which are not preventable. *Environmental factors* include such variables as the type of hospital admission, intensive care, the number of prescribers, look-alike drug packaging, look-alike and sound-alike drug names, sloppy prescribing, dispensing, and medication administration errors, and willful violations in following policy and procedures. There may also be interactions between host and exposure factors.

THE CURRENT STATE OF COMPUTERIZED MEDICATION-USE SYSTEMS

Computerized medication-use systems should be able to help prevent ADEs. However, a field test of computerized medication-use systems at 307 hospitals found that only four of the hospital systems were able to detect and prevent all ten specific, lethal medication orders entered into the hospital system.[2] According to the report, 87 percent of the systems tested failed to detect toxic doses of antibiotics for patients with reduced kidney function, and 87 percent did not detect single or cumulative lethal doses of colchicine, a drug used for gout. Despite a flurry of activity since 1999 to improve these systems, little has changed.[3]

THE IDEAL ADVERSE DRUG EVENT SYSTEM

The ideal electronic adverse drug event (ADE) system would: (1) classify patients according to their degree of risk for experiencing a serious adverse drug event, (2) have hard stop signs to prevent a practitioner from prescribing, dispensing, or administering a drug that has high potential to cause harm in a patient, and (3) produce a signal when an ADE may have just occurred. Work is progressing on the second component of the ideal system in the form of decision-support software that should be built into computerized physician order entry (CPOE) systems (see Chapter 15). Work is also progressing on the third compenent of the ideal system in the form of automatic signal generation for ADEs (see Chapter 12). However, little work has been done on developing the first component of the ideal system—identifying a patient at "high risk" for an ADE.

In 1999, one group of active medication safety researchers used basic patient information available electronically and a nested case-control study within a cohort study to develop a risk-stratification model.[4] The conclusion was that "adverse drug events occurred more often in sicker patients who stayed in the hospital longer. However, after controlling for the level of care and the length of stay, few risks emerged."

This study was a good start, but had two limitations. First, and most important, the study was limited to information that was available electronically. Second, studies like this need a larger number of patients. This study was limited to two institutions. As this is only one of a few studies on risk factors for ADEs and it had these two limitations, the conclusion may be overstated.

IDENTIFYING RISKS FOR ADVERSE DRUG EVENTS

The process of identifying risk factors for ADEs involves studying populations of patients, some of whom experienced an ADE and some who did not experience an ADE. Because serious ADEs are rare, large populations of patients must be studied using cohort or case-control designs to be statistically sound.

Making sure the study group (those with the ADEs) and the control group (those without ADEs) are drawn from the same population of patients is critical. In addition, there must be a valid way of ascertaining that an ADE has occurred, and the ADE must be assessed for causality (definite, probable, possible, or doubtful) using objective measures. Only those ADEs found to be definite or probable should be used to discover ADE risk factors. In addition, criteria for preventable ADEs should be established since only preventable ADEs should be used in discovering risk factors.[4,5] Focus should be on ADEs that are serious (organ damage), fatal, life threatening, or permanently disabling.[4,6] Unfortunately, few studies have been performed to discover ADE risk factors, and those that have been done have failed to adhere to all the previous criteria. Most studies failed to study enough patients.

Table 14.1 displays potential risk factors for ADEs. Many variables have been suggested as risks for ADEs, but few have been adequately studied. An adverse drug reaction (ADR) is a function of the biology of the patient and the chemistry of the drug, or the interaction between the two factors. The lower the incidence of the adverse drug reaction, the more likely the reaction is based on individual factors rather than exposure factors.[7] Errors occur independent of the individual or the chemistry of the drug.

POTENTIAL RISK FACTORS
FOR ADVERSE DRUG EVENTS

Host Factors

Many variables within individuals may predispose them to an ADE, some of which are controllable, many of which are not.

Age

Age has long been debated as a factor in ADEs. Many articles have been written about the very young (because of immature organ system development) and the very old (because of organs wearing out). However, the data on age as an independent risk factor for ADEs are mixed.[8,9,10] A potential problem in deciding the effect of age on ADEs involve potentially confounding variables such as renal function and polypharmacy in older patients.[4,11] One cohort analysis sug-

TABLE 14.1 Variables That May Be Predictive of a Potential ADE

Variables	References Suggested	Found Predictive*	Not Found Predictive*
Host Factors			
Age	a,b,c,d,e,f,g	d,f	e
Gender	a,d,e,f,h,i	h,f	a,d,e
Ethnicity	a		a
Body weight	b		
Mental status/dementia	a,e		e
History of allergy	i,j,k	j	i
History of ADEs	d,i	d,i	
Severity of illness	a,e	e	
Comorbidity score	a,e	e	
Comorbidities	d		d
GI Disease	i		i
Infection	i		
Social history			
Social-economic status	d		d
Alcohol use	d		d
Drug abuse	e		
Tobacco use	d,e		
Laboratory			
Low serum albumin	a,c		
Low serum bilirubin	a		
Low renal function	a,c,i,f,j	f,i,j	
Low liver function	c,i	i	
Low platelets	a	a	
Exposure Factors			
Drug category			
Alzheimer drugs	e		e
Anticoagulants	e,j	e,j	a
Antigout drugs	e		e

TABLE 14.1 *(continued)*

Variables	Suggested	Found Predictive*	Not Found Predictive*
Anti-infective agents	e	e	
Antiseizure drugs	a,e	e	a
Antidepressants	a,e	a,e	
Antihypertensives	a	a	
Antihistamine drugs	e		e
Anti-Parkinson's drugs	e		e
Cancer drugs	a,e		a,e
Cardiovascular agents	a,e	a,e	
Cholesterol-lowering drugs	e		e
Diuretics	a,e	a	e
Drugs monitored by serum levels	j,k	j	
Electrolyte concentrates	a	a	
Gastrointestinal drugs	e		e
High alert drugs†	l		
Hypoglycemics	e	e	
Investigational drugs	l		
Muscle relaxants	e	e	
Opioids	e	e	
Psychoactive drugs	a,e	a,e	
Thrombotics	j	j	
Dose	l		
Route	l		
Duration of use	l		e
Number of drugs	a,d,f,i	i,f	d
No. of regularly scheduled meds	e	e	
High drug serum levels	l		
Unapproved uses	l		

TABLE 14.1 *(continued)*

	References		
		Found	Not Found
Variables	Suggested	Predictive*	Predictive*
Environmental Factors			
Intensive care	a		a
No. of prescribers	m		
Type of admission	a	a	

a: Bates DW, Miller EB, Cullen DJ, Burdick L, Williams L, Laird N, Petersen LA, Small SD, Sweitzer BJ, Vander Vliet M, Leape LL. (1999). Patient risk factors for adverse drug events in hospitalized patients. *Arch Intern Med* 159:2553-2560.
b: Park BK, Pirmohamed M, and Kitteringham NR. (1992). Idiosyncratic drug reactions: A mechanistic evaluation. *Br J Clin Pharmac* 34:377-395.
c: Hoigne R, Lawson DH, and Weber E. (1990). Risk factors for adverse drug reactions – epidemiological approaches. *Eur J Clin Pharmacol* 39:321-325.
d: Hutchinson TA, Flegel KM, Kramer MS, Leduc DG, King HH. (1986). Frequency, severity, and risk factors for adverse drug reactions in adult outpatients: A prospective study. *J Chron Dis* 39(7):533-542.
e: Field TS, Gurwitz JH, Avorn J, McComrick D, Jain S., Eckler M, Benser M, Bates DW. (2001). Risk factors for adverse drug events among nursing home residents. *Arch Intern Med* 161(13):1629-1634.
f: Hoigne R, Maibach R, Maurer P, Jaeger MD, Egli A, Galeazzi R, Hess T, Muller U, Kuenzi UP. (1991). Risk factors for adverse drug reactions communication of the CHDM. *Bratislavske Lekarske Listy* 92(11):564-567.
g: Gurwitz JH and Avorn J. (1991). The ambiguous relation between aging and adverse drug reactions. *Annals of Internal Med* 114(11):956-966.
h: Montastruc JM, Lapeyre-Mestre M, Bagheri H, Fooladi A. (2002). Gender differences in adverse drug reactions: Analysis of spontaneous reports to a regional pharmacovigilance centre in France. *Fundamental and Clinical Pharmacology* 16(5):343-346.
i: Smith JW, Seidl LG, and Cluff LE. (1966). Studies on the epidemiology of adverse drug reactions. *Ann Intern Med* 65(4):629-640.
j: Pearson TF, Pittman DG, Longley JM, Grapes ZT, Vigliotti DJ, Mullis SR. (1994). Factors associated with preventable adverse drug reactions. *Am J Hosp Pharm* 51:2268-2272.
k: Popescu IG, Popescu M, Man D, Ciolacu S, Georgescu M, Ciurea T, Aldea GS, Stancu C, Badea M, Ulmeanu V. (1984). Drug allergy: Incidence in terms of age and some drug allergens. *Rev Roum Med – Med Int* 22(3):195-202.
l: Kelly WN. (2001). Potential risks and prevention, part 4: Reports of signicant adverse drug events. *Am J Health-Syst Pharm* 58:1406-1412.
m: Saltsman CL and Hamilton RA. (1999). Risk factors for patient hospitalization. *Am J Health-Syst Pharm* 56:450-732.

*By controlled analysis (use of a control group). ADE may or may not have been preventable, and may have included all or just preventable ADEs
†For errors, interactions, adverse reactions, and allergic drug reactions

gests that "the effect of advancing age may be modest at best," probably because many prescribers adjust drugs and drug dosages in older patients to account for the patient's age.[4]

Gender

More ADEs are reported for females than for males. However, is gender an independent risk factor for ADEs? The data are not consistent—some studies say yes while others say no.[4,8,9,10,12] However, it may be that one gender may be more susceptible to the adverse effects of one drug class or another. For example, one study found that females were more susceptible to the adverse effects of neuropsychiatric drugs and men more susceptible to the adverse effects of cardiovascular drugs.[12] The reasons for this remain elusive.

Ethnicity

Certain ethnic groups are known to be deficient in certain enzymes that metabolize drugs or other enzymes that affect cells. For example, African Americans, people of Jewish descent, and other darker-skinned Caucasian groups have a greater incidence of glucose-6-phosphate deficiency in erythrocytes, which causes weaknesses in cell membrane. When these patients are exposed to certain drugs, the cell membrane is disrupted causing hemolytic anemia.

Although there are good data on poor therapeutic responses of certain ethnic groups to certain categories of drugs, the data on ethnicity and adverse drug reactions is sparse. One controlled study was unable to show that ethnicity is a risk factor for ADEs.[4]

Body Weight

Body weight (and sometimes ideal body weight) sometimes decides the accurate dosing of medication. This has to do with the drug's distribution throughout various compartments in the body. Therefore, weight should be investigated as a potential risk factor for ADEs. However, this variable has not been adequately studied.

Mental Status/Dementia

Most of the studies investigating mental status/dementia are in nursing home patients. Mental status is not an independent risk factor for ADEs.[9]

History of Allergy

It seems logical that patients with a history of allergy (drug or otherwise) are more likely to experience adverse drug reactions. However, two studies show differing results. [5,13]

History of Previous Adverse Drug Reactions

Although ADRs need more study, two studies have shown that prior drug reactions may be predictive of future drug reactions.[8,13]

Severity of Illness

Many doctors feel the sicker the patient, the more likely the patient will experience an adverse effect. However, only one controlled study has shown this to be true.[9]

Comorbidity Score

The burden of disease for patients can be determined by calculating a comorbidity score based on the number and types of disease states for the patient. In one study, high Charlson comorbidity scores were correlated with a higher incidence of ADEs.[9] Some believe certain disease states such as congestive heart failure, infection, and GI disease may contribute to a higher incidence of ADEs, but this is yet to be proven.

Social History

Some have proposed that socioeconomic status, alcohol use, tobacco use, and a history of drug abuse may play important roles in promoting a higher incidence of ADEs, but this is yet to be shown. Of these, alcohol abuse, which can lead to liver decline and failure, is the likely candidate as an independent risk factor for ADEs.

Abnormal Laboratory Tests

Some feel that patients with low serum albumin levels may be more susceptible to the adverse effects of some drugs versus patients with normal serum albumin levels. This is because of less binding of the drug to albumin making more drug available to cause harm. However, this is yet to be proven. Reduced renal function is a risk factor for ADEs associated with renally cleared drugs, and this has been shown in controlled studies.[5,10, 13] Reduced liver function is a risk factor for those drugs metabolized by the liver.[13] Serum total bilirubin levels can be used as a proxy for hepatic insufficiency.[4] Patients with already low platelet levels are vulnerable to further lowering of their platelets by drugs that cause thrombocytopenia.[4]

Drug Factors

Several drug factors may be independent risk factors for ADEs.

Drug Category

The inherent toxicity of a drug may be one of the strongest predictors of a future ADE. Each category of drugs, and each drug within each category, has its own potential for causing an ADE. Those drug categories shown by controlled studies to produce the most ADEs are shown in Table 14.1. The most evidence is for anticoagulants, antidepressants, cardiovascular agents, and psychoactive drugs.

Dose, Route, and Duration of Use

The higher the dose, the more likely an ADE will occur. Also, drugs administered perenterally are more toxic than oral or topically administered drugs. Also, the longer a drug is used, the more likely an ADE will occur. Although it makes sense that these variables are independent risk factors for ADEs, there have been few studies on them.

Number of Drugs Used

The more drugs used concurrently, the more likely ADEs would result. However, studies are conflicting.[8,10,13] One study shows that the number of drugs did not change the risk of a reaction in ambulatory patients.[13] Why this occurred is unknown. The risk may vary by the drug used, the age of the patient, or the renal function. The other studies clearly show a relationship. [10,13] One study shows a relationship when only the number of regularly scheduled drugs was tested.[9]

High Drug Serum Levels

Almost always, when a drug's serum level is above normal, the potential for toxicity increases. Drugs that can be monitored by serum levels should be monitored in this fashion. However, one study shows that this is not always the case.[14]

Unapproved Uses

Some fear that the unapproved use of an approved drug leads to an increased risk of an ADE. This practice is lawful, allows practitioners flexibility in treating patients, and often benefits patients if the drug is monitored carefully. There is no evidence that this practice is unsafe.

Environmental Factors

Other factors may influence an increased risk of an ADE.

Intensive Care

At first blush, the intensive care of a patient is related to severity of illness and perhaps comorbidity, rather than the geographic location of the patient. However, some studies have shown that there are more medication errors in intensive care units versus medical-surgical units, and in some studies, when adjusted for the number of drugs, the error rate was still higher.[15] ADEs in intensive care, in general, are also higher.[4] This may be a reflection on the drugs used rather than the level of care.

Number of Prescribers

Although more investigation is needed, one study suggested that the number of prescribers may influence the risk of hospitalization.[16] It may also influence the risk of ADEs, especially errors due to "one hand not knowing what the other hand is doing." One study found the most common factors associated with medication errors were: a decline in renal or liver function requiring adjustment of drug therapy; a patient history of allergy; using the wrong drug name, dosage form, or abbreviations; wrong dosage calculations; and atypical or unusual and critical-dosage frequency considerations.[17]

Type of Admission

One controlled study found that type of admission correlated with higher ADE rates.[4] The odds of an ADE were much higher for patients admitted to an internal medicine unit than to other types of inpatient units. This may be a reflection of the number of medications used in these patients versus other types of patients.

Other

Other factors also increase the risk of an ADE, especially errors, look-alike drug packaging, look-alike and sound-alike drug names, sloppy prescribing, dispensing, and drug administration, and willful violations in following policies and procedures.

PREDICTING ADVERSE DRUG EVENTS

The idea that ADEs can be predicted using prognostic criteria is not new. In 1990, one investigator developed a bleeding index for estimating the probability of major bleeding in hospitalized patients starting anticoagulant therapy.[18] This index provides valid estimates of the probability of major bleeding and complements doctors' predictions. Another investigator has worked over a long period to develop a method to estimate the individual risk of breast cancer.[19,20] This model has been validated.[21,22,23,24] In 2001, a prognostic index for estimating the risk of dying after being discharged from a hospital was developed.[25] The index uses six risk factors known at discharge and a simple additive point system to stratify medical patients 70 years or older according to one-year mortality after hospitalization. The index had good discrimination and calibration and generalized well in an independent sample of patients at a different site.

The first study to distinguish which patients may need special monitoring by pharmacists occurred in 1974.[26] The objectives of the study were: (1) to discover a discriminate function for selecting acute-care patients who should be monitored by pharmacists, (2) to validate the discriminate function in a prospective study, and (3) to estimate the number of clinical pharmacists required to monitor the patient population of the hospital studied.

The equation for the discriminate function stemmed from a multivariate statistical analysis of variables or characteristics obtained from samples of different populations. The function can be used for prediction, classification, or discrimination. The discriminate function correctly classified 78 percent of the "contribution" patients and 86 percent of the "no contribution" patients in a retrospective study of 150 patients, and 61 percent and 54 percent respectively, in a prospective study.[27]

In 1989, one group of investigators developed indicators for selecting ambulatory patients who warrant pharmacist monitoring.[28] Six prognostic indicators were identified:

1. Five or more medications in present drug regimen.
2. Twelve or more medication doses per day.
3. Medication regimen changed four or more times during past 12 months.
4. More than three concurrent disease states present.
5. History of noncompliance.
6. Presence of drugs that require therapeutic drug monitoring.

Although no mathematical formulas were used to develop a prediction and the validation of a model, the study showed that the likelihood that a patient would develop an adverse outcome increased as the number of prognostic indicators present increased.

In 1990, a therapeutic risk-assessment model for identifying patients with adverse drug reactions was developed.[29] Theoretical risk factors for ADRs to digoxin and theophylline were identified through a literature search. The records of patients who experienced an ADR to either of the two drugs were compared with matched controls of patients who did not experience an ADR to either drug. The ADRs were verified using the Naranjo algorithm.

Seven risk factors for each drug were found to be significantly statistically associated with ADRs. A serum digoxin concentration greater than 2.5ng/mL and high blood urea nitrogen (BUN) were the best two predictors (94.1 percent) of an ADR to digoxin. A serum theophylline concentration greater than 25 mcg/mL was the greatest predictor (85.2 percent) of an ADR to theophylline. The sensitivity and specificity of the therapeutic risk-assessment model were 92.9 percent and 61.8 percent, respectively, for digoxin and 95.8 percent and 84.0 percent, respectively, for theophylline.

BUILDING A MODEL

The best way to build a model to predict the high-risk patient for an ADE is to use pharmacoepidemiologic methods.[19,26,27,29,30] The best estimates of risk (odds ratios and relative risks with confidence intervals) are derived from controlled, population-based studies. Building a model for all drugs will be more difficult than building a model for specific drugs, based on the difficulty of obtaining the point estimates of risk for all drugs. However, this should not be discouraging. Point estimates can be estimated and tested, not only for categories of drugs, but for the other important variables as shown in Table 14.1. For example, if females are more likely than males to experience an ADE, then an odds ratio (e.g., an OR of 1.2) can be tested for females versus an OR of 1.0 for males.

Once a model is built to estimate the individualized risk for ADE, it can be tested for sensitivity and specificity against retrospective populations of patients who experienced a definite or probable, serious, and preventable ADE.

APPLICATION OF RISK MODEL

Applying risk models for ADEs is dependent on the patient setting. The two major settings are acute care and ambulatory care. The mathematical basis for each model will be different for each setting based on the different types of drugs used in each setting and types of patients.

Acute Care Model

A prognostic prediction model for ADEs in the inpatient setting would run in the background of the hospital's total information system. Each time (or on a scheduled basis) a drug is ordered or discontinued for a patient, a new laboratory result is known, or an important variable changes, the model would recalculate the patient's ADE risk rate. The risk rate could be posted in the patient's record for the doctor to see or the pharmacy could run a report each shift to see which patients have the highest risk factors for an ADE.

Ambulatory Care Model

In this setting, the prognostic prediction model for ADEs would run on the pharmacy's computer. Each new patient would complete a short, machine-readable form that would capture risk-associated demographic information, insurance information, and answers to the most important risk-assessment questions such as "have you ever been told that your kidneys don't work well?" All of this information would be uploaded to the pharmacy's computer system using a facsimile machine saving valuable time for the pharmacist.

Once the prescriptions are entered into the computer system, the risk model for ADEs would run and produce a risk-assessment score. For high-risk patients, the system would generate possible negative patient outcomes, and ask the pharmacist what actions he or she will take to reduce the risk. Pharmacists should take extra time to counsel these patients, be sure to interview the patients when they return for the first refill, and document how the patients are handling their medications. These are necessary steps to ensure patient safety, an opportunity for the pharmacists to show they provide value-added services and to gain payment for these services.

GENOMICS

Despite the scientific and statistical credibility of a computer model to predict ADEs, the sensitivity and specificity of such models may be low. This is because many ADEs are idiosysncratic and unpredictable. Much of the unpredictability is based on biological differences between individuals, in other words, a person's genetic makeup. Recent advances in molecular biology have led to modern pharmacogenetics that have focused on examining drug metabolizing enzymes and genetic determinants of pharmacokinetic variability.[31]

Various enzymes metabolize drugs (convert them from active to inactive drugs, or make them ready for excretion), and some people either do not have the enzyme or enough of the enzyme to metabolize the drug. When they take additional doses of the drug, it builds up in the body in toxic levels, as it is not eliminated as fast as it should.

Even before the secrets of the human genome were discovered, phenotyping and genotyping of individuals were used to discover if they had major deficiencies to the most common drug-metabolizing enzymes (cytochrome p-450 enzymes).[32] At least one commercial company tests patients for the presence of these enzymes and provides "report cards" to patients of the results to take to their doctors as a helpful tool. Most of the work so far has been done on which drugs to avoid. The flip side is that certain patients will have a genetic profile that metabolizes the drug too quickly, resulting in a therapeutic failure.

One vice president of a commercial company offering pharmacogenetic testing stated that its testing can identify about 70 percent of adverse drug reaction risks, and that traditional pharmacoepidemiology methods can supplement and strengthen these results (i.e., the use of an ADE prediction model).[33]

Despite the enthusiasm and potential for genomics to help reduce the risk of ADRs, progress has not gone as fast or as smoothly as some would like. [34,35] In 2003, one author said that tests to anticipate and decrease individual risk for ADRs are not expected to become available to the practicing clinician for at least five to ten years.[34]

However, a 2004 article was more positive.[36] The article reports on "genetic chips" that can be used to identify the form of the gene a person has and how well he or she will metabolize certain drugs.

SUMMARY

Although most drug therapy is safe, at times it can be devastating. Too many patients experience morbidity and mortality from their medication, even when it is prescribed correctly. Why some patients experience serious adverse effects of medication and some do not needs further investigation. Risk factors for ADEs need to be identified and quantified, and a risk model needs to be developed to predict the high-risk patient for an ADE. Once the high-risk patient is identified, added measures need to be taken to protect the patient from harm.

Chapter 15

Preventing and Reducing
Medication Injury

Since the 1999 Institute of Medicine's (IOM) report on medical errors, various organizations have been working to decrease the number of medication errors. Unfortunately, most of the activity has been uncoordinated and much work has been duplicated. One of the IOM's key recommendations was creating a national center for patient safety. It was envisioned that this Center would have the proper funding, staffing, and resources to set a national agenda and coordinate activities for patient safety. This has not happened. Until it does, health care institutions and practitioners will need to do the best they can to carry out strategies to reduce and prevent medication injuries in their centers.

This chapter discusses local strategies that may have the most impact at reducing preventable adverse drug events (ADEs). Thus, it is a micro view of ADE prevention. Macro issues on ADEs will be addressed in Chapter 18.

WHAT IS THE GOAL?

The best results are achieved when the end is in mind.[1] Before embarking on a program to reduce medication errors or ADEs, practitioners should ask—"What will the medication system look like when we achieve our goals?" Good baseline data are needed to set such goals. What are the incidence rates of ADRs and medication errors now? Were the numbers determined correctly? What was the morbidity and mortality associated with those ADEs?

Prescribed Medications and the Public Health
© 2006 by The Haworth Press, Inc. All rights reserved.
doi:10.1300/5688_15

When setting goals for preventing and reducing ADEs remember that not all ADEs are preventable. Second, a goal of reducing *all* medication errors is not attainable. Medication errors will always take place. So what is attainable? How about no medication-related injury as a long-term goal, and cutting the medication injury rate in half each year until there are no medication-related injuries? These are merely suggestions. What is important is that realistic short- and long-term goals be established, once baseline data have been collected.

The recommendations to help health care institutions and practitioners prevent and reduce medication injury are: evidence-based safe medication practices, best practices, and innovative practices.

EVIDENCE-BASED SAFE MEDICATION PRACTICES

In general, people do what they think is correct, yet sometimes there is little evidence to support what they do. It is ironic (and shameful) that despite evidence that certain medical procedures or drug therapies work, the procedures or therapies are not used. Examples are duodenal ulcer patients not being treated with triple antibiotic therapy; high-risk, male, cardiac patients not taking small prophylactic doses of aspirin; and postmyocardial infarction patients not being treated with a beta-blocker.

Evidenced-based safe medication practices were established through an interdisciplinary effort contracted by the Agency for Healthcare Research and Quality (AHRQ) with the University of California at San Francisco-Stanford Evidence-based Practice Center.[2]

Computerized Physician Order Entry with Clinical-Decision Support

The most promising evidenced-based strategy to reduce ADEs is a physician (prescriber) order entry system with clinical-decision support software in all health care settings (critical, acute, ambulatory, home, and long-term care).

Definitions

A *computerized physician order entry* (CPOE) system enables the direct entry of orders (diagnostics tests, medications, patient care instructions, and referrals) into a computer by a doctor or other authorized prescriber.[3] A *clinical decision support system* (CDSS) is computer software that uses rules to either stop or suggest drug doses, routes of administration, and frequencies based on patient information, laboratory values, or other drugs the patient is taking, all in real time.

Background

The problems and errors associated with handwritten prescriptions are legendary. In 1998, two academic researchers suggested that computerized prescribing could have a positive impact on eight important areas of the medication-use process and was long overdue.[4] These areas included:

1. drug selection,
2. a patient role in pharmacotherapy risk-benefit decisions,
3. screening for interactions (drug-drug, drug-laboratory, drug-disease),
4. linkages between the pharmacy and the laboratory,
5. dosing calculations and scheduling,
6. coordination between team members,
7. monitoring and documenting adverse events, and
8. postmarketing surveillance of therapy outcomes.

More important, most errors would be intercepted before they occur.

CPOE should be seen as a redesigned infrastructure for prescribing.[5] Conceptually, CPOE systems should be implemented to change how medications are prescribed and used, and to track and link patient outcomes. Other parts of the medication-use process need to be addressed using other strategies discussed later in this chapter.

The different levels of electronic prescribing are as follows:

- Level 1: basic electronic reference only
- Level 2: stand-alone prescription writer
- Level 3: supporting information is included
- Level 4: medication management
- Level 5: connectivity with MD's office, pharmacy, pharmacy benefits management (PBM) companies, and intermediaries
- Level 6: integration with electronic medical record[6]

CPOE systems function best at level 6. At a minimum, the laboratory should be linked to the pharmacy.[7]

How CPOE Works

A CPOE works in the following way: The medical staff approves the medication safety rules by consensus and these are programmed into the rule editor.[8] As data are written into the patient database (for example, new orders or new lab results), a copy of the data is sent to the inference engine for evaluation (Figure 15.1). The inference engine examines a knowledge base to discover if any rules concern this new piece of data and then performs the evaluations. The inference engine may have to examine other patient data to discover if the rules are true.

If a rule is found to be true, an *annunciator* is called to communicate the message. The knowledge base contains information about how the event should be communicated. If a clinician needs to be contacted, the

Event Monitor Architecture

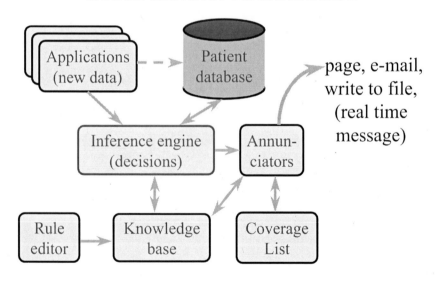

FIGURE 15.1. Event Monitor Architecture (*Source:* Reprinted with permission from a presentation by DW Bates to USP, 2003.)

coverage list database tells who is covering and the doctor can be paged or sent an e-mail. Other events, such as possible adverse drug events, are simply written to a file for later review. Also, if this process occurs in the middle of an interactive session, a message can be presented to the user in real time (Figure 15.2).

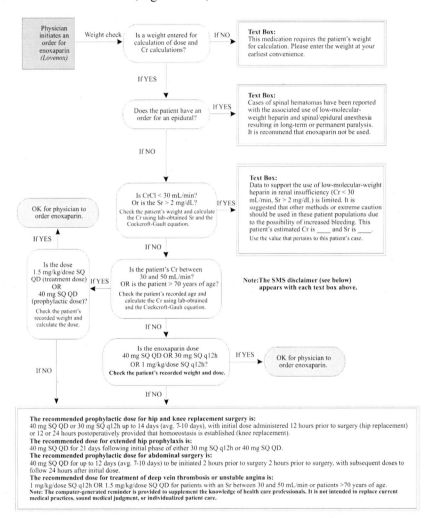

FIGURE 15.2. Exampled of a CPOE Rule's Algorithm (*Source:* Adapted with permission from *Hospital Pharmacy*, 2002:37:414.)

Clinical Decision Support

Rules are flags that remind the prescriber about a characteristic of a patient, other drug orders, or a laboratory result. Examples of triggers are shown in Table 15.1. These rules are the basis of the clinical decision support system (CDSS) that supports CPOE. Without CDSS, CPOE is simply an order entry system.

A CDSS can alert doctors to out-of-range laboratory values, remind the clinician to schedule a test, critique or stop an errant order, interpret an electrocardiogram, predict risk of mortality from a severity-of-illness score, list a differential diagnosis for a patient with chest pain, tailor antibiotic choices for liver transplant and renal failure, and produce suggestions for adjusting the mechanical ventilator.[9] Alerts are programmed as hard (cannot continue) or soft (may proceed if you wish after reading) stop signs.

CDSSs can prevent the most preventable ADEs such as excessive anticoagulation from overdoses of heparin or warfarin, excessive sedation or respiratory arrest from overdose of opiates or drug-drug interactions, and hypoglycemic events from insulin overdoses.[10] Using CDSS is an evidence-based safe medication practice.[11,12,13,14,15] To be effective, the CDSS must be continually reviewed and updated. For example, the FDA periodically requires new "black box warnings" for FDA-approved drugs. Black box warnings are safety warnings in a black box required in the drug's product labeling (package insert). These warnings can include newly discovered drug interactions, contraindications between a drug and a disease, or new adverse effects. New black box warnings should be programmed into CDSSs.

TABLE 15.1. Examples of Triggers and Corollary Orders

Trigger	Corollary Orders
Warfarin	Prothrombin time each morning
Aminoglycosides	Peak and trough levels after dosage changes and every week
Narcotics (class II)	Docusate if not taking other stool softener or laxative
Intravenous fluids	Place a saline lock when IV fluids are discontinued

Source: Adapted from Randolph AG, Haynes RB, Wyatt JC, Cook DJ, Guyatt GH (1999). Users' guide to the medical literature: XVIII. How to use an article evaluating the clinical impact of a computer-based clinical decision support system. *JAMA* 282(1):67-74. Copyright ©1999. American Medical Association.

Developing the rules for a CDSS can be difficult. Which rules should be chosen? What should the trigger point be for each rule? How many rules should there be? Gaining medical staff consensus on what is needed can be challenging but not impossible.[14]

Benefits of CPOE

CPOE is an evidenced-based safe medication practice.[13,16] Many studies have shown the positive impact CPOE has on error reduction. At one community teaching hospital, a computer alert system fired 1,116 times over a six-month period and 596 alerts were considered true-positives (positive predictive value of 0.53).[17] The alerts identified opportunities to prevent patient injury secondary to ADEs at a rate of 64 for every 1,000 admissions. Of 596 true-positive alerts, 265 (44 percent) were unrecognized by the doctor before alert notification.

At one large teaching hospital in Boston, the use of CPOE reduced serious medication errors by 55 percent in one study, and reduced errors (excluding missed doses) by 81 percent over four and a half years in another study.[18] In the second study, prescribing practices, such as the use, dose, and frequency of use of drugs improved.[19]

CPOE and linked computerized systems have also been tested in specialty populations of patients. In one pediatric critical care unit, the use of CPOE resulted in almost an elimination of medication prescribing errors and rule violations, and a significant, but less dramatic effect on potential ADEs.[20] A computerized system linking doctors and pharmacists in telepharmacies resulted in alerts to change to a more appropriate drug 24 percent of the time for patients 65 years and older throughout the United States.[21] Further studies on the value of using CPOE in the ambulatory environment are underway.[22] It has been estimated that the United States could save roughly $44 billion with nationwide implementation of advanced ambulatory CPOE.[22]

In one study, combining CPOE and team interventions was not shown to confer added benefit over CPOE alone.[23] In a study of pharmacist interventions after setting up CPOE, CPOE was effective in addressing many, but not all, of the problems associated with manual order writing.[24] There was an increase in the overall number of pharmacist interventions related to medication orders after implementing CPOE and the interventions were notably different.

One study using simulation modeling estimated that computerized information systems that detected 26 percent of medication errors and prevented associated ADEs could save 1,226 days of excess hospitalization and $1.4 million in hospital costs yearly.[25]

Status of CPOE

Despite the proven benefits of CPOE, the results of a 2002 survey showed that only 9.6 percent of U.S. hospitals had CPOE available.[26] In roughly half of those hospitals, more than 90 percent of the doctors used the system; in one-third of the hospitals, more than 90 percent of orders were entered using CPOE. Information is available about successful strategies used at ten community hospitals to implement CPOE.[27]

Hurdles and Barriers

Setting up CPOE is a big change and change can be difficult. The challenges to using CPOE include:[3, 28-30]

- *Commitment:* The organizational impact of CPOE systems, effort, and resources needed to set up the system are great.
- *Cost:* For any hospital, CPOE is a sizable investment, but not as large as some equipment and new building costs. It is a matter of making patient safety a priority. The return on the investment on CPOE includes improved patient care, reduced patient injury, a decrease in liability associated with ADEs, and annual cost savings. However, does patient safety need cost justification?
- *Doctors' work practices:* Some doctors are reluctant to give up long-established and comfortable manual processes for prescribing.
- *Current technology:* Unlike other industries, health care has long underinvested in information technology. Most hospitals have computer systems that support administrative and financial functions, but few that support patient care.
- *CPOE takes longer:* Some doctors feel that CPOE systems are too slow and provide too much information. Possibly, some doctors lack computer and keyboarding skills. Touch screen and voice-activated technology would improve this.

- *Status of commercial systems:* Most of the leading CPOE systems in place are "homegrown." None of the commercially available systems function as well as "homegrown" systems.
- *Lack of financial incentives:* The cost of completing a CPOE system depends on several factors, but is in the millions of dollars. Of course there are cost savings, but these may not accrue to doctors and hospitals under current reimbursement arrangements.
- *Weak CDSS or too many rules:* A CPOE system is only as good as the data that are fed into it and the rules it possesses. Some systems are not fine-tuned and too many alerts are firing. This slows processing orders and frustrates doctors.
- *Lack of data on how much CPOE systems improve patient outcomes:* Studies need to go to the next step. Rather than only showing a decrease in errors, they need to show improvement in patient outcome, declined inpatient stays, earlier return to work or school, and improved quality of life.

Mandates and Incentives

Several mandates are in place for CPOE. The first was the Leapfrog Group, a consortium of health care payers (major employers who buy health care for their employees), who early on saw the benefits of CPOE and put forth the following standards for hospitals:[31]

- Require doctors of patients in hospitals to enter medication orders via a computer system that is linked to prescribing-error-prevention software.
- Require documented acknowledgment by the prescribing doctor of the interception before any override.
- Demonstrate that their CPOE system can intercept 50 percent of common serious prescribing failures using the Leapfrog Evaluation Tool.
- Post the Leapfrog CPOE Evaluation Tool results on a Leapfrog site.

The California Senate passed a bill (Minimization of Medication-Related Errors) in 2000 requiring urban hospitals to implement a plan to reduce medication errors, and to address technology implementation such as CPOE by January 2005.[3] The bill required California hospitals to create medication error reduction plans, focusing on reducing medical errors, and submit those plans to the State Department of Health Services. Of 344 plans submitted, 46 percent would employ CPOE by January 1, 2005.[32] Estimates show advanced ambulatory CPOE systems could prevent 249,000 ADEs each year in California and save the state $3.2 billion.[33]

Cautions

Some say this excitement for CPOE needs to be tempered and put into perspective. In March 2002, testimony before Congress revealed the following about new health care technologies: [34]

- Many commercial CPOE systems have not been tested in typical community hospitals.
- CPOE systems do not provide a complete solution to drug prescribing problems.
- CPOE systems are not standardized.
- A lot of technical and clinical resources are needed to set up CPOEs.
- CPOE systems require large commitments among hospital personnel.

Krizner states, "There is concern that people think technology is the final answer. But, technology is only as good as the people behind it. Nothing can be done if the software package is written wrongly."[35] Three pharmacists intimately involved in the early stages of CPOE development recently offered eleven realities and cautions about CPOE:[36]

1. CPOE systems take more time and are more complex than manual systems.
2. Pharmacists should be intimately involved in CPOE development and implementation.
3. Order entry is a new skill for many doctors and adds to the learning curve and a potential increase in early errors.

4. Sometimes nurses, ward clerks, and pharmacists are being asked or are needed to enter doctors' orders. This defeats the purpose of CPOE.
5. Many existing CPOE systems do not have bidirectional interface with the pharmacy and other areas, and some are stand-alone.
6. CDSS is often limited or gets turned off because alerts go off too much or are irrelevant.
7. Most institutions have not fully integrated CPOE with other medication components (such as automated dispensing devices, robots, bar code point-of-care systems, or infusion technology).
8. CPOE systems are not "plug and play." Without a systematic approach to redesigning existing processes, shortcuts will eventually occur, resulting in increases in workload and possibly new sources of error.
9. The transferability of internally developed CPOE systems has not been studied.
10. CPOE systems are yet to be developed to fully support the needs of high-risk populations (e.g., neonates and geriatric patients).
11. CPOE systems, so far, do not allow for the complexity of orders.

Grissinger and Globus stated, "computer order-entry systems and other technologies are supposed to make medication administration safer. But if poorly designed or used wrongly, they can introduce errors."[37] The point about still making errors was reinforced by a pharmacist who documented the types of medication errors post-CPOE implementation in an ambulatory clinic.[38] The most common prescription errors were: wrong directions (21 percent), wrong dosage form (19 percent), and wrong quantity (15 percent).

Getting Started

Previous CPOE implementations have offered suggestions for those about to embark on the CPOE path. CPOE implementation requires:

- first, and far most important, a strong and honest commitment to improve safety;[39]
- strong leadership,[39]
- a committed team;[40]
- each team educated and committed to CPOE;[39]
- getting "buy-in" from the medical staff;[39] and
- being patient.[41]

Help is available for those setting up a CPOE system. First, a series of articles on each step of setting up CPOE is available in *Hospital Pharmacy*.[40,42] Second, a published record is available of a round table discussion by several early implementers of CPOE.[43] The ISMP Web site has a guide titled "Land mines and pitfalls of computerized prescriber order entry."[44]

Summary

In 1995, a study showed that the most common systems problems in hospitals were associated with the dissemination of patient drug information.[45] The inadequate availability of patient information, such as laboratory test results, was associated with 18 percent of errors. CPOE systems help solve this problem.

The evidence reveals that CPOE can improve patient safety and lessen variation in care and cost.

Unit-Dose Drug Distribution Systems

In unit-dose distribution systems, most medication is dispensed from the pharmacy in single-unit or unit-dose packages, with enough medication dispensed for 24 hours or less at one time. Unit-dose packages are labeled and ready to administer to the patient.

Using the unit-dose drug distribution method is an evidenced-based, safe medication practice.[46] The first study to prove that medication errors were lessened (from 8.3 to 3.5 percent) with unit-dose distribution was in 1970.[47] Another study in 1975 showed a decrease from 7.4 to 1.6 percent using a multiward drug distribution system with a unit-dose system.[48] Despite unit-dose drug distribution being the safest means of distributing medication in an organized health care setting, still some organizations do not use it. Reasons for not using a unit-dose system need to be investigated.

Bar Coding

Bar coding and scanning systems are used to speed processing and to avoid error. Bar coding has been used for over 20 years in grocery stores, but their use in the health care industry has been minimal. In a recent survey of pharmacists, bar coding was the number one choice for preventing medication errors.[49] Thirty-nine percent of respondents selected bar-code scanning over CPOE.

Using bar-code scanning in the prescription or drug distribution process allows matching prescriptions and drug orders with drug products, and checks the dispensed medications. Using bar-code scanning in organized health care settings allows checking the medication dispensed, identifies the patient (scan patient's wristband) before medication is administered, checks to make sure it is the right time to give medication, identifies who administered the medication (e.g., by scanning the nurse's ID badge), and charges for the medication.

Hospitals have been slow to buy equipment for bar coding. Until 2004, drug manufacturers were not required to bar code their unit-dose medications. Most drug manufacturers did not want to retool their production lines to put bar codes on single-unit doses until more hospitals used them, and, bar-coded unit doses cost more (pennies). However, now (as of June 2004), the FDA requires pharmaceutical companies to use bar codes on most drugs used in hospitals. The FDA estimates medical savings could total $93 billion during the next 20 years. Currently, only 2 percent of U.S. hospitals have bedside scanning systems to read bar codes.[50]

Point-of-Care Systems

Bar coded point-of-care systems (BPOC) provide the closed loop needed in bar-coded unit-dose systems to decrease errors associated with medication dispensing and administration. BPOC is sometimes referred to as bedside charting. Optimally, BPOC requires three bar codes—the unit dose of medication, the nurse's name badge, and the patient's wristband. When it is time to administer a medication, the nurse scans the unit-dose medication with a portable bar-code reader, then scans his or her name badge, and then scans the patient's ID wristband. The scanned information is sent (wirelessly) to the hospital's computer system to verify that the nurse has the correct patient, correct medication, and if it is the correct time to give the medication. If something is wrong, a red light glows on the bar-code reader. If everything is correct, a green light glows on the bar-code reader. Once the nurse signals on the bar-code reader that the medication has been given, the hospital computer system charts the time the medication was given, by whom, and sends a charge to the patient's bill. In some hospitals, the point-of-care system uses bedside or handheld computers. In a round table discussion of pharmacists involved with the early implementation of CPOE, many felt that setting up BPOC was more important than setting up CPOE.[43]

A study performed on BPOC in 2002 reported a 87 percent decline in medication errors.[51] The prevalence of wrong dose, wrong dosage form, and omission errors dropped 90 percent, while medications given at the wrong time dropped by over 75 percent. Similar results were seen in another study.[52] Nurses love BPOC.[51,52,53] One nurse said, "I never realized how vulnerable I was to the possibility of committing a serious error before the system began documenting all of my near-misses."[53]

Automated Dispensing

Hospital pharmacists have been experimenting with automated dispensing for some time, based on their need to improve safety and efficiency. Automated dispensing comes in three forms: (1) robotic dispensing machines (RDMs) used in inpatient pharmacies, (2) automated dispensing machines (ADMs) located on patient care units, and (3) automatic prescription dispensing machines (PDMs) used in outpatient pharmacies.

Robotic Dispensing Machines

Several studies have been presented on robotic dispensing machines.[54,55] These authors found that the RDM they were using increased the accuracy of filling and checking medication, reduced personnel costs, and had an early cost savings estimate of $300,000 over the eight-year life of the system. Another study comparing manual unit-dose cart filling versus using RDM, found dispensing error rates to be low with both systems.[56] Dispensing errors for the manual system were 1 percent and for the RDM 0.65 percent.

Automated Dispensing Machines

ADMs are like automatic teller machines (ATMs), only they are located in a patient care area. The user (usually a nurse) inserts identification of the patient and the user, and signals the medication needed. If the information is consistent with data stored in the pharmacy computer system, a drawer opens to allow the user access to the medication. The system records the person who gave the medication, what medication was given, and the time the medication was given.

Several studies have been conducted on ADMs and dispensing errors. One observational study showed a unit-dose dispensing error rate of 15.9 percent versus an error rate of 10.6 percent using ADMs.[57] In another observational study using the before-and-after format, the medication administration errors before ADMs was 16.9 percent and 10.4 percent after using ADMs. This is a statistically significant difference.[58] The most prevalent problems were wrong-time errors, and these occurred in both parts of the study. In another study, medication errors decreased after using ADMs on a cardiovascular surgery unit, but increased on the cardiovascular intensive care unit.[59]

Automatic Prescription Dispensing Machines

More community and outpatient pharmacies are investigating the advantages of using APDMs. These devices use patient and prescription data entered into the pharmacy's computer system. The information is sent to a canister holding the medication needed. While the patient prescription vial is centered under the canister, the exact amount of medication is dropped into the vial. The vial is then automatically labeled and sent to an area where a pharmacist views a computer screen with a picture of the medication that is supposed to be in the vial. Once checked, the vial is ready for dispensing to the patient. A literature search in 2004 failed to find a study on medication error rates of these devices versus error rates using manual dispensing.

Automated medication dispensing devices are designed to reduce medication errors and improve efficiency. Although bar-coding technology and other safeguards have been included in these devices, and there are some data that show these devices reduce medication errors, data are limited and need expansion.[60,61] This may be because the use of automated dispensing devices is so limited, especially in the ambulatory setting.

The Use of Clinical Pharmacists

Evidence shows that the use of clinical pharmacists—those clinically involved with the patient's care—lessens the number of potential ADEs. Many studies, some as early as 1987, show that pharmacists working with other health care providers reduces preventable ADEs such as medication errors.[62,63,64] However, data on whether this involvement and ADE decline improves patient outcomes are scant.[65]

One 1999 study showed that pharmacist participation in hospital rounds in an intensive care unit reduced preventable ADEs by 66 percent.[66] In another study, the use of clinical pharmacists in the inpatient, outpatient, and nursing home settings improved patient outcomes by 44.6 percent, 34.1 percent, and 33.3 percent, respectively.[67] Another study of community pharmacists' interventions to correct prescribing problems found that 28.3 percent of the identified problems could have resulted in patient harm if the pharmacist had not intervened to correct the problem.[68]

Protocols for High-Risk Drugs

Published studies on ADEs have consistently identified certain classes of drugs as serious threats to patient safety. These "high-risk" or "high-alert" medications include anticoagulants, intravenous opioid analgesics, concentrated electrolyte solutions, insulin, and chemotherapeutic agents. Protocols for the storage, distribution, and use of high-risk drugs is an evidence-based, safe medication practice.[69] For example, a policy to keep concentrated electrolyte solutions off patient care areas (only used in the pharmacy) and stored away from the same diluted product, reduces medication errors associated with this practice.

Order templates for chemotherapeutic agents, a policy for pharmacists to double-check all calculations for preparing neonatal products, protocols for reviewing the settings of intravenous pumps delivering continuous or intermittent doses of opiates, and automated selection of drugs and drug dose in patients with renal insufficiency, all help reduce errors.

Several practices about managing anticoagulant therapy have been studied extensively and found to be evidenced-based, safe practices.[69] These include: heparin-dosing protocols, inpatient anticoagulation clinics, outpatient anticoagulation clinics, and patient self-monitoring using a finger-stick device.

Evidence-Based Practice

Shortly after the first IOM report on patient safety, the Agency for Healthcare Research and Quality (AHRQ) shared a list of best safety practices for all clinicians. The AHRQ requested that the National Quality Forum (NQF) use a consensus process of experts to define the list. This list was eagerly anticipated by health care leaders and published in 2002.[70] However, it provoked surprise and confusion as some improvements in safety practice were not mentioned in the report.[71]

BEST PRACTICES TO IMPROVE MEDICATION SAFETY

Following are examples of best practices that may not have enough data to make them evidence based or may be hard to study. Yet there is consensus that they probably reduce preventable ADEs.

Organizational Commitment to Improving Safety

Little improvement in medication safety, if any, occurs without a commitment from the CEO of a health care organization to improve patient safety. Patient safety needs to be more than just being "the right thing to do."[72] Creating a culture of safety takes commitment, leadership, and resources. It also takes a zero-based assessment of the medication-use system, with no areas being held sacred. Medication safety must start with the top hierarchy: the board of trustees, then the organization's top management, then the medical staff leadership. For corporately owned pharmacies, it means the company's officers and managers.

A Nonpunitive Approach for Solving Medication Mishaps

Health care workers do not purposely make errors and are trained to "first do no harm." Doctors, nurses, and pharmacists continually worry about making errors. Severe punishment or termination for making a serious error only compounds the self-punishment that already has taken place. It wrecks people's careers, and sends a loud message and incentive to other health care workers to bury the medication errors they and others make.

Health care workers who make serious medication errors need to be counseled and perhaps more closely supervised, but not punished. Fortunately, new ways of dealing with the consequences from serious medication errors are being used.[73]

An Emphasis on Documenting All ADEs

All potential ADEs (PADEs) and ADEs should be documented. No picture is complete without seeing all of its parts. Thus, which parts of the medication-use system are broken may not be obvious without good documentation. Continuous enforcing of the need for documentation is needed.

Appoint a Medication Safety Officer

The idea that there should be a single point of accountability for medication errors has recently been advanced, and the American Society of Health-System Pharmacists (ASHP) has a model job description available on its Web site (www.ashp.org). The medication safety officer (MSO) does not have to be a pharmacist, but should be full-time, and may report to the Office of Quality Assurance, Risk Management, or an organizational part of the medical staff.

Enforce the Verbal Order Policy

Verbal orders should be used only in emergencies. When it is an emergency, the verbal order policy should state that the recipient of the verbal order must immediately record and echo what they heard to the person giving the verbal order. This is so simple, yet violated all the time. Most community pharmacies do not have a verbal order policy on who can take verbal orders (only the pharmacist and pharmacy intern, not a pharmacy technician) and from whom (only a doctor or a nurse, not a clerk working in a doctor's office).

Have a War on the Use of Abbreviations

Medical Abbreviations: 24,000 Conveniences at the Expense of Communications and Safety states "abbreviations in medical practice are sometimes not understood, misread, or interpreted wrongly."[74] They sometimes result in patient harm so abbreviations should not be used.

Manage the High-Risk Patient for ADEs

Until genetic testing mechanisms become inexpensive, fast, and readily available, it makes sense to take extra precautions and efforts to monitor patients who may be at high risk for an ADE. These populations include: pediatric patients, elderly patients, and patients who are renally, hepatically, or immunologically compromised.[75,76,77] Management mechanisms to handle the high-risk patient include the use of decision-support software, medication protocols, and clinical pharmacists to actively monitor the patient's therapy. One study using clinical pharmacists to help manage medication used in patients at high risk for a medication-related problem showed a decrease in the side effects of the medications.[78]

A Major Effort to Reduce Polypharmacy

Studies consistently show that the number and severity of ADEs increases with the number of medications prescribed and used. The etiology of *polypharmacy* has not been studied well. However, a contributing reason may be patients going to more than one doctor or to more than one pharmacy. Thus, the real culprit is lack of one, central, electronic medical record for the patient. Pharmacists who have experienced patients bringing them "brown bags" full of medications can relate their surprise on how much medication some patients take— sometimes more than 15 medications daily. One clinic for identifying and addressing polypharmacy discovered overprescribing, underprescribing, drug interactions, inappropriate dosages, and overlapping therapy.[79]

Use Failure Mode and Effects Analysis

Failure mode and effects analysis (FMEA) in medication error prevention is the process of examining each step of the medication-use process and identifying the weaknesses and measures to overcome these weaknesses.[80] FMEA is a preventative process that every health care organization should undertake at least once a year.[81,82] However, data on how many health care organizations use FMEA and how often they use it are unknown. The American Hospital Association (AHA) and the Institute for Safe Medication Practices (ISMP) recently launched a nationwide survey to hospital pharmacy directors to assess the safety status of the medication-use system. Hospitals using FMEA will be able complete this survey easily.

Perform a Root Cause Analysis on All Serious Errors

When a serious error occurs, a root cause analysis (RCA) should be performed by an interdisciplinary team to identify: (1) failure points, (2) root cause of the failure points, (3) system failures, and (4) the prevention strategies with the highest leverage.[83,84] Health care organizations accredited by the Joint Commission on Accreditation of Healthcare Organizations (JCAHO) must perform a RCA for all sentinel events—an unexpected instance involving death or serious physical or psychological injury, or the risk of it.

Proper Staffing

The past ten years have seen a shift from acute care to ambulatory care. Patients in hospitals today are much sicker and this increases the time it takes to care for a patient. Shifting patients to the ambulatory environment, and the aging population have increased the number of prescriptions being filled dramatically. Medication dispensing and administration safety can be threatened and the margin of safety decreases without proper staffing.

USP's national medication error reporting system for hospitals is a good barometer of staff contributions to medication errors. In its 2002 MEDMARX report, USP reported that four of the top six factors contributing to medication errors were: workload increase, inexperienced staff, inadequate staffing, and the use of agency or temporary help.[85]

A shortage of nurses and pharmacists has been documented over the past five years. However, evidence shows increased pressures by health care employers to increase productivity, and some chain pharmacies have even provided incentives for pharmacists to fill prescriptions faster.[86] Nurses and pharmacists who work in places they think are unsafe have a duty to make it safer. If this cannot be done, they should leave, otherwise, they are contributing to compromised care and risking their professional license.

Provide Patient Counseling

Patients should be counseled about their medication by the prescriber and by the pharmacist who dispenses the medication. At a minimum, patients should know:

- what medication they are taking,
- why they are taking it,
- how much to take,
- how often to take it,
- how long to take it, and
- when they should contact their pharmacist or doctor about a side effect they are experiencing.

Unfortunately, some patients do not receive this information from their doctor or pharmacist.

When OBRA 90 legislation was enacted, pharmacists suddenly were required to offer counseling to patients about their medication. Most states' boards of pharmacy required pharmacists to offer to counsel all patients about their medication.[87] In 1994, one study found only four of ten patients were offered counseling by their pharmacist.

Today, observation suggests that the rate of pharmacists offering counseling may be much lower than in 1994. Instead, a clerk makes the offer (illegally), or the patient is asked to "sign here." A study shows that patients have no idea why they are signing their name. Some think it is for insurance reasons or to verify that they picked up their medication. However, what they are doing by signing is indicating that they do not want counseling by the pharmacist. Some pharmacy companies think they are within the law by including information on the medication in the prescription bag.[88]

Many pharmacists probably do not realize that patient counseling detects and reduces medication errors. In one study over an 18-month period, 323 errors were discovered.[89] Of these, pharmacist counseling caught 89 percent of the errors before the patient left the pharmacy. Today's new pharmacy graduates are taught how to counsel all patients (prescription and OTC), and know that they are required to offer counseling, but many are prevented or do not have enough time to do this. Unfortunately, enforcement of the law is almost nonexistent.

Provide Patient Education

Most patients need help to understand their medication and understand alternatives about medication. This extends to over-the-counter (OTC) medication. Many patients wander around the OTC aisles wondering what they should be getting, and most pharmacists are oblivious, or under pressure from management to fill more and more prescriptions faster and faster. They stay behind the counter with their heads buried in their computers. It is no wonder that patients often select the wrong OTC or misuse it.[90]

INNOVATIVE PRACTICES TO IMPROVE MEDICATION SAFETY

Many new ideas have been put forth for improving medication safety. Some have had limited testing, and some, no testing at all, but each has potential to have a significant effect on reducing ADEs.

Use of Smart Infusion Pumps

"Free flow" used to be a problem with intravenous infusion pumps. When the nurse opened the door to the pump and did not close the roller clamp on the IV tubing, the IV fluid "free flowed" into the patient. Some companies have been experimenting with smarter pumps. These pumps use a modular point-of-care platform that integrates patient information, care-specific protocols, and safeguards to avoid medication errors.[91]

Improve Reporting ADEs in Non–Acute-Care Settings

ADEs outside the hospital setting need better reporting about the incidence, severity, type of ADE, and how to identify contributing factors. USP is working on this problem as are others. The National Coordinating Council for Medication Error Reporting and Prevention (NCC MERP) recently released recommendations to reduce medication errors in non-health care settings such as day care centers, assisted living facilities, and correctional facilities.[92]

Fast-Track E-Prescribing

The problems and errors associated with handwriting are well-known. The practice of handwritten prescriptions is archaic and needs to be replaced with electronic prescribing (e-prescribing) and decision support (e.g., CPOE). In early 2002, Giant Food announced that it had signed on to offer e-prescribing for doctors in the Silver Spring, Maryland, area.[93] Doctors could access the system using a desktop computer, handheld PC, or a cell phone. In January 2003, this system was expanded through a partnership with Dr First.[94] In the fall of 2002, it was announced that two-thirds of the chain pharmacy market had signed on to provide connectivity between their pharmacies and doctors' offices.[95]

The problem with e-prescribing is in getting doctors to use it. Who will pay for the equipment and software is an issue. In February 2003, some doctors in the Boston area started using and evaluating e-prescribing.[96] Investigators found that patients love it and recognize that it removes mistakes and decreases time in the pharmacy. However, the barriers to wider acceptance by doctors are: (1) the cost of buying and setting up e-prescribing technology (81 percent), (2) the time it takes to learn and use the technology (40 percent), and (3) lack of awareness of the benefits of the system (22 percent). Chain pharmacies may consider the primary benefit of e-prescribing (increased efficiency and lower costs), while doctors and pharmacists are seeking improved safety and ease of use.[97] Nevertheless, it looks like e-prescribing will happen.[98] It is hoped that standards on how information should be communicated electronically will be established to avoid errors.[99] It is also hoped that prescribing prescriptions electronically is just the first step, that decision support will be added to the system soon, and that improvements in safety are documented. The Centers for Medicare & Medicaid Services (CMS) drafted guidelines on electronic prescribing and hopes to make this a requirement for their prescription benefit program.

Address Human Factors That Contribute to Errors

Most attention has been focused on system improvements that are needed to reduce medication errors, while little attention has been given to why people make mistakes and what can be done to help them be less prone to making errors.[100] Improving performance can be achieved through human factor analysis (HFA). HFA is defined as the study of the interrelationships among humans, the tools they use, and the environment in which they live and work.[101]

Some of the problems of people making errors can be traced to the way behavior is managed in the workplace. The focus is usually away from the cause and toward the symptoms. Often, corrective action is taken against a nurse or other health professional, yet the most common cause of errors is found in supervision.[102]

What the practitioner does is usually the result of management's acts of commission or omission, yet the common-sense approach rarely sees that result. The best ways to manage behavior in the health care environment are to:

- focus on the solution rather than the problem,
- train workers to fluency,
- pay attention to the details of behavior, and
- use positive reinforcement for procedure compliance.[102]

Require the Use of the Medication in the Directions for Use or on the Prescription

Many drug names look alike if the prescription is handwritten. Also, many drugs have more than one indication. For example, there are at least four indications for Inderal. Because of the way prescriptions are written, the pharmacist is in the dark about why the drug is being used. Sometimes, because of poor handwriting, Inderal may look like Indocin. If the use of the medication is in the directions or somewhere on the prescription, the pharmacist will have a better chance of: (1) knowing for sure what is needed, (2) avoiding unsafe combinations of drugs, and (3) offering more information to educate, counsel, and help the patient.

SUMMARY

The IOM "rang the bell" on medical and medication errors. The number and severity of preventive ADEs is unacceptable. Current systems and approaches to managing behavior need improvement. Every medication-use system should set achievable goals for improving medication safety and employ all evidenced-based safe medication practices that apply. In addition, best practices in medication safety should be pursued. Leading health care providers should test and evaluate innovative practices that might potentially and substantially improve safety. The first step is to gain commitment from the hierarchy of organizations to make patient safety a top priority and to budget resources.

Chapter 16

What's a Patient to Do?

Being a patient can be scary. The origin of this fear may be a bad experience, but usually stems from lack of medical knowledge, a high level of respect for health professionals, and being timid. Patients are often bewildered and confused by the terms used by health professionals, and because they sometimes do not understand, they feel they must trust the professionals who are treating them.

Most health care professionals do not recognize the communication chasm between themselves and the patient. Most health care professionals will never be able to understand and recognize what patients endure unless *they* become a patient.[1] No wonder many patients do not take their medications correctly and some patients tolerate serious side effects because they do not connect the problem to their medication. Some patients do not know the name of their medication or why they are taking it because their doctor is too busy with the next patient or their pharmacist is too busy filling other prescriptions.

This chapter is about patients and the changes that are needed to improve how practitioners relate to patients, and how better communication is needed to improve medication safety.

PATIENT NEEDS

In the film *The Doctor,* William Hurt plays a cardiovascular surgeon who says to his surgical residents, "patients feel frightened, embarrassed, vulnerable, and sick, and most of all they want to feel better. Because of this, they place their total faith in us. I can explain that until I am blue in the face, but you will never get it until you experience it for yourself."[1]

Prescribed Medications and the Public Health
© 2006 by The Haworth Press, Inc. All rights reserved.
doi:10.1300/5688_16

Patients are often frightened because they do not understand what the health care providers are saying—the information is too technical or is told to them too quickly. Terms are used that are common to the health care professional because of years of training, but are foreign to the average person. An example is that hospitals use the term "radiology department" while patients look for the "X-ray department." Medical care is far from being "user friendly."

Patients are embarrassed because they are often asked to undress, are placed in revealing hospital gowns, and must discuss confidential matters. Many feel vulnerable because they know so little about health care. Health care to the average patient is like a foreign language. Because of the high level of education needed to be a health care professional, most patients are in awe of those who care for them. This lack of understanding and high respect for doctors often causes patients to surrender their bodies, minds, and sometimes dignity. Patients commonly present themselves "here I am, do whatever it is you are going to do to me" without questioning their medical treatment.

Patients have names—they are not the cabdriver with the gastric ulcer or the married woman with the Southern accent. They come from many cultural backgrounds and have differing attitudes about being sick. Patients can be passive, compliant, demanding, challenging, questioning, or cooperative. Most of all, they are sick and usually worried. They are real people.

Most patients want to demystify health care, have more control over their own destiny, and be treated like an individual. They want their health care professionals to connect with them, care about them, not treat them like a number, and to do their best at getting them well. They need understanding, reassurance, and education.

Patients' fears run deep about medication. In a 2002 national survey of patients, it was discovered that a vast majority of the public is concerned about medication-related issues.[2] The most frequent medication concerns were:

- being given two or more medicines that interact in a negative way (70 percent),
- being given the wrong medicine (69 percent),
- the cost of treatment (69 percent), and
- the potential harmful side effects from taking a medication (67 percent).

The most common medication errors patients make in their home are taking the wrong dose of medication or forgetting to take their medication.[3] Twenty-one percent of patients reported communication problems and 19 percent reported recurring causes of error because of lack of knowledge. Another cause of error was lack of patient-specific labeling on how to take the drug samples provided by doctors' offices. Patients reported that these samples are typically given out without any information on the drug's use, side effects, or warnings.

Federal and state laws require pharmacists to offer counseling personally to patients about their medication. Unfortunately, this duty is seldom fulfilled. Corporate pharmacy attorneys have found a way of skirting the law. They have told pharmacy clerks to ask the patient to "sign or initial here," and provide written take-home information about the drug that patients seldom read. What the patient signs is a waiver that they were offered counseling but did not want it, even though they were not offered it. When asked to sign, most people think they are signing for insurance reasons or to verify that they picked up the medication.[4]

FULFILLING PATIENTS' NEEDS

All health professionals need to look at themselves in the mirror and try to remember why it was they went into health care. Most will answer that it was to help patients, and most will say that is what they are doing. They are helping patients, except many are not doing it in a user-friendly way, nor are they working to demystify the system for patients.

Doctors, pharmacists, and nurses should be working inside the hospital to make the environment user friendly. Take down the "radiology" signs and replace them with signs that read "x-ray." Remove the gowns that cause patient embarrassment. In short, remember your oath and return to your roots of working in the best interest of the patient, rather than in the best interest of the hospital or corporate pharmacy. Practitioners should take the proper time, try to connect emotionally, and counsel each patient about their disease and treatment.

William Hurt may be correct when he said "I can explain that until I am blue in the face, but you will never get it until you experience it for yourself."[1] Most health care workers (doctors, nurses, pharmacists) will never understand, appreciate, or be able to transcend the chasm between themselves and the patient because of ego, pride, or self-imposed or externally applied time pressures. Other than becoming a patient in a hospital or nursing home for at least 72 hours, their next best chance is to read *Becoming a Good Doctor,* and focus on the chapter on beneficence.[5]

Even if health care workers are honest and able to remember why they entered health care, other pressures will prevent them from becoming more attuned to patients' needs, fears, and anxieties. Organizations (e.g., hospitals, HMOs, and corporately owned pharmacies) advertise how the patient is "number one," yet behind closed doors make it known that the organization is number one. They even say, "remember, if we are not successful, we will not be here to employ you and to help patients."

The merit system for health care workers within patient health care organizations—even not-for-profit ones—is geared toward more market share and a successful bottom line. Most health care workers would not argue with this, but should argue how this should be accomplished. They should always fight for quality care that is provided by enough qualified health workers, using the most affordable equipment, which improves health outcomes. Patients treated under such a system will be loyal and return for care when they need it.

Unfortunately, most health care employers (hospitals, HMOs, and corporately owned pharmacies) will use numbers to improve their bottom line. They exert pressure to see more patients, increase admissions, and fill more prescriptions. Doctors, nurses, and pharmacists are expected to care for more patients with less help than ever before. The priority of many organizations is to build more additions, more labs, and more pharmacies, but administrators often tell their employees that they cannot afford more help.

Today, there are documented shortages of nurses and pharmacists, and more and more people are approaching retirement age. The baby boomers will soon crush the health care system that is already in poor shape. Who will lead us out of this mess? The only hope to improve patient care is within the health professions. It will not come from the government or the health care industry. Traditionally, developing models for restructuring such important and complex areas rests with the academic medical professions. However, leadership for this critical issue is nonexistent.

PATIENT AND PRACTITIONER EDUCATION

Practitioners and patients need education on what is missing in the health care worker-patient relationship and how this relationship can improve. This can be done using mass media or on a one-on-one basis. There is also a need to discover what educational methods work best in helping patients understand their medication, and helping doctors and pharmacists know how to best communicate with patients about their medication.

Most programs that educate patients about the safe use of their medication share a weak link in evaluating success and affecting behavior change.[6] The same can be said for changing doctor behavior to improve drug therapy. Simply learning about poor medication practices does not change practice. For instance, a message flashed on a computerized physician order entry (CPOE) system indicating that what a doctor is about to do may be dangerous is too often ignored.

For patients, it may take both mass media messages and working one-on-one to affect change. More public service announcements (PSAs) are needed to help improve the public's health. The contrast in the number of public health PSAs between Canada and the United States is striking—with Canada in the lead.

All doctors should explain to patients:

1. the name of the medication they are prescribing,
2. why it is the preferred treatment,
3. alternative treatments and their advantages and disadvantages,
4. how the medication should be taken,
5. the medication's common side effects,
6. any warnings, and
7. when the patient should contact his or her doctor or pharmacist about any adverse effects.

The pharmacist has a professional and legal duty to make sure patients know about their medication, despite what their employer may say or want them to do. The best way of doing this is to use the Indian

Health Service (IHS) method of counseling patients about their medication.[7] Three prime questions form the foundation for the medication consultation: (1) What did your doctor tell you your medication was for? (2) How did your doctor tell you to take your medication? and (3) What did your doctor tell you to expect? This method is efficient and probes the patient's knowledge and understanding that is needed to self-medicate. The pharmacist can reinforce what patients know and fill in the gaps on what they need to know.

Then we come to practitioner education. Although education about how to improve communication with patients can be provided to health professionals through journal articles, newsletters, and conferences, these methods seldom effect much change. The information just does not stick. It goes in one ear and out the other. The audience just does not get it. Most doctors and pharmacists do not count this as a primary responsibility yet it reduces their legal liability should a medication injury occur.

One-on-one education to improve practitioner sensitivity and medication safety would probably work if there were consequences for not listening or not trying new methods. However, what would the consequences be and who would do the training?

Behavior-based safety coaching (BBS) is essentially an interpersonal process of one-on-one observation and feedback which can improve an individual's safety record. One person (the coach) systematically sees the behaviors of another person, then provides constructive feedback related to those behaviors."[8] This may work well for training future health care practitioners such as students in the health professions, but is too threatening for most seasoned practitioners.

TIPS FOR PATIENTS

Patients can improve their understanding of health care, health outcomes, and reduce the likelihood of experiencing an adverse drug event (ADE):

- First, and most important, is to take more responsibility for your health. Be on the team![9]

- Do not allow health care practitioners to "snow you" with terminology you do not understand. Speak up and ask what something means. Don't be embarrassed—you are the customer!
- Know that everything being said by your health care practitioner is a recommendation, no matter how it is stated. You have choices.
- Always ask about alternatives and the pros and cons of everything.[10]
- Question everything that is being done to you or a loved one.
- For your medication, ask the following questions:[11]
  —What are the brand and generic names of the medication?
  —What is the purpose of the medication?
  —What is the strength and dosage?
  —What are the possible side effects? What should I do if they occur?
  —Are there any other medications I should avoid while using this product?
  —How long should I take this medication? What outcome should I expect?
  —When is the best time to take the medication?
  —How should I store the medication?
  —What do I do if I miss a dose?
  —Should I avoid any foods while taking this medication?
  —Is this medication meant to replace any other drug that I am already taking?
  —May I have written information about this drug?

Patients should also know everything about their illness and the medication they need to take for the illness. There are many excellent sources of such information. Attend health fairs and "brown bag" programs offered at health fairs or pharmacies. Pharmacists review the medicines brought to them in a brown bag, search the internet for information (from reliable sources), and answer questions. Several health care organizations produce excellent and free educational materials for patients about medication.

NCPIE

The National Council on Patient Information and Education (NCPIE) is solely dedicated to improving patient understanding of medication, improving health outcomes, and reducing medication misadventures. NCPIE has information for patients and practitioners located at its Web site: http:/www.talkaboutrx.org/resources.html. Following are samples of information available:

- "Prescription Pain Medicines: What You Need to Know"
- "Your Medicine: Play It Safe"
- "Tips on Safe Medication Storage"
- "Buying Prescription Medication Online"
- "Think It Through: A Guide to Managing the Benefits and Risks of Medicines"
- "Managing Side Effects"
- "Alcohol and Medicines: Ask Before You Mix"

USP

The United States Pharmacopeia (USP) has information about medication safety available for patients and practitioners at its Web site: http://www.usp.org. Examples of information available include:

- "Guide to Help Consumers Manage the Benefits and Risks of Medication"
- "Ten Ways Consumers Can Help Ensure That Medication Errors are Avoided"
- "The Personal Medication Organizer"
- "Tips to Seniors to Help Reduce Medication Errors"

FDA

The U.S. Food and Drug Administration (FDA) has a list of materials for patients at its Web site: htpp://www.fda.gov/cder/consumer info/DPAdefault.htm. Examples include:

- "Don't Buy These Drugs Over the Internet or from Foreign Sources"
- "Drug Interactions: What You Should Know"
- "Over-the-Counter Drug Products"
- "When Using Medicine, Sometimes Two Rights Make a Wrong"

ISMP

The Institute for Safe Medication Practices (ISMP) (http://www.ismp.org) has a consumer newsletter with information for patients such as:

- "Why It's Important to Read the Labels of Your Medication"
- "How You Can Help Ensure Your Safety When Receiving Cancer Treatments"
- "How to Take Your Medications Safely"
- "Treat Medicine Samples with Respect"

TIPS FOR PRACTITIONERS

All practitioners need to remember who is number one—the patient—not themselves, and not those who employ them. You work for the good of the patient. Feeling the patient's vulnerability is part of your job as is doing your best for that patient. Avoid thinking about the next patient. Caring for the patient is what you vowed to do and you have a duty to carry this out.

Doctors also need patient safety information and education. The American Medical Association (AMA) has "Guidelines for Physicians for Counseling Patients About Prescription Medication" available at: http://www.ama-assn.org/ama/pub/article/2036-2401.html.

Pharmacists need to follow the law in counseling patients about their medication. The law (OBRA 90) states the pharmacist *will personally offer* to counsel the patient about his or her medication. Counseling patients about their medication does not mean telling them everything you know about the medication, nor does it take much time if you use the IHS method of counseling patients. This method informs patients, prevents errors, and fulfills your legal and professional duty to the patient.

Although nurses do not have a legal or professional duty to educate or inform patients about their medication, many nurses take on this role and perform this added responsibility admirably.

SUMMARY

Patients often feel frightened, embarrassed, and vulnerable, mostly because of their lack of understanding of health care, the unknowns about their illness, and the possibilities of harm from treatment. Many patients are intimidated by the health care system or are threatened by health care practitioners who are insensitive to patients' concerns and lack of understanding. This can lead to patients not taking their medication properly and to medication errors.

Most patients need to take more control of their health care and ask questions. Practitioners need to be more sensitive, more patient, or educate patients more about their medication. This will improve patient relationships, reduce medication errors, reduce practitioner liability, improve patient outcomes, and fulfill the practitioner's duty to the patient.

Chapter 17

Developing National and Local Plans to Improve Medication Safety

The Institute of Medicine (IOM) has published three books since 1999 with clear recommendations to improve patient safety.[1,2,3] Even though it was controversial regarding the number of medical errors, the first book, *To Err Is Human—Building a Safer Health System,* galvanized strong reaction from both the private and public sectors. During the years since this report, there has been a flurry of activity by many health care centers, by various professional health care organizations, and by the government to improve patient safety.

Although all the effort to improve patient and medication safety is to be commended, success is far from being achieved. This is most likely because of a haphazard and overlapping effort. Without a more coordinated effort, progress is hampered and we may be just "spinning our wheels." This chapter addresses the national landscape for improving medication safety and what needs to be done. It also addresses an organized approach to improving medication safety on a local level.

THE NATIONAL LANDSCAPE FOR IMPROVING MEDICATION SAFETY

Response to the First IOM Report

Although the seven recommendations in the first IOM report were well thought out, critics immediately focused on a micro issue in the report—the number of fatal medical errors estimated to occur yearly

Prescribed Medications and the Public Health
© 2006 by The Haworth Press, Inc. All rights reserved.
doi:10.1300/5688_17

(44,000 to 98,000)—instead of stepping back and seeing the big picture.[4] The report concluded that:

- The extent of harm that results from medical errors is great.
- Errors result from system failures, not people failures.
- Achieving acceptable levels of patient safety will require major system changes.
- A concerted national effort is needed to improve patient safety.

The IOM suggested a goal of a 50 percent decrease in medical errors within five years and laid out the following recommendations:

- Create a national center for patient safety.
- Mandate a reporting system for medical errors.
- Encourage voluntary reporting.
- Provide greater protection for data collected on patient safety and quality improvement purposes.
- Promote performance standards for people and organizations that emphasize safety.
- Emphasize the safe use of drugs through the FDA.

The public sector's response to the first report was swift. Within two weeks the U.S. Congress began a series of hearings, the president ordered a government feasibility study that resulted in affirming the IOM goals of a 50 percent decrease in medical errors within five years, and, the Agency for Healthcare Research and Quality (AHRQ) received $50 million to fund error-reduction research. Some state governments also responded by passing legislation, and a bill titled "The Medication Errors Reduction Act of 2001" was authored. The U.S. Food and Drug Administration (FDA) also stepped up its effort to improve medication safety and issued final rules for requiring bar coding on all pharmaceuticals down to the unit-of-use with few exceptions. Also, the U.S. Department of Health and Human Services (HHS) started developing the structure for a proposed national patient safety database.

The private sector's response was mostly confined to one well-organized and financed organization—the Leapfrog Group. This group is a coalition of many of the nation's leading companies. It identified three initial patient safety standards: (1) reduce medication prescribing errors using computerized physician order entry (CPOE) with decision support; (2) refer patients undergoing certain high-risk procedures to high-volume hospitals; and (3) staff intensive care units (ICUs) with intensivists—doctors certified in critical care medicine.

The Leapfrog Group recommends a plan to encourage compliance with its standards by presenting financial awards to providers who meet the safety standards.[5]

Many professional health care organizations have responded to the first IOM report as well.

American Hospital Association

Although (at the time of this writing) there is nothing on the American Hospital Association's (AHA) Web page (http://www.aha .org), to indicate that patient safety is a priority, the AHA (in partnership with Institute for Safe Medication Practice) has an extensive document titled "Pathways for Medication Safety: Leading a Strategic Planning Effort."[6]

American Medical Association

Information about patient safety legislation and an interest in rebuilding the faltering health care system in the United States is prominent on the American Medical Association's (AMA) Web site (htpp:// www.ama-assn.org).

American Nurses Association

The American Nurses Association (ANA) includes patient safety and advocacy as one of its five core initiatives (http://www.nursing world.org).

American Pharmacists Associations

The American Pharmacists Association (APhA) Foundation has an interest and notable resources on patient safety available for their members and for patients. For example, a Medication Safety Self Assessment Tool is available for community and ambulatory pharmacies, and a comprehensive, authoritative book to help those working in health care to improve safety. These are available at http://www.aphafoundation.org/Quality_Center/SafeMedication.htm.

American Society of Health-System Pharmacists

The American Society of Health-System Pharmacists (ASHP) has developed a Patient Safety Resource Center. The mission of the center is to foster fail-safe medication use in health systems with the leadership of pharmacists. The center fulfills its mission through advocacy, education, and research. A resource for patients is available at http://www.safemedication.com.

Healthcare Information and Management Systems Society (HIMSS)

HIMSS is the health care industry's membership organization that focuses on providing leadership for the best use of health care information technology and management systems for bettering human health. HIMSS has many patient safety resources on its Web site, such as position papers on improving the infrastructure of health care, implementing computerized physician order entry (CPOE), and an electronic medical record (http://www.himss.org/asp/abouthimss_homepage.asp).

Institute of Medicine

The Institute of Medicine (IOM) of the National Academy of Science has been the stimulus for many of the discussions and best thinking on how to improve the health care system in the United States. Its Web site is loaded with projects and position papers about improving patient safety (http://www.iom.edu/projects.asp).

Institute for Safe Medication Practices

The Institute for Safe Medication Practices (ISMP), which came into existence long before the first IOM report, focuses on improving the safety of medication practices. Many resources are available from ISMP's Web site (http://www.ismp.org). One important service ISMP provides is periodically distributing safety alerts about medication.

The Joint Commission on Accreditation of Healthcare Organizations (JCAHO)

JCAHO sets standards for health care organizations and inspects these organizations using these standards. In 2002, JCAHO (http://www.jcaho.org) approved the first National Patient Safety Goals. JCAHO established Patient Safety Goals for accredited organizations to address specific patient safety concerns. These goals can change from year to year. In 2004, the seven goals included:

1. To improve the accuracy of patient identification
2. To improve the effectiveness of communication among caregivers
3. To improve the safety of using high-alert medications
4. To eliminate wrong-site, wrong-patient, and wrong-procedure surgery
5. To improve the safety of using infusion pumps
6. To improve the effectiveness of clinical alarm systems
7. To reduce the risk of health-care-acquired infections

National Coordinating Council for Medication Error Reporting and Prevention (NCC MERP)

The NCC MERP was started in 1995 as a way for all health care organizations to meet quarterly to collaborate and cooperate in addressing the interdisciplinary causes of medication errors and to promote the safe use of medications. The NCC MERP Web site has recommendations about improving medication safety (http://www.nccmerp.org/) including a guideline on comparing medication error rates between institutions and recommendations to reduce medication errors in non-health care settings.

National Council on Patient Information and Education (NCPIE)

The NCPIE is a diverse coalition of over 130 organizations committed to safer, more effective medicine use through better communication. NCPIE's Web site www.talkaboutrx.org is designed to help consumers decide soundly about the use of their medicines.

National Patient Safety Foundation

The National Patient Safety Council (NPSF) states that they are the indispensable resource for organizations committed to improving the safety of patients. The NPSF research program's objective is to promote research on human and organizational error and to prevent accidents in health care. Located at NPSF's Web site (http://www.npsf.org/) are materials such as "Talking to Patients About Health Care Injury" and "The Impact of Staffing Shortages on Patient Safety."

The National Quality Forum (NQF)

The NQF (http://www.qualityforum.org) was created in 2000 to develop and carry out a national strategy for health care quality measurement and reporting. The NQF does its work through developing voluntary consensus standards. One project of the NQF was to set up a compendium of evidence-safe medication practices that can and should be widely implemented to reduce the likelihood of health care errors. This report was completed in 2003 and its executive summary is available at: http://www.qualityforum.org/txsafeexecsumm+order 6-8-03PUBLIC.pdf.

The United States Pharmacopeia (USP)

The USP has a long history of improving medication safety. Some current and prominent safety initiatives of USP include: two national medication error reporting systems, two medication error reporting systems (MER and MEDMARX), and an Expert Committee on Safe Medication Use. USP's Web site on patient safety (http://www.usp.org/patientSafety) has various resources to improve patient safety.

Organized health care settings responded to the first IOM report by trying to comply with new standards on patient safety set by JCAHO. Because the standards are comprehensive, many organizations have had a difficult time interpreting what JCAHO wants and find the standards ambitious. Many hospitals complained, especially smaller ones, that they did not have the resources and staffing to meet the standards. JCAHO has since clarified what is needed.

Response to the Second IOM Report

The second IOM report—*Crossing the Quality Chasm—A New Health System for the 21st Century*[2]—describes the current medical system in which doctors, other health professionals, hospitals, and other health care systems act as "silos, often providing care without the benefit of complete information about the patient's condition, medical history, services provided in other settings, or medications prescribed by other physicians."[2] An example of a major "silo" in health care is the community pharmacist who has no link to the patients' medical information. The IOM's silo theory led to a fourth report—*Health Professions Education: A Bridge to Quality.*[7] A major recommendation in this report is for the health professions to integrate a core set of competencies into their curricula.

The IOM went on to say that patient safety problems are caused by a system that "relies on outmoded systems to work." The solution, says the IOM, is to "redesign systems of care, including the use of information technology to support clinical and administrative processes."

The response to the second IOM report has been muted, probably because few people working within the health care system in the United States disagree with the IOM's diagnosis.

Response to the Third IOM Report

The IOM released its third report titled *Patient Safety—Achieving a New Standard for Care.*[3] This is the most comprehensive report of the three and is more prescriptive. Some areas in this report include: the elements of a health system infrastructure, a public-private partnership for setting data standards, an action plan for setting those standards, patient safety systems in health care settings, and patient safety reporting.

PROGRESS SINCE THE FIRST IOM REPORT

No one can argue that little work has been done to improve patient safety since the IOM report in 1999. The challenge to reduce medical errors by 50 percent in five years was taken up by many organizations.

The efforts of the IOM and AHRQ to promote developing standards applicable to the collection, coding, and classification of patient safety data are commendable. So are JCAHO's standards to improve patient safety in the organizations it accredits. The NQF effort to identify evidenced-based safe medication practices is a help to practitioners and the organizations where they work. Leapfrog's standards to improve patient safety provide incentives for health care organizations to improve their safety records. The USP's efforts to improve patient safety are commendable. However, is there any proof the IOM goal is being met?

Most health care professionals would probably say that the incidence and severity of medication-related morbidity and mortality has changed little. A 2004 report stated, "the number of hospital patients who die of preventable errors may be twice as high as previously estimated and shows no sign of decreasing."[8] The article went on to report that "the findings would make medical mistakes the third leading cause of death in the country. There is little evidence that patient safety has improved in the last five years."

To be fair, this small amount of progress is because the problem is an abyss and is complex. It has taken more time than expected to diagnose the problem, to make real fixes, and to carry out the changes. For example, work on the national electronic medical record started late. Some states started to develop their own medical error reporting systems ("silos" the IOM recommends should be avoided); the Senate (after five years) finally passed patient safety legislation to shield patient safety organizations (PSOs) and protect information sent to national reporting systems (there stills needs to be agreement with a House bill). Hospitals continue to deal with culture issues and lack of interdisciplinary cooperation, which limits progress.

However, much work has been done and there is optimism that the IOM goal will be met, not in five years, but maybe ten. Breakthroughs are needed to change patient safety culture in organizations, rebuild the health care infrastructure, appoint a national center on patient safety, protect medical error information sent to national reporting systems, and build a national electronic health record. Many feel this latter effort is the tipping point to improve patient safety. Challenges in developing a national electronic health record include developing a common terminology, data standards, privacy and security of patient data, and to show a return on investment for health care organizations.[9] HIMSS has provided a call-to-action position statement on changing the national health information infrastructure.[10]

LOCAL PLANS TO IMPROVE MEDICATION SAFETY

Health care facilities that need to improve patient safety need to think nationally, but act locally. Thinking nationally means keeping tuned into what is happening nationally about patient safety. Acting locally means implementing or improving procedures that are in line with (or at least not opposed to) national efforts that substantially improve patient safety.

The AHA's publication titled "Pathways for Medication Safety: Leading a Strategic Planning Effort" is a good place to start, even if you do not work in a hospital.[6] The document is comprehensive, yet easy to understand and follow. Another helpful resource is "Pharmacists Building a Safer Health System."[11] Recommendations in this article for hospital pharmacists to improve medication safety include:

- setting up an administrative structure for improving the medication-use system,
- helping create an environment of improvement,
- carrying out best practices,
- measuring performance of the medication-use system, and
- testing proposals that have the potential to improve medication use.

Although the steps are good, it is important to develop a process for an entire organization to improve patient safety. Such efforts may include:

1. taking the lead,
2. organizing the effort,
3. keeping the end in mind,
4. deciding on what's important,
5. developing the plan,
6. implementing the plan, and
7. assessing progress.

Taking the Lead

In every worthwhile effort there must be leadership. This leadership must come from the top of the organization if the effort is going to be successful. The leader must make it clear that improving patient safety is a top priority and must "walk the talk" by providing the resources and tools to carry out the goal. Simply talking about improving patient safety does not get it done. Employees and outside observers must see action, not just talk.

The management and supervisory climate decides how important patient safety is in an organization, how careful workers do their work, and how often they report violations in safety procedures or errors.[12] In 1995, a leading health care facility in Boston experienced two tragic medication errors resulting in one well-publicized death. After the error was discovered, the media, the public, and many health care professionals were riveted on the event. Once the dust settled, personnel at this hospital took a serious look at the way they were handling medication and performed a root cause analysis of the error. Two of their major findings included creating and committing to a culture of safety in their organization, and their health care executives needed to play an essential role in leading the patient safety initiatives.[13]

Organizing the Effort

Once the priority is set, the next step is to create an integrated patient safety team. A good way to learn how to build such a team is to study the way the Brigham and Women's Hospital (Boston) did this in 2001. "The team should work with individual departments and preexisting quality structures to drive changes to the systems of care that enable health care to become as safe as possible."[14]

Keeping the End in Mind

One of the most important principles of being effective is to keep the end in mind.[15] When it comes to patient safety at your health care facility, what will improved safety look like? What will be different? Another way to approach seeing the end is for the patient safety team to select one major determinant of success—such as no medical error deaths, or cutting medication errors in half each year until there are almost none, or reducing harmful medication errors by a certain percent each year.

Deciding What Is Important

Once the goal is set, it is time to write objectives to achieve the goal. This requires thinking about what an ideal medication-use system looks like. There are many good ways to do this.[16,17] One way is to ask those working in the medication-use system daily what the problems are and how they can be corrected. Once this is done, it is time to think about building a new medication-use system. The best form of planning is to develop a vision of what the ideal system would look like. This needs to be done with no restrictions.[18] Next, the patient safety team needs to look back at how the system is constructed now, then work toward making the current system into the ideal system.

Developing the Plan

The patient safety plan needs broad input both within and outside the patient safety team, wide distribution, thorough discussion, adjustments, and commitments before a plan is implemented. This may be the most difficult part of the process as it takes time and there will be many different opinions on what the problems and solutions are. Reaching consensus on the plan may be difficult, but if needed can be achieved by using *nominal group technique*.[19]

Implementing the Plan

Once the patient safety plan is approved, the real work begins. To do this effectively, the plan should be prioritized and funds budgeted to get the expected results. To be most effective, an implementation team should be appointed and this should be a full-time job for some of the team members. The team leader should be titled the "Patient Safety Officer," and he or she should be given the authority to do whatever it takes to get the job done. Also, the team needs to provide effective and frequent communication.

Assessing Progress

Progress needs to be checked against predetermined targets and any targets not being met should be assessed to discover why the intended progress was not met. Report cards need to be posted to display to all how the effort is going. At the top of the report card list should be progress on the overall goal.

TOOLS FOR IMPROVING MEDICATION SAFETY

Several good tools are available for helping to improve patient and medication safety. One is from MEDSTAT.[20] Another helpful tool for hospitals is available from Southeastern Pennsylvania's Regional Medication Safety Programs for Hospitals (RMSPH).[21] Community pharmacists interested in improving medication safety may be interested in a self-assessment tool from ISMP (http://www.ismp.org).[22] Another publication is HCPro's *Briefings on Patient Safety.*

The USP has a wonderful publication titled *Advancing Patient Safety in U.S. Hospitals.*[23] This publication contains "real world" case studies of how a diverse number of hospitals are working to improve patient and medication safety. Other published case studies are also available.[24,25]

SUMMARY

In 1999, the IOM rang the warning bell on the problem of medical and medication errors and many heard the loud ring. Two other IOM publications have followed. These publications document how and why the United States health care system is in need of major repair, and what might be done to fix it. The response to these reports, both public and private, has been striking and a commendable effort is taking place to improve patient and medication safety. The IOM's challenge of reducing medical errors by 50 percent in five years has not been met, not because of lack of effort, but because the problem is so deep and so complex. It has taken five years to assess and reach consensus on how to get the job done. Therefore, the IOM's goal may be off by five years.

Health care organizations and professionals need to think nationally, but act locally. This can be done by knowing what is going on nationally in the patient safety arena and identifying a major goal for patient safety, assessing their patient safety environment, making a plan for dramatically improving safety, and assessing progress against the goal.

Chapter 18

Improving Medication Safety: Pursuing Optimization or Perpetuating Illusions?

The previous chapters have shown that medication safety is a complex and widespread problem not only in the United States but in other nations as well. Many of these medication-use safety issues were identified as early as 1987.[1] However, there was little notice until 1999 when the first IOM report showed the extent of medical errors.[2] Despite all the publicity, data indicating that drug-induced mortality and morbidity have been reduced since 1987 are sparse. Given the population growth alone, it might not be surprising to learn these numbers could have increased. This perplexity begs the question—why isn't this important problem being corrected? The more powerful question though would focus on why society and health professionals have failed to adopt methods that facilitate self-correction as an integral part of the health care delivery system.

This final chapter addresses some of the macro issues associated with the medication safety problem, considers some public policy issues that merit closer examination, and offers a brief explanation why shortcomings persist.

SOME MACRO ISSUES AND PROPOSED SOLUTIONS

The problems associated with medication safety problems can be divided into six general areas: manufacturing, regulation, distribution, practice, drug use, and the health care environment.

Prescribed Medications and the Public Health
© 2006 by The Haworth Press, Inc. All rights reserved.
doi:10.1300/5688_18

Manufacturing

The pharmaceutical industry needs to support constructive efforts to improve safer use of the medications they manufacture. Past behavior, though, cautions us that more rigorous methods of surveillance by the FDA will be required to help close the gap between ideal use patterns and contemporary practices.

Drug Packaging

Many medication mix-ups and errors occur because of how drugs are packaged and named.[3] The sales component of most pharmaceutical companies is so strong that it often overpowers the good science and the good sense of the company. The marketing department wants the drug packaging to be recognized to make a statement about the company. This management strategy means that information about the drug and its strength becomes a subordinate element in designing containers. Each company's "cloned" packaging has led to errors. Look-alike packaging, and small, less prominent placement of drug strengths on packaging may contribute to enhanced patient risk. Pharmaceutical companies point out the more fundamental problem lies in trained health personnel failing to read labels. Nevertheless, the evidence seems persuasive that critical limits in packing procedures still account for many preventable drug safety problems.

The pharmaceutical industry should explore the contributions its packaging makes to serious medication errors. USP's large hospital error reporting database (MEDMARX) could help drug manufacturers undertake this task.

Look-Alike and Sound-Alike Drug Names

The literature is filled with reports in which a drug either looked like or sounded like another drug and an error occurred that harmed or killed a patient. This problem has persisted for over 40 years and little progress has been made in correcting it. The major problem is that pharmaceutical companies think trade naming their products provides a competitive edge. However, the proof for this hypothesis is lacking. Because there are no regulations that require pharmaceutical companies to test prospective names for new products against existing product names, drugs continue to be introduced that look like or sound like other drug products.

Medication morbidity and mortality associated with sound-alike and look-alike drug name errors represent a long-standing problem meriting scrutiny federally. At a minimum, manufacturers should voluntarily compare their proposed product names with existing products to see if they sound alike or look like another product. However, the most effective remedy would be abolishing trade names. Yet pharmaceutical firms that have developed sophisticated methods of subverting policy intervention can be expected to reject such a proposal. One alternative might allow exclusive use of the brand name until the patent expires. After that, however, nomenclature could revert to either the established name or trade name followed by name of the labeler.

Drug Strengths

In his 2001 book, Jay S. Cohen accused drug companies of recommending starting doses that are much higher than needed.[4] One clear example is documented with antihypertensive medications. The recommended starting doses for 23 antihypertensive drugs are commonly twice as high as what is recommended by the Joint National Committee on Prevention, Detection, Evaluation, and Treatment of High Blood Pressure. Cohen concludes that using starting doses recommended by pharmaceutical companies leads to more side effects and adverse drug reactions that cause some patients to stop taking their medication.

The pharmaceutical industry could make a major contribution to the national welfare if it sponsored scientific studies that examine why patients are splitting their solid oral medication, the need for lower strength at the initial dosing, as well as the special requirements of pediatric and elderly patients.

Lack of Standardized Imprint Codes on Tablets and Capsules

Drug companies are allowed to put any identifying marks on their tablets. The problem is that this coding is not standardized and the tablets from one company may have the same imprint code as tablets from another company. Yet the products may not be the same drug or strength. Thus identification of a single tablet or capsule becomes problematic.[5]

Imprint codes on solid oral medications (tablets and capsules) should be standardized. The USP has been studying this issue and has formulated methods for controlling this problem. Unfortunately, the pharmaceutical industry is fighting this idea vigorously by charging that it will cost too much. However, the cost of introducing this safety measure is likely to be insignificant as the social and safety gains should be great.

Misleading Marketing

Cohen accuses drug manufacturers of slanting their research, skewing their findings to make their drugs look more favorable than they are, manipulating the publishing process, and threatening researchers planning to publish negative findings.[4]

A 2003 study of 100 promotional claims for blood pressure and cholesterol-lowering drugs in medical journals found that 44 percent of the references to research studies did not support what the advertisements were claiming.[6] Several drug companies have been accused of (and some have admitted to) minimizing the safety risks and making misleading claims about some of their drugs.[7] The FDA is finally starting to monitor what drug companies say about their products.[8,9]

Pharmaceutical manufacturers may have promotional budgets 10 to 50 times greater than quality control resources allocated to ensure the manufacturing quality of the same products. The implication seems clear—a national study might be indicated to discover the prevalence and significance of this concern throughout the pharmaceutical industry. This may be a problem of great significance. One wonders what additional problems lurk in the manufacturing and drug-use process that have never been identified. How big is this iceberg that represents negative social outcomes?

The sales hustle is so intense that big companies can contact 150,000 doctors every week to pitch a new drug.[10] The direct-to-consumer television advertising used by pharmaceutical companies makes it seem like there is a drug for every ill and that only the new and expensive "blockbuster" drugs will work. Pill popping may be replacing healthy habits.[11] Therefore, permission for direct-to-consumer advertising by the pharmaceutical manufacturers should be rescinded.

Drug companies fund about 80 percent of medical research. Thus, studies that raise doubts about a medicine's safety and effectiveness are rarely published.[12] Medical journals often focus on studies of medical breakthroughs rather than on negative or confirmatory studies. Drugs companies have resisted making such information public. Such cavalier attitudes keep prescribers in the dark and place patients at risk. If the drug companies do not make such information available, remedial legislation or regulation should be enacted to make it compulsory.

Overbearing Influence on Practice

Dr. Arnold Relman, editor emeritus of the *New England Journal of Medicine,* published an essay on the pharmaceutical industry in which he contends, "The American health care system cannot live without the pharmaceutical industry, but it may not be able to live with it either, unless the industry is greatly reformed."[13] Relman goes on to say the pharmaceutical industry "uses its great wealth and influence to ensure favorable government policies," and that it has "with acquiescence of the medical profession addicted to drug company largesse, assumed a role in directing medical treatment, clinical research, and physician education that is totally inappropriate for a profit-driven industry." In a commentary, one well-known academic and national health insurance consultant said Relman's critique of the drug industry "tends to be more understated than exaggerated."[14] Unfortunately, nothing in this arena seems likely to change without some form of social regulation.

Regulation

Regulations can often provide broad and dramatic improvements or can hinder positive developments.

The FDA

The United States Food and Drug Administration has an awesome responsibility to ensure the drug supply is safe and effective. This is not an easy process.[15] The scientific rigor with which randomized controlled trials are conducted is the first line of social defense to ensure the safety and efficacy of medications intended for public consumption. The FDA represents the nation's control system to confirm these claims.[16] How well do they do this? According to some—not well.[17]

"Industry-supported reforms have provided the FDA major resources to focus on the approval of new drugs, but once these drugs are out in the market, the picture changes dramatically."[18] Thomas Moore reported that the FDA is in crisis and even the approval process is in question.[19] Between September 1997 and April 2000, nine drugs had to be removed from the market for safety reasons. Moore says, "in the words of Carol Scheman, an FDA deputy commissioner in the 1990s, the nation's system for keeping track of the bad effects of prescription drugs is appallingly bad." Moore later quotes a former FDA commissioner as saying the FDA's system for keeping tabs on how and when drugs hurt people is "terrible, and when we know enough, it takes a lot to get the drug off the market."

Some feel that the FDA has many times acted "too little, too late." For example, the dangers of ephedra in over-the-counter (OTC) drugs has been known for a long time.[20] It has been linked to more than 150 deaths and dozens of heart attacks and strokes, and was finally banned by the FDA in April of 2004.[21] Often, a state will have enough sense and courage to ban a dangerous drug before the FDA gets around to it. For example, the state of New York banned ephedra in OTC drugs in 2003.[22]

Another danger known for some time is the possibility of suicidal thoughts and actions when taking antidepressants. It has taken a long time to admit and accept this and only recently has the FDA required suicidal warnings on antidepressant labels.[23] One wonders how long it will take for the FDA to act on teenage cough syrup abuse,[24] and remove OTC products long known to be purchased for their pseudoephrine content which is the starting ingredient for home-cooked methamphetamine, a CNE stimulant.

Again, it took a state (New York) to uncover that a major drug company made false claims about the safety of one of its products by excluding negative data.[25] Other problems with the FDA include:

1. not following up on more than half of the product research that drug companies routinely promise as a condition of sales approval,[26]
2. not acting for 78 days after it was decided that an ad by a drug manufacturer was misleading,[27]
3. approving a drug despite negative votes by one of its advisory panels, and
4. no long-term testing of drugs after approval for marketing.[28]

The FDA is staffed with well-qualified, dedicated experts. It may be that they do not have the resources to get the job done or political interference overwhelms scientific findings, or both. The FDA is no match for the deep pockets of the drug industry that has increased promotion for its products from a little over $8 billion in 1995 to over $15 billion in 1999.[8] Moreover, the drug industry in the past has had the ears of many in Congress.

Strengthening the FDA should be a priority of Congress. Following are a few ways in which the responsibilities of the FDA might be improved:[13,29]

- The FDA's dependence on user fees from the pharmaceutical industry should be replaced by government support.
- New drug applications should include the drug's effectiveness with existing products.
- FDA advisory committee members should be required to declare any conflicts of interest.
- Direct-to-consumer advertising of prescription drugs should be eliminated.
- The drug industry should not be the sole evaluator of its own products.
- New drug applications should be required to contain genome-based drug data.
- All new drug names and drug packaging should undergo "failure mode analysis" before being approved.

National Center for Patient Safety

One of the major recommendations of the first IOM report was that Congress should create a center for patient safety. This addition to our clinical and social armamentarium has yet to happen. However, most practitioners seem unaware of the nature and power of this function and the status of this recommendation.

A national center would make patient and medication safety a national priority, in the same way as the National Transportation Safety Board (NSTB) did for aviation safety.[17] The IOM recommends the center be responsible for setting "the national goals for patient safety, track progress in meeting these goals, and issue an annual report to the President and Congress on patient safety."[2] It was further recommended that the center "develop knowledge and understanding of errors in health care by developing a research agenda, funding Centers of Excellence, evaluating methods for identifying and preventing errors, and funding dissemination and communication activities to improve safety."

Unfortunately, the IOM recommendations reveal at least one drawback—they focus solely on medical errors. If maximum benefits for patients and society are to be achieved, a more comprehensive management model is essential.[3] All cases of iatrogenic morbidity or mortality associated with any form of treatment should be reported. Why not include adverse drug reactions? Why not include other forms of treatment such as vaccines, medical gases, and medical devices?

The primary roles of a national center for patient safety should be to:

- Receive patient safety reports: The center should be the central repository for reports from all health care settings on any serious morbidity and mortality events associated with medical intervention. The reports should:
  —be standardized and anonymous;
  —include mechanisms—medical errors, adverse drug reactions, allergic drug reactions and drug interactions;
  —include all interventions—drugs, vaccines, medical devices, medical gases, surgery and invasive techniques; and
  —be received from all health care settings—hospitals, emergency rooms, clinics, managed care organizations, long-term care, home care, community pharmacies, and doctors' offices, regardless of health insurance coverage.
- Conduct patient safety research
- Identify evidence-based safe medication practices

- Disseminate information and issue safety alerts
- Educate practitioners and consumers
- Set patient safety standards
- Recommend rules to the FDA and CDC
- Recommend public policy

To achieve these objectives, a national center for patient safety will depend on a model electronic medical record system for the nation and strong funding as a public health unit in the private sector. A model organization may be derived from more intensive study of the National Transportation Safety Board (NTSB). Since 1975, this agency has focused extensively on exploring why things go wrong in transportation and on building safer systems. "Between 1990 and 1994, the U.S. airline death rate was less than one-third the rate experienced in mid-century. In 1998, there were no deaths in the United States in commercial aviation."[2]

The NTSB is organized to perform at "arms length" from the Department of Transportation and other government agencies despite being a federally funded agency. This minimizes conflicts of interest. Recent breakdowns in systems developed to serve as a double-check at NASA and Wall Street highlight the importance of separating risk assessment from risk management. Based on this, vaccine safety should be separated from vaccine promotion (e.g., the CDC), drug safety should be separated from drug approval (e.g., FDA), and both should be made the responsibility of a national center for patient safety.[30]

Start-up funds and most operating expenses would come from public funds for public health. Furthermore, other funds would be generated to offset operating expenses by charging for "extra services" provided by the center such as allowing academic researchers access to its anonymous databases.

An Electronic Health Record

We will never get to the truth about medical and medication errors and ADEs until we have national electronic health records. The IOM has recommended eight core functions that electronic health records (EHRs) should perform:

1. health and information data,
2. result management,
3. order management,
4. decision support,
5. electronic communication and connectivity,
6. patient support,
7. administrative processes, and
8. reporting.[31]

The eHealth Initiative has authored recommendations on how EHRs should be designed and implemented.[32]

President George W. Bush has been trying to drag medicine into the twenty-first century by offering the challenge of making EHRs available for most Americans within ten years.[33,34] However, doubters worry that this push could be an unfounded mandate, and some doctors worry that rigid guidelines for treating patients would be imposed. Yet the social deficit continues. The need for computerized prescribing and an electronic infrastructure for better medication use was clearly recognized in the mid-1990s yet is ignored.[35]

Require the Mandatory Reporting
of All Fatal Medical Errors

Only a tiny proportion of ADEs is ever documented and reported. Thus, reported ADEs represent only the visible portion of an iceberg. There are many reasons for this, namely: being too busy, not making this a priority, not wanting to get someone else in trouble, and fear of retribution. Lack of information about ADEs restricts analysis and forming preventive measures.

Only better reporting will help uncover what's below the surface of the iceberg, but this will only happen if reporting fatal medical errors and ADEs becomes compulsory. Such reporting, if protected from liability, seems likely to yield meaningful data from which meaningful patient-care solutions can be formed.

Distribution

Among others, current public health safety issues on drug distribution include:

1. drugs from other countries,
2. counterfeit drugs,
3. drugs ordered by means of the Internet,
4. potentially harmful drugs being introduced as a possible means of a terrorist threat, and
5. not using unit-dose and closed-loop drug distribution systems.

Drugs from Foreign Countries

The principal debate about using drugs from other countries regards cost versus safety. It is unreasonable, but fashionable, to bash the FDA and the current administration for not allowing foreign drugs to enter the United States. The FDA acts within the constraints placed on it by Congress through legislation. Yet the FDA clearly is looking the other way when U.S. citizens buy small supplies of drugs from, e.g., Canada. This finesse policy may be expected to prevail until Congress makes up its mind about the legality of drug importation.

The public and media are concerned about the cost of drugs in the United States versus the cost in other countries, especially Canada, where the government controls the cost of medication. The difference in cost (i.e., savings) is often 40 to 50 percent less than in the United States. This controversy has been heightened by recent Medicare legislation that claims to save most Medicare recipients an average of 10 to 25 percent of their medication costs. However, recent information from the American Association of Retired Persons (AARP) showed the average price to wholesalers for the 200 most-used brand name drugs increased 7.2 percent during the 12 months ending March 31, 2004. This increase is more than triple the inflation rate of 2 percent.[36] This difference has fueled the call for letting foreign drugs into the country, especially from Canada.

Former FDA Associate Commissioner, John M. Taylor III, recently testified in drug importation hearings before the Senate Commerce Committee. Mr. Taylor said that a recent study by the FDA of cross-border prescription drug shipments found that 88 percent of the parcels entering the United States from abroad "contained unapproved drugs that could pose significant safety problems" for patients in the United States.[37] Thus, the scope of the problem extends beyond the ostensible cost of medication.

Counterfeit Drugs

In July 2004, the FDA uncovered counterfeit drugs that several Americans had purchased in Mexico.[38] One claiming to be the cholesterol drug Zocor contained no active drug, and one claiming to be a generic muscle relaxant was subpotent. Counterfeit drugs thus constitute a growing problem when they enter community or institutional pharmacy inventories or are purchased over the Internet.

In May 2000, thousands of vials of epoetin (Procrit), a drug used to treat anemia associated with chronic renal failure, were labeled as containing 40,000 units. The drugs were found to contain only 2,000 units.[39] Later, other vials were found that contained nothing but Miami tap water. There have been similar findings with the drug atorvastatin (Lipitor) and contraceptive patches sold under the Ortho Evra brand name. Although the economic issues for public policy are more complex than implied, the potential for public health safety alone seems enough to warrant systematic congressional examination.

Internet Drugs

In mid-2004, researchers at the Government Accountability Office (GAO) bought 11 different drugs from 68 Internet pharmacies in 12 countries. The GAO concluded that "many drugs are mishandled, missing warning information, or sold without proper prescriptions."[40] Some of the Internet pharmacies where GAO purchased drugs without a prescription sold narcotics, and most asked buyers to complete an online questionnaire, but did not require any examination by a doctor.[41]

The Institute for Safe Medication Practices (ISMP) advises patients to look for the National Association of Boards of Pharmacy (NABP) Verified Internet Pharmacy Practice Sites (VIPPS) seal on the Web site to ensure proper licensing and safety.

Drugs Used for Terrorism

Perhaps the greatest drug threat to public safety is a potential terrorist attack using drugs adulterated with poisons or pathogens.[42] One only needs to consider the anthrax scare after the September 11 tragedy (with still no culprit apprehended) to see the major ramifications for the nation if a similar event should occur. Terrorists could use Web sites as points of distribution then disappear quickly without a trace.

To help nullify this scenario all drug products should have radio frequency identification tags (RFID) for tracking, be easily identified with standardized imprints and bar codes, and have clearly identified names and strengths on all packages. Such a strategy should yield social benefits over cost. Unfortunately, regulation, based on good data, may be our only real hope.

Not Using Unit-Dose and Closed-Loop Drug Distribution Systems

All organized health care settings should use evidence-based safe-drug distribution systems. JCAHO should require the unit-dose drug distribution system in all health care institutions it accredits. This proven drug distribution system should also be required for HMOs that care for inpatients, and for all nursing homes. All medication-use systems should be required to be "closed looped," that is, the drug, the patient, the time, and the nurse are identified and checked before the medication is administered to the patient.

Practice

Many practice issues need to be addressed to improve medication safety. The following problems require prompt social and professional attention.

Blame

It is easy to blame someone for making a medication error, especially if you or someone you love is harmed. However, to err is human—everyone makes errors.

Although blame may be emotionally rewarding for the person doing the blaming, it does little to prevent error reoccurrence. Medication errors will remain frozen in the iceberg model until people feel safe in reporting their errors as well as the errors of others.

When policy relies on the blame model, we run the risk of significant adverse drug events going underground and thus avoiding reporting. This outcome results in not enough data on what contributes to medication errors and what could be done to prevent them in the future. Health professionals who make errors already blame and punish themselves. Rarely does a medication error occur because of the omission or commission of one individual, but is usually a combination of system errors.[43] Thus, blame does more harm than good.

Society needs to develop more effective control mechanisms that transcend this myopic solution. Federal regulations should be put in place to protect those who report medication errors. Recent congressional actions, however, may raise the likelihood that this reluctance can be overcome.[44]

Shortages of Nurses and Pharmacists

There has been a chronic shortage of nurses and pharmacists in the United State since the late 1990s. Schools of nursing and pharmacy have pushed their enrollments to the maximum, and many colleges and universities have started new nursing and pharmacy programs. However, the shortage continues, largely because of the increased intensity of care, new roles for pharmacists and nurses, and the baby boom generation that is starting to reach the age of 60. Without significant gains in professional productivity via computerization of medical records and related functions, and if more useful means are not found to augment health labor supply, the graying of the American population can be expected to produce significant shortages among health professionals.

Low-cost student loans could stimulate admissions to nursing and pharmacy schools and grants to schools would help develop the infrastructure needed to train these future practitioners. Government subsidies also could facilitate efforts by health professional schools to improve their curricula in medication safety.

The shortage of health care workers is already producing negative effects in the form of more errors. A recent IOM study reported that "tired and grumpy nurses forget to wash their hands, give the wrong medication, and waste hours on paperwork."[45] A study in 2004 showed that when nurses work shifts longer than 12 hours, the chance of an error nearly triples.[46] Most errors in this study—about 58 percent—involved administering medication.

Not Enough Technology

Although technology support for those who care for patients is available and is a significant help in preventing adverse drug events (ADEs), it is expensive and therefore its use is minimal. Computer alerts that signal a possible dangerous situation when a drug is prescribed are lacking in most hospitals. Lack of linkage between pharmacy and laboratory information represents another barrier. All prescription pads and paper medication order forms should be outlawed and destroyed. Only those electronic medication orders verified as being authored by a practitioner licensed to prescribe medication should be honored.

Lack of clinical information about patients is a disaster waiting to happen. Software programs to detect potentially harmful drug interactions are deficient and appalling. "Some grocery stores have better technology than our hospitals and clinics."[37]

Implementing some of the most rewarding evidence-based safe-medication practices (such as computerized physician order entry with decision support and closed-loop medication systems) can be expensive but cost effective. Providing incentives for health care facilities to set up evidence-based safe-medication practices will improve patient safety. One incentive may be to increase government reimbursement for Medicare and Medicaid patients. Providing low-cost loans to health care institutions to invest in technology to improve patient safety also might work.

Reliable Drug Information

Doctors and pharmacists need reliable computer systems and accurate, unbiased, and up-to-date drug information when prescribing and dispensing. The current system of allowing pharmaceutical sales representatives to sway doctors to use their products is unacceptable and shortchanges patients who need medicines that are most likely to optimize patient outcomes, not what a drug company wants the patient to receive.

A model for providing unbiased and up-to-date drug information to doctor and pharmacists has been proposed that would far surpass the way drug information is provided now.[48] This basic measure, coupled with computer support for clinical decisions, should help provide and improve the drug information now provided to doctors and pharmacists. This proposal calls for the "establishment of a National Drug Education Foundation that would employ some 4,000 therapeutic consultants, subsidize professional journals and schools, develop regional drug information centers, and conduct various related functions."[48] The cost of this model system is estimated to be well under one-seventh of current drug outlays for drug promotion and information.

Medication Use

Various problems are associated with the use of medication. The following problems need systematic study and satisfactory resources.

Tablet Splitting

Some people split tablets into halves or quarters. Two reasons for doing this are to titrate the dose, or, the smallest-strength tablet is an excessive quantity for some patients.[4] Another reason to split tablets is to save money. Several insurance plans have promoted splitting double-strength tablets to reduce medication costs. Furthermore, sometimes tablets meant for adults are split because the proper pediatric dose is not available.

A 2002 study by the United States Pharmacopeia (USP)—the organization that sets drug standards in the United States—found that of 11 razor-split products, eight failed uniformity testing.[49] The USP concluded that "the general practice of splitting tablets is not recommended, particularly for narrow therapeutic index drugs, because of lack of dose uniformity in the resulting fragments."

The obvious solutions are for the pharmaceutical manufacturers to: (1) make the dosage strengths needed by patients, and (2) price the products in such a way so that patients are not forced to split tablets to save money.

Improper Use of Medications in the Elderly

According to a study of 1999 insurance claims, one in five elderly Americans filled prescriptions for drugs considered inappropriate and harmful for older patients.[50] At a series of screenings in Atlanta in the fall of 2003, 54 of 420 senior adults were found to have a medication problem, ranging from unnecessary medications to expired drugs.[51] One study of medication-related reasons elderly patients are readmitted to the hospital found the most common issues to be:

1. unexpected adverse drug reactions,
2. not taking the medication as prescribed,
3. overdose,
4. lack of necessary drug therapy, and
5. underdosing.[52]

A review of records over a two-year period from more than 5,300 assisted living facilities in seven states found common medication errors. These included failure to follow prescription orders, neglecting to make sure residents take their medication, and inappropriate drug administration.[53] A well-written commentary describing the problems associated with medication use among the elderly is available.[54]

Additional problems include patients not taking their medication as prescribed. Many studies report that less than 50 percent of patients take their medication as prescribed. Paternalism is a lingering problem that can be dichotomized into health professionals thinking "I am the expert and know what is best for you," and, many patients become submissive in the presence of medical authority. Patients who fail to take an active role in their care are more vulnerable and therefore more likely to experience medication misadventures.

Health care practitioners can improve the quality of treatment when they bring their knowledge and skill to help patients achieve positive health outcomes. Implementation of this requires intensive, research-based support to show the most effective means of such integration. Doctors, pharmacists, and nurses need to be sensitive to their patients' lack of knowledge about medical conditions and terminology, as well as their fears and desires. Health care practitioners should include patients on the health care team, let them ask good questions, and take responsibility for their health and care.

The Hospital Environment

Some important changes are needed in the hospital environment to improve medication safety. Hospital pharmacists and risk managers have worked to ensure that medication errors are documented, reported, and studied, however, their findings and recommendations often don't receive much support from hospital administration. Since the IOM report, JCAHO has strengthened its standards on medication errors. This has put pressure on nurses and pharmacists to do more reporting. Unfortunately, many nurses and pharmacists say they have not been given satisfactory resources to deal with these new standards.

IS PROGRESS BEING MADE?

It is approaching the seven-year mark since the IOM warned about patient safety, and it is time to assess its progress. Five well-known experts working in medication safety were asked to comment on progress since the first IOM report. All comments were similar and best summed up by the comments of one person (who would like to remain anonymous) who said:

> We have made small but real progress in creating awareness, and with some regulatory levers, especially JCAHO and Leapfrog, have gotten the attention and activity in every institution and sector which is a big deal. Measurable gains in actual safety are less palpable.

Furthermore, several public critiques about progress since the first IOM report have been less favorable.[55,56] In addition, many books published over the past 25 years corroborate various aspects of our national problem of medication safety. Selected examples include:

- *Confessions of a Medical Heretic.* Robert S. Mendelsohn, Contemporary Books, Inc., Chicago, IL: 1979.
- *The Wrong Kind of Medicine?* Charles Medawar, Social Audit, Ltd., London: 1984.
- *Tragedies from Drug Therapy.* Ronald B. Stewart, Charles C Thomas Publisher, Ltd., Springfield, IL: 1985.
- *Bitter Pills: Inside the Hazardous World of Legal Drugs.* Stephen Fried, Bantam Books, New York: 1998.
- *Worst Pills—Best Pills.* Sid M. Wolfe, Pocket Books, New York: 1999.
- *Demanding Medical Excellence.* Michael L. Millenson, The University of Chicago Press, Chicago, IL: 1997, 1999.

- *Overdose—The Case Against Drug Companies.* Jay S. Cohen, Jeremy P. Tarcher, Putnam, New York: 2001.
- *Escape Fire.* Donald M. Berwick. The Commonwealth Fund, New York: 2002.
- *Preventing Medication Errors and Improving Drug Therapy Outcomes.* Charles D. Hepler and Richard Segal, CRC Press, Boca Raton, FL: 2003.
- *Medicines Out of Control?: Antidepressants and the Conspiracy of Goodwill.* Charles Medawar, Aksant Academic Press, Amsterdam: 2004.
- *Powerful Medicines: The Benefits, Risks, and Cost of Prescription Drugs.* Jerry Avorn, Random House, Inc., New York: 2004.
- *The Truth About the Drug Companies: How They Deceive Us and What to Do About It.* Marcia Angell, Random House, New York: 2004.

POCKETS OF RESISTANCE

Why Has There Not Been More Progress?

Most of the problems and potential solutions to the medication-error problem have been known long before the 1999 IOM report. Medication error rates have been what they have been for years. Retarded progress can be attributed chiefly to four reasons:

1. stubborn, unconvinced hospital administrators,
2. unbelieving doctors,
3. an overpowering, and at times, arrogant pharmaceutical industry, and
4. a love affair with haphazard incrementalism.

Stubborn, Unconvinced Hospital Administrators

The increased safety associated with the gold standard of institutional drug distribution—unit dose—has been known since the early 1960s. Yet there are still hospitals in this country that do not use this evidence-based medication system. Moreover, bar codes have been available for over 20 years—every supermarket uses them. The increased safety offered by bar coding and automated medication dispensing devices has been public knowledge for over ten years, yet most hospitals lack these technological solutions. Studies have shown a dramatic drop in preventable medication errors when CPOE with CDSS is implemented, yet only a few hospitals have chosen to employ this basic safety strategy.[57]

Studies also show that the use of clinical pharmacists in patient care areas reduces morbidity, mortality, and cost of medication. Nevertheless, most pharmacists perform their professional functions in hospital basements. One reason for these managerial shortfalls is that few hospital administrators today have patient care backgrounds—most have training in business. They do not relate to patient care as much as they do to financial ledger sheets. A second reason is that these techniques have not been shown to be cost effective. Patient safety should be a cost consideration. A third reason is that patient safety is a lower priority than equipment, brick and mortar, new catheterization laboratories, and buying MRIs. Hospital accounts claim these yield a return on investment whereas patient care outlays just increase the cost of doing business.

Unbelieving Doctors

Soon after the IOM report was published a blistering letter to the editor was published in *JAMA*.[58] The essence of the critique was the extent of morbidity and mortality from medical errors could not possibly be correct. This critique was followed by a recent report stating that only 5 percent of doctors viewed medical errors as one of the nation's most important health care issues.[59] The number one health care issue in the eyes of doctors was the cost of medical malpractice insurance and lawsuits. Medication errors seldom surfaced on the radar screen of professional perception.

An Overpowering and, at Times, Arrogant Pharmaceutical Industry

Despite making drugs that improve the quality of health, the pharmaceutical industry often is uncooperative and self-serving.[4] Obstacles include:

1. eliminating look-alike and sound-alike drug names,
2. eliminating or having a time limit on the use of trade names,

3. changing packaging and labeling to be safer,
4. using standardized imprint codes on oral tablets and capsules, and
5. making recommended doses higher than they need to be.

Common arguments the pharmaceutical industry uses for not making these changes include:

1. huge investments in research (clinical, but also marketing),
2. high retooling costs to change packaging, labeling, and imprint codes on drugs, and
3. lack of data that any change will result in better safety.

Haphazard Incrementalism

Haphazard incrementalism is defined as applying Band-Aids on a problem where major surgery is indicated. This phenomenon is the cause of many problems in the U.S. health care system, especially the infrastructure. A prime example is the medication-use system, which needs to be reviewed, questioned, and overhauled, but instead is merely "patched up."[60]

WHAT IS NEEDED?

Several immediate actions are required to speed improvement in medication safety. *First* is a political, professional, and public "buy-in" that medication errors are a real social problem that can negatively impact over 100 million Americans who enter the delivery system each year. *Second,* we need system redesign. Every hospital should employ a medication safety officer (a clinician) and a health safety engineer. Failure mode and human factor analyses should be routine funtions in health care business. *Third,* continuous quality improvement (CQI) is needed. The medication-use system should be continually monitored and improvements made without major cost-effective analyses and negotiations through layers of administrative approval. The *fourth* need, and the most important, is leadership. Who will lead the way on improving medication safety? It is doubtful that it will be the government or private enterprise. Our greatest hope lies in a coalition of health care practitioners, patient safety engineers, and concerned consumer groups.

The *last* action needed to start a blaze of passion for improving medication safety is what Malcolm Gladwell talks about in his book, *The Tipping Point.*[61] A "tipping point" is that magic moment when an idea, trend, or social behavior crosses a threshold, tips, and spreads like wildfire.

Gladwell discusses three rules for tipping points: (1) the law of a few; (2) the stickiness factor; and (3) the power of context. The law of a few says that only a few people are needed to achieve a tipping point, but these people have special skills. The *maven* knows something good when he or she sees it. The *connector* networks the idea with many people, and, the *salesman* sells the good idea. Yet the idea must also be *sticky*—there must be a way to package the idea to make it irresistible. Last, ideas are exquisitely sensitive to the power of context. The idea must come at the right time and at the right place for people to take notice of, interest in, and act, or the idea will not tip.

Was the IOM report the tipping point for medication safety? The idea that medication errors happen much too often and need to be prevented has been picked up by many mavens, and many connectors have been networking about the idea. Have the answers to this critical problem made so little progress because we don't have enough salesmen? Or is the idea not sticky enough? It should be—adverse drug events are harming and killing people, and many of these negative consequences can be prevented.

SUMMARY

Although most medication use is safe, it can be much safer. Most of the medication-related morbidity and mortality is a direct effect of a broken medication-use system that has been broken for a long time, is in need of more support, and thus is preventable. However, the broken medication-use system is part of a larger problem—a broken health care system.[62,63] Evidenced-based safe-medication practices and model systems have been identified and need to be broadly implemented.[64] A business case for quality has been proven.[65] Health professionals and political leaders need to seek and stimulate catalysts that can capture the scientific and technological power for improved drug usage whose foundation is readily visible on the horizon of American health care.

My goal for writing this book is singular—to help stimulate society to come to grips with a pandemic that is giving rational drug therapy a bad name. Moreover, ADEs, such as medication errors and ADRs, are probably preventing some individuals or even doctors from using appropriate medication therapy when this resource clearly represents the therapy of choice.

Notes

Chapter 1

1. The U.S. Department of Health and Human Services. Substance Abuse and Mental Health Services Administration. (2003). *Results from the 2002 National Survey on Drug Use and Health: National Findings.* http://www.samhsa.gov/oas/nhsda/2k2nsduh/Results/2k2results.htm. Accessed October 6, 2003.

2. U.S. Department of Health and Human Services. National Institutes of Health. National Institute on Drug Abuse. (2003). NIDA InfoFacts. Hospital Visits. http://www.nida.nih.gov/Infofax/hospital.html. Accessed October 6, 2003.

3. U.S. Department of Health and Human Services. National Institutes of Health. National Institute on Drug Abuse. (2003). NIDA InfoFacts. Costs to Society. http://www. nida.nih.gov/Infofax/costs.html. Accessed October 6, 2003.

4. U.S. Department of Health and Human Services. Agency for Healthcare Research and Quality. (2003). Statistical Brief #21: Trends in Outpatient Prescription Drug Utilization and Expenditures: 1997-2000. July 2003. http://www.meps.ahrq.gov/papers/st21/stat21.htm. Accessed August 8, 2003.

5. Rucker NL (2003). Risk, respect, responsibility: Educational strategies to promote safe medication use. *J Medical Systems* 27(6):519-529.

6. NDC Health. (2004). The top 200 drugs for 2003 by U.S. States. http://www.rxlist. com/top200_sales_2003.htm. Accessed July 1, 2004.

7. Kaufman DW, Kelly JP, Rosenberg L, Anderson TE, Mitchell AA (2002). Recent patterns of medication use in the ambulatory adult population of the United States. *JAMA* 287(3):337-344.

8. Manasse HR (1989). Medication use in an imperfect world: Drug misadventuring as an issue of public policy, part 1. *Am J Hosp Pharm.* 46:929-944.

9. Manasse HR (1989). Medication use in an imperfect world: Drug misadventuring as an issue of public policy, part 2. *Am J Hosp Pharm.* 46:1141-1152.

10. Kohn LT, Corrigan JM, and Donaldson M (1999). *To Err Is Human: Building a Safer Health System.* Washington, DC: Institute of Medicine.

11. Johnson JA and Bootman JL (1995). Drug-related morbidity and mortality: A cost-of-illness model. *Arch Int Med.* 155:1949-1956.

12. Ernst FR and Grizzle AJ (2001). Drug-related morbidity and mortality: Updating the cost-of-illness model. *J Am Pharm Assoc.* 41(2):192-199.

13. Griffin JP. Editorial (2000). Medical errors major killers in UK and USA. *Adverse Drug React. Toxicol. Rev.* 19(1):9-16.

14. McDonald CJ, Weiner M, and Hui S (2000). Deaths due to medical errors are exaggerated in Institute of Medicine Report. *JAMA* 284(1):93-95.

Prescribed Medications and the Public Health
© 2006 by The Haworth Press, Inc. All rights reserved.
doi:10.1300/5688_19

15. Kohn L. (2001). The Institute of Medicine report on medical error: Overview and implications for pharmacy. *Am J Health-Sys Pharm.* 58:63-66.

16. Mendelsohn RS (1979). *Confessions of a Medical Heretic* (p. x). Chicago, IL: Contemporary Books, Inc.

17. Medawar C (1984). *The Wrong Kind of Medicine?* London: Social Audit, Ltd.

18. Stewart RB (1985). *Tragedies from Drug Therapy.* Springfield, IL: Charles C Thomas.

19. Medawar C (1992). *Power and Dependence.* London: Social Audit Ltd.

20. Wolfe SM (1999). *Worst Pills—Best Pills.* New York: Pocket Books.

21. Rucker TD (1987). Prescribed medications: System control or therapeutic roulette? In *IFAC Monograph: Control Aspects of Biomedical Engineering,* Nalecz Maciej (Ed.). Oxford: Permamon Press, 167-175.

22. Hepler CD and Segal R (2003). A model of the medication use system. In *Preventing Medication Errors and Improving Drug Therapy Outcomes* (pp. 35-62). Boca Raton, FL: CRC Press.

23. U.S. Food and Drug Administration (2002). Safety-based drug withdrawals (1997-2001). *AGENCY Consumer Magazine.* www.agency.gov/cder/features/2002/chrtWithdrawls.html. Accessed May 19, 2003.

24. Moore TJ (2000). FDA in crisis. Adapted from the *Boston Globe,* Sunday Focus Section. April 2, 2000. http://www.thomasjmoore.com/pages/fda_crisis. html. Accessed June 25, 2000.

25. Prescription drugs: What you don't know can kill you. (2003). *The Montel Show.* October 16, 2003. http://www.montelshow.com/show/upcoming_detail.htm?index=3. Accessed October 17, 2003.

26. Rashed SM, Nolly RJ, Robinson L, and Thoma L (2003). Weight variability of scored and unscored split psychotropic drug tablets. *Hosp Pharm.* 38:930-934.

27. Polli JE, Kim S, and Martin BR (2003). Weight uniformity of split tablets required by a Veterans Affairs policy. *J Man Care Pharm.* 9(65):401-407.

28. Welch WM (2002). Once just a trickle, Canada's Rx drugs pouring into the USA. *USA Today.* Newsline section (pp. 1A-2A), October 7.

29. Frommer FJ (2003). Drugmaker lobby spends $8.5M amid fight against imports. *USA Today* (AP). Newsline section (p. 1A), October 13.

30. Eban K (2003, October). It's a fake, and your pharmacist doesn't know it. *Reader's Digest.* 126-133.

31. Appleby J (2003). U.S. drug supply a terrorism target? *USA Today.* Money section (p. 2B), September 25.

32. Bacon J (2003). Crackdown nets plethora of dangerous drugs, FDA say. *USA Today.* Newsline section (p. 8A), September 30.

33. Gaul GM and Flaherty MP (2003). U.S. Prescription drug system under attack. *Washington Post* (p. A01, Parts 1-4), October 19-22.

34. FDA counterfeit task force continues work on wholesaler "best practices." (2003). *The Pink Sheet* 65(40):5.

35. FDA counterfeit report seeks "electronic pedigree" to aid drug tracking. (2003). *The Pink Sheet.* 65(40):3.

36. Lipton HL and Lee PR (1988). *Drugs and the Elderly.* Stanford, CA: Stanford University Press.

37. Kratz AM (1977). The senescent drug "abuser": A new sociologic problem. *Am J Pharm.* 149:119-124.

38. Lipscomb WR (1976). Geriatric drug abuse said virtually ignored problem. *Psychiatric News* 11:15.

39. Kurtz H (2003). Limbaugh goes off the air to battle painkiller habit. *The Washington Post* (p. A01), October 11.

40. Cohen JS (2001). *Overdose—The Case Against the Drug Companies.* New York: Jeremy P. Tarcher/Putnam.

41. Institute of Medicine (2001). *Crossing the Quality Chasm: A New Health System for the 21st Century.* Washington, DC: Author.

42. Leading hospitals drop the ball. *USA Today* (p. 3D), September 30.

43. Millenson ML (1997, 1999). *Demanding Medical Excellence.* Chicago, IL: The University of Chicago Press.

44. Berwick DM (2002). *Escape fire: Lessons for the future of health care.* New York: The Commonwealth Fund.

45. British Medical Association (1909). *Secret Remedies: What They Cost and What They Contain.* London: Author.

46. Cook J (1957, 1958). *Remedies and Rackets.* New York: W.W. Norton and Company.

47. Boodman SG (2002). No end to errors. *Washington Post* (p. HE01), December 3.

Chapter 2

1. Kelly WN (2002). How drugs are discovered. In *Pharmacy: What It Is and How It Works* (pp. 41-56). Boca Raton, FL: CRC Press.

2. Manasse HR (1989). Medication use in an imperfect world: Drug misadventuring as an issue of public policy, part 1. *Am J Hosp Pharm.* 46:929-944.

3. U.S. Department of Health and Human Services, the Food and Drug Administration, Center for Drug Evaluation and Research. (2002). *2002 Report to the Nation: Improving Public Health Through Human Drugs.* Rockville, MD: Author.

4. Thomas EJ, Studdet DM, Burstin HR, Orav EJ, Zeena T, Williams EJ, Howard KM, Weiler PC, Brennan TA (2000). Incidence and types of adverse events and negligent care in Utah and Colorado. *Med Care* 38:261-271.

5. Brennan TA, Leape LL, Laird NM, Hebert L, Localio AR, Lawthers AG, Newhouse JP, Weiler PC, Hiatt HH (1991). Incidence of adverse events and negligence in hospitalized patients: Results of the Harvard Medical Practice Study 1. *N Engl J Med* :370-376.

6. Classen DC, Pestotnik SL, Evans RS, Lloyd JF, Burke JP (1997). Adverse drug events in hospitalized patients: Excess length of stay, extra costs, and attributable mortality. *JAMA* 277(4):341-342.

7. Bates DW, Cullen DJ, Laird N, Petersen LA, Small SD, Servi D, Laffel G, Sweitzer BJ, Shea BF, Hallisey R, et al. (1995). Incidence of adverse drug events and potential adverse drug events. *JAMA* 274(1):29-34.

8. U.S. Government Accounting Office (2002). *Adverse Drug Events: The Magnitude of Health Risk Is Uncertain Because of Limited Incidence Data.* GAO/HEHS-00-21. Washington, DC: Author.

9. Dennehy CE, Kishi DT, and Louie C (1996). Drug-related illness in emergency department patients. *Am J Health-Syst Pharm* 53:1422-1426.

10. Schneitman-McIntire O, Farnen TA, Gordon N, Chan J, Toy WA (1996). Medication misadventures resulting in emergency department visits at an HMO medical center. *Am J Health-Syst Pharm* 53:1416-1422.

11. Patel P and Zed PJ (2002). Drug-related visits to the emergency department: How big is the problem? *Pharmacotherapy* 22:915-9923.

12. Gurwitz J, Field S, Avorn J, McCormick D, Jain S, Eckler M, Benser M, Edmondson AC, Bates DW (2002). Incidence and preventability of adverse drug events in nursing homes. *Am J Med* 109:87-94.

13. MacKinnon NJ and Hepler CD (2003). Indicators of preventable drug-related morbidity in older adults. Use within a managed care organization. *J Managed Care Pharm* 9(2):134-141.

14. Rothschild JM and Leape LL (2000). The nature and extent of medical injury in older adults. Washington, DC: AARP Public Policy Institute.

15. Jick H (1974). Drugs—remarkably nontoxic. *N Engl J Med* 291(16):824-828.

16. Jick H (1984). Adverse drug reactions: The magnitude of the problem. *J. Allergy and Clin Immunology* 74:555-557.

17. Hafner JW, Belknap SM, Squillante MD, and Bucheit KA (2002). Adverse drug events in emergency department patients. *Ann Emergency Med* 39(3):258-267.

18. Kelly WN (2001). Can the frequency and risks of fatal adverse drug events be determined? *Pharmacotherapy* 21(5):521-527.

19. Kelly WN (2001). Potential risks and prevention, part 1: Fatal adverse drug events. *Am J Health-Sys Pharm* 58(14):1317-1324.

20. Kelly WN (2001). Potential risks and prevention, part 3: Drug-induced threats to life. *Am J Health-Sys Pharm* 58(15):1399-1405.

21. Kelly WN (2001). Potential risks and preventions, part 2: Drug-induced permanent disabilities. *Am J Health-Sys Pharm* 58(14):1325-1329.

22. Peach H and Charlton JRH (1986). Illness, disability, and drugs among 25 to 75 year olds living at home. *J Epidemiology and Community Health* 40:59-66.

23. Senst BL, Achusim LE, Genest RP, Cosentino LA, Ford CC, Little JA, Raybon SJ, Bates DW (2001). Practical approach to determining costs and frequency of adverse drug events in a health care network. *Am J Health-Sys Pharm* 58:1126-1132.

24. Bates DW, Spell N, Cullen DJ, Burdick E, Laird N, Petersen LA, Small SD, Sweitzer BJ, Leape LL (1997). The costs of adverse drug events in hospitalized patients. *JAMA* 277(4):307-311.

25. Moore N, Lecointre D, Noblet C, and Mabille M (1998). Frequency and cost of serious adverse drug reactions in a department of general medicine. *Br J Clin Pharmacol* 45:301-308.

26. Bootman JL, Harrison DL, and Cos E (1997). The health care cost of drug-related morbidity and mortality in nursing facilities. *Arch Intern Med* 157:2089-2096.

27. Johnson JA and Bootman JL (1995). Drug-related morbidity and mortality: A cost of illness model. *Arch Intern Med* 155:1949-1956.

28. Ernst FR and Grizzle AJ (2001). Drug-related morbidity and mortality: Updating the cost-of-illness model. *J Am Pharm. Assoc* 41(2):192-199.

29. Zoppi M, Braunschweig S, Kuenzi UP, Maibach R, Hoigne R (2000). Incidence of lethal adverse drug reactions in the comprehensive hospital drug monitoring, a 20-year survey, 1974-1993, based on the data of Berne/St. Gallen. *Eur J Clin Pharmacol* 56(5):427-430.

Chapter 3

1. Nash DB, Koening JB, and Chatterton ML (2000). Why the Elderly Need Individualized Pharmaceutical Care. Philadelphia: Thomas Jefferson University.
2. Hanlon JT, Shimp LA, and Semla TP (2000). Recent advances in geriatrics: Drug-related problems in the elderly. *Ann Pharmacother* 34:360-365.
3. Moore TJ (2000). FDA in crisis. Adapted from the *Boston Globe,* Sunday Focus Section, April 2, 2000. http//www.thomasjmoore.com/pages/fda_crisis.html. Accessed June 25, 2000.
4. USP Quality Review (2003). PPR at a second glance No. 55. Issued 8/96. The United States Pharmacopeia. http://www.usp.org/patientSafety/briefsArticles Reports/qualityReview/qr551996-08-01a.hmtl. Accessed November 12.
5. Pomper S (2000). Drug rush: Why the prescription drug market's unsafe at high speeds. http://www.washingtonmonthly.com/features/2000/0005.pomper.html. Accessed November 2003.
6. Cohen JS (2001). *Over Dose.* New York: Most Tarcher/Putnam Books.
7. Public Citizen (2000). Myths about generic drug use. http://www.worstpills. org/public/myths.cfm.worstpills.org.
8. U.S. Food and Drug Administration. Center for Drug Evaluation and Research. (2003). Questions and Answers. Over-the-Counter Drug Products Public Hearing. June 28 and 29, 2000. http://www.fda.gov/cder/meeting/otcqa-600.htm. Accessed November 14.
9. Gunn VL, Taha SH, Liebelt EL, and Serwint JR (2001). Toxicity of over-the-counter cough and cold medications. *Pediatrics* 108(3):1-5.
10. U.S. Food and Drug Administration. Center on Drug Evaluation and Research. (2003). Over-the-Counter Medicines: What's Right for You? http://www. fda.cder/consumerinfo/WhatsRightForYou.htm. Accessed November 14.
11. Bates DW, Cullen DJ, Laird N, et al. (1995). Incidence of adverse drug events and potential adverse drug events. *JAMA.* 274(1):29-34.
12. Leape LL (1995). Preventing adverse drug events. *Am J Health-Syst Pharm* 52:379-382.
13. Kelly WN (1995). Pharmacy contributions to adverse medication events. *Am J Health-Syst Pharm.* 52:385-390.
14. Marcellino, K (2001). What do Georgia's patients expect from their pharmacist? *Georgia Pharmacy Journal* 23(10):22-23.
15. Pepper GA (1995). Errors in drug administration. *Am J Health-Syst Pharm* 52:391-395.
16. Kelly WN (2001). Potential errors and prevention, part 4: Reports of significant adverse drug events. *Am J Health-Syst Pharm* 58:1406-1412.
17. Rucker, TD (1987). Prescribed medications: System control or therapeutic roulette? In *IFAC Monograph: Control Aspect of Biomedical Engineering,* Nalecz (Ed.). Oxford: Permamon Press, 167-175.

18. Naik R and Kelly WN (2002). The identification and documentation of significant patient risk problems in Florida pharmacies. *Florida Pharmacy Today* 67:19-22, 26.

19. Schneider PJ (2002). Applying human factors in improving medication-use safety. *Am J Health-Syst Pharm* 59:1155-1159.

20. Pihl R (2002). Predicting who will make a medication error. Presented to the Safe Medication Use Expert Committee of the USP. Rockville, MD. September 30.

21. Daniels J and Kelly WN (2003). Managing behavior can reduce medical and medication errors. *Modern Healthcare*. In press, December, 2005.

Chapter 4

1. Benjamin DM (1998). Pharmaceutical risk management: Special problems encountered in the hospital setting. *J Health Risk Manag* Spring 18(2):5-17.

2. WHO Collaborative Center for International Drug Monitoring. Uppsala, Sweden. (2004). http://www.who-umc.org/defs.html. Accessed September 8, 2004.

3. Royer RJ (1997). Mechanism of action of adverse drug reactions: An overview. *Pharmacoepi and Drug Safety* 6(Suppl.3):S43-S50.

4. Manasse HR (1989). Medication use in an imperfect world: Drug misadventuring as an issue of public policy, part 1. *Am J Hosp Pharm* 46:929-944.

5. Lazarou J, Pomeranz, BH, and Corey, PN (1998). Incidence of adverse drug reactions in hospitalized patients: A meta-analysis of prospective studies. *JAMA* 279:1200-1205.

6. Gotti EW (1974). Adverse drug reactions and autopsy. *Arch Pathol* 97:201-204.

7. Gurwitz JH, Field TS, and Avorn J, McCormick D, Jain S, Eckler M, Benser M, Edmondon AC, Bates DW. (2000). Incidence and preventability of adverse drug events in nursing homes. *Am J Med* 109:87-94.

8. Bowman L, Carlstedt BC, Hancock EF, and Black CD (1996). Adverse drug reaction (ADR) occurrence in elderly inpatients. *Pharmacoepi and Drug Safety* 5:9-18.

9. Kelly WN (2001). Potential risks and prevention, part 4: Reports of significant adverse drug events. *Am J Health Syst Pharm* 58:1406-1412.

10. U.S. Department of Health and Human Services. Food and Drug Administration. (1997). Annual adverse drug experience report: 1996. October 30, 1997. http://www.fda.gov/cder/dpe/annrep96/index.htm.

11. Generali JA (2002). Drugs with black box warnings. *Hospital Pharmacy*. Facts and Comparisons. chart.

12. Koch-Weser J, Sellers EM, and Zacest R (1977). The ambiguity of adverse drug reactions. *Europ J Clin Pharmacol* 11:75-78.

13. Hill AB (1965). The environment and disease association or causation? *Proc R Soc Med* 58:295-300.

14. Naranjo CA, Busto U, Sellers EM, Sandor P, Ruiz I, Roberts EA, Janecek E, Domecq C, Greenblatt DJ (1981). A method for estimating the probability of adverse drug reactions. *Clin Pharmacol Ther* 30(2):239-245.

15. Naranjo CA, Lane D, Ho-Asjoe M, and Lanctot KL (1990). A Bayesian assessment of idiosyncratic adverse reactions to new drugs: Guillain-Barre syndrome and zimeldine. *J Clin Pharmacol* 30:174-180.

16. Lanctot KL and Naranjo CA (1995). Comparison of the Bayesian approach and a simple algorithm for assessment of adverse drug events. *Clin Pharmacol Ther* 58(6):692-698.

17. Busto U, Naranjo CA, and Sellers EM (1982). Comparison of two recently published algorithms for assessing the probability of adverse drug reactions. *British J Clin Pharmacol* (2):223-227.

18. Macedo AF, Marques FB, Ribeiro CF, and Teixeira F (2003). Causality assessment of adverse drug reactions: Comparison of the results obtained from published decisional algorithms and from the evaluation of an expert panel, according to different levels on inputability. *J Clin Pharmacy and Therapeutics* 28:137-143.

19. Last JM (2001). *A Dictionary of Epidemiology,* Fourth Edition. New York: Oxford University Press.

20. Council for International Organizations of Medical Sciences (CIOMS). (1997). World Health Organization. Definitions of terms and minimum requirements for their use: Respiratory disorders and skin disorders. *Pharmacoepi and Drug Safety* 6:115-127.

21. Study shows that genetic differences in minorities may cause varied reactions to medicines (2002). *PR Newswire—Healthcare/Hospital News.* http://www. prnewswire.com/cgibin/stori . . . 1806487&EDATE=WED+Sep+25+2002,+09:30+ AM. Accessed October 31, 2002.

22. Beaty TH and Khoury MJ (2000). The interface of genetics and epidemiology. *Epidemiologic Reviews* 22(1):120-125.

23. Rioux PP (2000). Clinical trials in pharmacogenetics and pharmacogenomics: Methods and applications. *Am J Health-Syst Pharm* 57:887-898.

24. Evans WE and McLeod HL (2003). Pharmacogenomics – Drug disposition, drug targets, and side effects. *N Engl J Med* (6):538-549.

Chapter 5

1. DiPiro JT, Ownby DR, and Schlesselman LS (2002). Allergic and pseudo-allergic drug reactions. In *Pharmacotherapy: A Pathophysiologic Approach,* 5th Ed., pp. 1585-1598, JT DePierro et al., (Eds.). Stamford, CT: Appleton Lange.

2. Royer RJ (1997). Mechanism of action of adverse drug reactions: An overview. *Pharmacoepi and Drug Safety.* 6(Suppl. 3):S43-S50.

3. Alkhawajah AM, Eifawal M, and Mahmoud SF (1995). Fatal anaphylactic reaction to diclofenac. *Forensic Science International* 60:107-110.

4. Hagen MD and White RD (1983). Thrombocytopenia secondary to trimetho-prim-sulfamethoxazole. *South Med J* 76:503.

5. Sakai H, Komatsuo S, Matsuo S, and Iizuka H (2002). Two cases of minocycline-induced vasculitis. *Japanese J of Allergology* 51(12);1153-1158.

6. Roman A and Pietrantonio F (1997). Delayed hypersensitivity to flurbi-profen. *J Internal Med* 241(1):81-83.

7. Ponte CD (1983). A suspected case of codeine-induced erythema multi-forme. *Drug Intell & Clin Pharm* 17:128-130.

8. Patterson R, DeSwarte RD, Greenberger PA, Grammer LC (1994). Drug allergy and protocols for management of drug allergies. *Allergy Proc* 15(5):243-244.

9. Demoly P and Bousquet J (2001). Epidemiology of drug allergy. *Curr Opinion in Allergy and Immunology* 1(4):305-310.

10. Jones TA and Como JA (2003). Assessment of medication errors that involved drug allergies at a university hospital. *Pharmacotherapy* 23:855-860.

11. Escolana F, Bisbe E, Castillo J, Lopez R, Pares N, Arilla M, Castano J. (1998). Drug allergy in a population of surgical patients. *Revista Espanola de Anestesiolologia y Reanimacion* 45(10):425-430.

12. Schneitman-McIntire O, Farnen TA, Gordon N, Chan J, Toy WA (1996). Medication misadventures resulting in emergency department visits at an HMO medical center. *Am J Health-Syst Pharm* 53:1416-1422.

13. The Boston Collaborative Surveillance Program (1973). Drug-induced anaphylaxis. *JAMA* 224(5):613-615.

14. Kelly WN (2001). Potential risks and prevention, part 4: Reports of significant adverse drug events. *Am J Health-Syst Pharm* 58:1406-1412.

15. Kelly WN (2001). Potential risks and prevention, part 1: Fatal adverse drug events. *Am J Health-Syst Pharm* 58:1317-1324.

16. Wedner HJ (1987). Allergic reactions to drugs. *Primary Care: Clinics in Office Practice* 14(3):523-545.

17. Marcellino K and Kelly WN (2001). Potential risks and prevention, part 3: Drug-induced threats to life. *Am J Health-Syst Pharm* 58:1399-1404.

18. Preston SL, Briceland LL, and Lesar TS (1994). Accuracy of penicillin allergy reporting. *Am J Hosp Pharm* 51:79-84.

19. Bouwmeester MC, Laberge N, Bussieres J-F, Lebel D, Bailey B, Toy WA. (2001). Program to remove incorrect allergy documentation in pediatrics medical records. *Am J Health-Syst Pharm* 58:1722-1727.

20. Cantrill JA and Cottrell WN (1997). Accuracy of drug allergy documentation. *Am J Health-Syst Pharm* 54:1627-1629.

21. Patterson R, DeSwarte RD, Greenberger PA, Grammer LC, Brown JE, Choy AC. (1994). Overview of adverse drug reactions. *Allergy Proc* 15(5):243-244.

22. Beyea SC (2003). Oops—the patient is allergic to that medication. *AORN Journal* 77:650-654.

23. Patterson R, DeSwarte RD, Greenberger PA, Grammer LC, Brown JE, Choy AC. (1994). General principles of prevention of allergic drug reactions. *Allergy Proc* 15:245-248.

Chapter 6

1. Abood RR and Brushwood DB (2005). Pharmacist malpractice liability and risk management strategies. In *Pharmacy Practice and the Law* (pp. 313-364). Gaithersburg, MD: Aspen Publications.

2. Lesser PB, Vietti MM, Clark WD (1986). Lethal enhancement of therapeutic doses of acetaminophen by alcohol. *Dig Dis Sci* 31:103-105.

3. Klimke A and Klieser E (1994). Sudden death after intravenous application of lorazepam in a patient treated with clozapine. *Am J Psychiat* 151(5):780.

4. Dean RP and Talbert RL (1980). Bleeding associated with concurrent warfarin and metronidazole therapy. *Drug Intell & Clin Pharm* 14:864-866.

5. Tatro DS (Ed.). (1992). *Drug Interaction Facts*. St. Louis: J.B. Lippincott Co.

6. Bjerrum L, Andersen M, Kragstrup J, and Petersen G (2002). Exposure to drug interactions in general practice. *Pharmacoepi and Drug Safety* 11(Supp. 1): S21.

7. Merlo J, Liedholm H, Lindblad U, Bjorck-Linne A, Falt J, Lindberg G, Melander A (2001). Prescriptions with potential drug interactions dispensed at Swedish pharmacies in January 1999: A cross sectional study. *BMJ* 32(7310):427-442.

8. Peng C, Glassman PA, Marks IR, Fowler C, Castiglione B, Good CB (2003). Retrospective drug utilization review: Incidence of clinically relevant potential drug-drug interactions in a large ambulatory population. *J Managed Care Pharm* 9(6):513-522.

9. Doucet J, Chassagne P, Trivalle C, Landrin I, Pauty MD, Kadri N, Menard JF, Bercoff E (1996). Drug-drug interactions related to hospital admissions in older adults: A prospective study of 1,000 patients. *J Am Geriatr Soc* 44(8):944-948.

10. Armstrong WA, Driever CW, and Hays RL (1996). Analysis of drug-drug interactions in a geriatric population. *Am J Hosp Pharm* 37:385-387.

11. Cooper JW, Wellins I, Fish KH, and Loomis ME (1975). Frequency of potential drug-drug interactions. *J Am Pharm Assoc* NS15(1):24-31.

12. Tamai IY, Strome LS, Marshall CE, and Mooradian AD (1989). Analysis of drug-drug interactions among nursing home residents. *Am J Hosp Pharm* 46:1567-1569.

13. Jankel CA and Fitterman LK (1993). Epidemiology of drug-drug interactions as a cause of hospital admission. *Drug Safety* 9(10):51-59.

14. Juurlink DN, Mamdani M, Koop A, Laupacis A, Redelmeier DA (2003). Drug-drug interactions among elderly patients hospitalized for drug toxicity. *JAMA* 289(13):1652-1658.

15. Hamilton R, Briceland LL, and Andritz MH (1998). Frequency of hospitalization after exposure to known drug-drug interactions in a Medicaid population. *Pharmacotherapy* 18:1112-1120.

16. Lisby SM and Hahata M (1987). Medication use and potential drug interactions in pediatric patients with infectious disease. *Hosp Pharm* 22:354-356.

17. Kelly WN (2001). Potential risks and prevention, part 4: Reports of significant adverse drug events. *Am J Health-Syst Pharm* 58:1406-1412.

18. Brown KE (2004). Top ten dangerous drug interactions in long-term care. The M3 Project. http:www.scoup.net/M3Projet/topten/. Accessed May 4, 2004.

19. Voiles KM and Kelly WN (2004). Potential interactions between oral contraceptives and other medications and natural substances. *U.S. Pharmacist* 29(1): 61-68.

20. Scott GN and Elmer GW (2002). Update on natural product-drug interactions. *Am J Health-Syst Pharm* 59:339-347.

21. Kelly WN (2001). Potential risks and prevention, part 1: Fatal adverse drug events. *Am J Health-Syst Pharm* 58:1317-1324.

22. Shad MU, Marsh C, and Preskorn SH (2001). The economic consequences of a drug-drug interaction. *J Clin Psychopharmaco* 21(1):119-120.

23. Hamilton RA and Gordon T (1993). Incidence and cost of hospital admissions secondary to drug interactions involving theophylline. *Ann Pharmacotherapy* 26:1507-1511.

24. Fulda TR, Valuck RJ, Zanden JV, Parker S, and Byrns PJ (2000). Disagreement among drug compendium on inclusion and ratings of drug-drug interactions. *Curr Ther Res* 61(8):540-548.

25. Abarca J, Malone DC, Armstrong EP, Grizzle AJ, Hansten PD, Van Bergen RC, Lipton RB (2004). Concordance of severity ratings provided in four drug interaction compendia. *Am J Pharm Assoc* 44(2):136-141.

26. Jankel AC and Martin BC (1992). Evaluation of six computerized drug interaction screening programs. *Am J Hosp Pharm* 49:1430-1439.

27. Greenlaw CW (1981). Evaluation of a computerized drug interaction screening program. *Am J Hosp Pharm* 38:517-521.

28. Headden S. Lenzy T, Kostyu P, Roebuck K, Locke K, Hordern BB, Beaven S, and Mullen R (1996, August 26). Danger at the Drugstore. *U.S. News and World Report* 121(8):46-53.

29. Hazlet TK, Lee TA, Hansten PD, and Horn JR (2001). Performance of community pharmacy drug interaction software. *Am J Pharm Assoc* 41(2):200-204.

30. Chrischilles EA, Fulda TR, Byrns PJ, Winckler SC, Rupp MT, Chui MA (2002). The role of pharmacy computer systems in preventing medication errors. *J Am Pharm Assoc* 42(3):439-448.

31. Dalton M, Chambers G, and Halvachs F (1999). Implementing an effective drug interaction reporting program. *Hosp Pharm* 34(10):31-42.

32. Chui MA and Rupp MT (2000). Evaluation of on-line prospective DUR programs in community pharmacy practice. *JMCP* 6(1):27-32.

33. Magnus D, Rodgers S, and Avery AJ (2002). GPs' views on computerized drug interaction alerts: Questionnaire survey. *J Clin Pharm Ther* 27(5):377-382.

34. Weingart SN, Toth M, Sands DZ, Aronson MD, Davis RB, Phillips RS (2003). Physicians' decisions to override computerized drug alerts in primary care. *Arch Intern Med* 163(21):2625-2631.

35. Housley SC and Kelly WN (2003). Drug-interaction monitoring: Good, bad, and ugly. *Drug Topics* 147:41-42.

36. Brushwood DB (1994). Expanding liability: Is the *Wall Street Journal* right? *Georgia Pharmacy Journal* 16(4):25.

37. Langdorf MJ, Fox JC, Marwah RS, Montaque BJ and Hard MM (2000). Physician versus computer knowledge of potential drug interactions in the emergency department. *Acad Emerg Med* 7:1321-1329.

38. Burns SB and Kelly WN (2002). 10 drug interactions every pharmacist should know. *Pharmacy Times* 68:46-48.

39. Howard T (1997). Ten drug interactions every pharmacist should know. *Southern J Health-Syst Pharm* 2:13-16.

40. Malone DC, Abarca J, Hansten PD, Grizzle AJ, Armstrong EP, Van Bergen RC, Duncan-Edgar BS, Solomon SL, Lipton RB (2004). Identification of serious drug-drug interactions: Results of the partnership to prevent drug-drug interactions. *J Am Pharm Assoc* 44(2)142-151.

41. Hartman C and Duong S (2004). Drug-food interactions. *Pharmacy Times* 70(2):insert.

42. Grapefruit juice and drugs (2004). http://emphysemafoundation.org/Grape Juice.aspx. Accessed January 19, 2004.

43. NAPRA (2004). Health Canada is advising Canadians not to take certain drugs with grapefruit juice. http://www.napra.ca/docs/0/509/513.asp. Accessed on January 19, 2004.

44. Brazier NC and Levine MAH (2003). Drug-herb interaction among commonly used conventional medicines: A compendium for health care professionals. *Am J Ther* 10(3):163-169.

45. Johnson L (2004). Common antibiotic tied to heart risk. *The Atlanta Journal-Constitution* (p. A-16), September 9.

46. Horn JR and Hansten PD (2004). Computerized drug-interaction alerts: Is anybody paying attention? *Pharm Times* 70(2):56,58.

Chapter 7

1. American Society of Health-System Pharmacists. (2002, July 17). Survey reveals patient concerns about medication-related issues. http://www.ashp.org/news/showArticle.cfm? cfid=2628430&CFToken=25465950&id=2996.

2. Schimmel EM (1964). The hazards of hospitalization. *Ann Intern Med.* 60: 100-110.

3. Steel K, Gertman PM, Crescenzi C, Anderson J (1981). Iatrogenic illness on a general medical service at a university hospital. *N Engl J Med* 304:638-642.

4. Brennan TA, Leape LL, Laird NM, Hebert L, Localio AR, Lawthers AG, Newhouse JP, Weiler PC, Hiatt HH (1991). Incidence of adverse events and negligence in hospitalized patients: Results of the Harvard Medical Practice Study I. *N Engl J Med* 324:370-376.

5. Leape LL, Brennan TA, Laird N, Lawthers AG, Localio AR, Barnes BA, Hebert L, Newhouse JP, Weiler PC, Hiatt H (1991). The nature of adverse events in hospitalized patients: Results of the Harvard Medical Practice Study II. *N Engl J Med* 324:377-384.

6. Thoreau HD (1999). *Civil Disobedience.* New York: Penguin Putnam, Inc.

7. Kohn LT, Corrigan JM, and Donaldson M (1999). *To Err Is Human: Building a Safer Health System.* Washington, DC: Institute of Medicine.

8. Conlan MF (2001). Check, please! *Drug Topics* 145:37-38, 43,45.

9. Stolberg SG (1999). The boom in medications brings rise in fatal risks: Death by prescription. *New York Times* (A1, A18), June 3.

10. Leape LL (1994). Error in medicine. *JAMA* 272(23):1851-1857.

11. Leape LL (1999). A systems analysis approach to medical error. In *Medication Errors: Causes, Prevention, and Risk Management* (pp. 2.1-2.14) M. C. Cohen (Ed.). Sudbury, MA: Jones and Barlett Publishers.

12. NCCMRP taxonomy of medication errors (2004). The National Coordinating Committee for Medication Error Reporting and Prevention. http://nccmerp.org. Accessed January 24, 2004.

13. United States Pharmacopeia (2003). Summary of information submitted to MEDMARX in the year 2002. November 18, 2003.

14. Cowley E, Williams R, and Cousins D (2001). Medication errors in children: A descriptive summary of medication error reports submitted to the United States Pharmacopeia 62(9):627-640.

15. Marcus J (1995). Hospital's error, not cancer, killed leading health writer. *The Charlotte Observer.* Main news (p. 13A), March 24.

16. Chandrasekaran R (1994). Prescription error claims dad's angel. *The Washington Post* (p. A11), October 31.

17. Bai M (1995). Children's Hospital admits giving wrong drug to child. *The Boston Globe* (p. 33), April 6.

18. Roberg, K (2000). Kelsey's story. *Am J Health-Syst Pharm* 58: 985-987.

19. National Coordinating Committee on Medication Error Reporting and/Prevention. (2002, June 11). Use of medication error rates to compare health care organizations is of no value. http://www.nccmerp.org/council2002-06-11.html. Accessed February 2, 2004.

20. Allan EA and Barker KN (1990). Fundamentals of medication error research. *Am J Hosp Pharm* 47:555-571.

21. Barker KN, Flynn EA, Pepper GA, Bates DW, Mikeal RL. (2002). Medication errors observed in 36 health care facilities. *Arch Intern Med* 162(16):1897-1903.

22. Kaushal R, Bates DW, and Landrigan C (2001). Medication errors and adverse drug events in pediatric inpatients. *JAMA* 285(16):2114-2120.

23. Lesar TS, Lomaestro BM, and Pohl H (1997). Medication-prescribing errors in a teaching hospital. *Arch Intern Med* 157:1569-1576.

24. Schumock GT, Guenette AJ, Keys TV, and Hutchinson RA (1994). Prescribing errors for patients about to be discharged from a university hospital. *Am J Hosp Pharm* 51:2288, 2290.

25. Deutsch N (2003). Medication errors more likely to reach patients in ER setting. *Medical Post Toronto* 39(14):63.

26. Lesar TS, Briceland LL, Delcoure K, Parmalee JC, Masta-Gornic V, Pohl H (1990). Medication prescribing errors in a teaching hospital. *JAMA* 263(17):2329-2334.

27. Barker KN, Mikeal RL, Pearson RE, Illig NA, Morse ML (1982). Medication errors in nursing homes and small hospitals. *Am J Hosp Pharm* 39(6):987-991.

28. Meredith S, Feldman PH, Frey D, Hall K, Arnold K, Brown NJ, Ray WA (2001). Possible medication errors in home healthcare patients. *J Am Geriatr Soc* 49(6):719-724.

29. National Coordinating Committee on Medication Error Prevention and Reporting (1998). Taxonomy of medication errors. http://www.nccmerp.org/pdf/taxo 2001-07-31.pdf Accessed February 5, 2004.

30. Siganga WW (1996). The role of Toledo pharmacists' documentation of interventions to correct prescribing errors. *Ohio Pharmacist* 45:17-19.

31. Flynn EA, Barker KN, and Carnahan BJ (2003). National observational study of prescription dispensing accuracy and safety in 50 pharmacies. *J Am Pharm Assoc* 43(2):191-200.

32. Friedman R (2002, September 9). Pharmacist-made products prone to error, FDA finds. *Reuters Health.* http://www.drbobmartin.com/2002k_09_24news08. html. Accessed February 9, 2004.

33. Romano MJ (2001). A 1000-fold overdose of clonidine caused by a compounding error in a 5-year old child with attention-deficit/hyperactivity disorder. *Pediatrics* 108:471-473.

34. Flynn EA, Pearson RE, and Barker KN (1997). Observational study of accuracy in compounding i.v. admixtures at five hospitals. *Am J Health-Syst Pharm* 54:904-912.

35. Kelly WN (2001). Potential risks and prevention, part 4: Reports of significant adverse drug events. *Am J Health-Syst Pharm* 58:1406-1417.

36. Trinkle R and Wu JK (1997). Sources of medication errors involving pediatric chemotherapy patients. *Hosp Pharm* 32(6):853-859.

37. Kelly WN (2001). Can the frequency and risks of fatal adverse drug events be determined? *Pharmacotherapy* 21(5):521-527.

38. Ebbesen J, Buajordet I, Erikssen J, Brors O, Hilberg T, Svaar H, Sandvik L. (2001). Drug-related deaths in a department of internal medicine. *Arch Intern Med* 161(19):2317-2323.

39. Kelly WN (2001). Potential risks and prevention, part 1: Fatal adverse drug events. *Am J Health-Syst Pharm* 58:1317-1324.

40. Phillips J, Beam S, Brinker A, Holquist C, Honig P, Lee LY, Pamer C (2001). Retrospective analysis of mortalities associated with medication errors. *Am J Health-Syst Pharm* 58:1835-1841.

41. Marcellino K and Kelly WN (2001). Potential risks and prevention, part 3: Drug-induced threats to life. *Am J Health-Syst Pharm* 58:1399-1404.

42. Kelly WN (2001). Potential risks and prevention, part 2: Drug-induced permanent disabilities. *Am J Health-Syst Pharm* 58:1325-1329.

43. Bates DW, Spell N, Cullen DJ, Burdick E, Laird N, Petersen LA, Small SD, Sweitzer BJ, Leape LL (1997). The costs of adverse drug events in hospitalized patients. *JAMA* 277(4):307-311.

44. Schneider PJ, Lee YL, Rotermich EA, and Sill BE (1995). Cost of medication-related problems at a university hospital. *Am J Health-Syst Pharm* 52:2415-2418.

45. Bootman JL, Harrison DL, and Cox E (1997). The health care cost of drug-related morbidity and mortality in nursing facilities. *Arch Intern Med* 157(18):2089-2096.

46. Johnson JA and Bootman LJ (1995). Drug-related morbidity and mortality: A cost of illness model. *Arch Intern Med* 155(18):19149-1956.

47. Rucker TD (1987). Prescribed medications: System control or therapeutic roulette? *Control Aspects of Biomedical Engineering.* Oxford, UK: International Federation of Automatic Control.

48. The Institute for Safe Medication Practices. (1999, February 10). Over-reliance on pharmacy computer systems may place patients at risk. ISMP Medication Safety Alert. htpp://www.ismp.org/MSAarticles/Computer.html. Accessed February 10, 2004.

49. Argo AL and Kelly WN (2000). The ten most common lethal medication errors in hospital patients. *Hosp Pharm* 35:470-474.

50. Joint Commission Resources (2001). *Preventing Medication Errors: Strategies for Pharmacists.* Oakbrook Terrace, IL: Author.

51. Opus Communications (1999). *First Do No Harm. A Practical Guide to Medication Safety and JCAHO Compliance.* Marblehead, MA: Author.

52. Leape LL, Bates DW, Cullen DJ, Cooper J, Demonaco HJ, Gallivan T, Hallisey R, Ives J, Laird N, Laffel G, et al. (1995). Systems analysis of adverse drug events. *JAMA* 274(1):35-43.

53. D'Arcy PF and Hadden DR (2000). Are drug proprietary names necessary? *Adverse Drug Reactions and Toxicologic Reviews* 19(2):117-121.

54. Ranii D (2003). Naming drugs an art form. Big bucks ride on picking memorable moniker. *The Atlanta Journal-Constitution* (p. 5), January 5.

55. American Association of Colleges of Pharmacy (2003). Pharmacy professor tackles drug-name confusion. *AACP News* 35(7):5.

56. Davis NM (2001). *Medical Abbreviations: 15,000 Conveniences at the Expense of Communications and Safety.* Huntingdon Valley, PA: Neil M. Davis Associates.

57. Kelly WN (1995). Pharmacy contributions to adverse medication events. Proceedings of the ASHP/AMA/ANA Conference on Understanding and Preventing Drug Misadventures. *Am. J. Hosp. Pharm.* 52:385-390.

58. American Society of Consultant Pharmacists (2004). Appendix A. Medication system: Potential breakdown points. http://www.ascp.com/public/pr/guidelines/appendixa.shtml. Accessed February 12, 2004.

59. Lesar TS, Briceland L, and Stein DS (1997). Factors related to errors in medication prescribing. *JAMA* (4):312-316.

60. Flynn EA, Barker KN, Gibson JT, Pearson RE, Berger BA, Smith LA (1999). Impact of interruptions and distractions on dispensing errors in an ambulatory care pharmacy. *Am J Health-Syst Pharm* 56:1319-1325.

61. United States Pharmacopeia (2003, September). Distractions contribute to medication errors. *USP Patient Safety CAPSLINK.*

62. Ukens C (1999). Errors linked to workplace by Massachusetts pharmacists. *Drug Topics* 143:35.

63. Schuman D (1999). Long hours, distractions raise potential for pharmacy errors. *The News-Sentinel* (p. 1A), November 16.

64. Fleming H (2000). Time bomb. *Drug Topics* 144:70, 73.

65. Landschoot RL (1997). Anatomy of an error. *Am Druggist* 214:47.

66. Talley CR (2001). Pharmacist shortage identified by government. *Am J Health-Syst Pharm* 58:108, 122.

67. Murray MK (2002). The nursing shortage: Past, present, future. *J Nursing Admin* 32(2):79-84.

68. Davis N (1996). Performance lapses as a cause of medication errors. *Hosp Pharm* 31:1524-1527.

69. Daniels JE, Kelly WN, and Malone JT (2004). Managing behavior can reduce medical and medication errors. In press, 2004.

70. Smetzer JL and Cohen MR (1998). Lesson from the Denver medication error/criminal negligence case: Look beyond blaming individuals. *Hosp Pharm* 33: 640-657.

71. Whitney, HAK (1989). Errors as a way of life. *J Pharm Tech* 5:1-2.

Chapter 8

1. Chen RT and Hibbs B (1998). Vaccine safety: Current and future challenges. *Pediatric Annuals* 27(7):445-455.

2. Centers for Disease Control and Prevention (1999). Achievements in public health, 1900-1999: Impact of vaccines universally recommended for children—United States, 1990-1998. *MMWR* 48:243-248.

3. Centers for Disease Control and Prevention (1999). Ten great public health achievements—United States, 1900-1999. *MMWR* 48:241-243.

4. Infant vaccine helps children, adults (2003). *USA Today.* Life section (p. D), October 13.

5. Centers for Disease Control and Prevention (2003). Surveillance for safety after immunization: Vaccine adverse event reporting system (VAERS)—United States, 1991-2001. *MMWR* 52(SS-1):15.

6. Chen RT (2003). Introduction. *Seminars in Pediatric Infectious Diseases* 14(3):187.

7. Chen RT, DeStefano F, Pless, R, Mootrey G, Kramarz P, Hibbs B. (2001). Challenges and controversies in immunization safety. *Infect Dis Clin N America* 15(1): 21-39.

8. Chen RT, Rastogi SC, Mullen JR, Hayes SW, Cochi SL, Donlon JA, Wassilak SG. (1994). The vaccine adverse event reporting system (VAERS). *Vaccine* 12(6):542-550.

9. Iskander JK, Miller ER, Pless RP, and Chen RT (2004). Centers for Disease Control. Vaccine safety post-marketing surveillance: The vaccine adverse event reporting system. Continuing Medication Education. http://www.phppo.cdc.gov/phtnonline. Accessed February 20, 2004.

10. Chen RT, Glasser JW, Rhodes PH, Davis RL, Barlow WE, Thompson RS, Mullooly JP, Black SB, Shinefield HR, Vadheim CM, Marcy SM, Ward JI, Wise RP, Wassilak SG, Hadler SC (1997). Vaccine safety datalink project: A new tool for improving vaccine safety monitoring in the United States. *Pediatrics* 99(6):765-773.

11. Centers for Disease Control and Prevention (2004). Vaccine side effects. http://www.cdc.gov/nip/vacsafe/concerns/side-effects.htm. Accessed February 20, 2004.

12. Chen RT, Mootrey G, and DeStefano F (2000). Safety of routine childhood vaccinations. *Paediatr Drugs* 2(4):273-290.

13. Chen RT and Hibbs B (1998). Vaccine safety: Current and future challenges. *Pediatric Annals* 27(7):445-455.

14. Hill AB (1965). The environment and disease: Association or causation. *Proc R Soc Med* 58:295-300.

15. Evans G (1997). Vaccine liability and safety revisited. *Arch Pediatr Adolesc Med* 152:7-10.

16. Wolfe RM, Sharp LK, and Lipsky MS (2002). Content and design attributes of antivaccination Web sites. *JAMA* 287(24):3245-3248.

17. Fisher BL (2004). Anti-science activists label pro-vaccine safety advocates "anti-vaccine" in June 26 *JAMA* article. http://www.909shot.com/Loe_Fisher/anti.htm. Accessed February 19, 2004.

18. CBC News Online Staff (2004, January 20). Anti-vaccine advice worries health officials. http://www.cbc.ca/stories/2004/01/19/Consumers/vaccine040119.

19. Park A (2002). Are the shots safe? *Time* 159(18):53.

20. Gangarosa REJ, Galazka AM, Wolfe CR, Phillips LM, Gangarosa RE, Miller E, Chen RT (1998). Impact of anti-vaccine movements on pertussis control: The untold story. *Lancet* 351(9099):356-361.

21. The Institute of Medicine (2001). *Immunization Safety Review: Measles-Mumps-Rubella Vaccine and Autism.* Washington, DC: Author.

22. DeStefano F and Chen RT (2001). Autism and measles, mumps, and rubella vaccination. *CNS Drugs* 15(11):831-837.

23. The politics of autism. *The Wall Street Journal online.* http://www.web reprints.djreprints.com/926640351653.html. December 29; Accessed February 20, 2004.

24. Manning A (2004). U.S. will pay for study to seek cause of autism. *USA Today* (9-D), February 25.

25. Autism and vaccines (2004). *The Wall Street JournalOnline.* http://www.webreprints.djreprints.com/926591461813.html. February 9; Accessed February 20, 2004.

26. The Institute of Medicine (2001). *Immunization Safety Review: Thiomerosal—Containing Vaccines and Neurodevelopmental Disorders.* Washington, DC: Author.

27. The Associated Press (2004). Medical journal regrets vaccine article. London. http://www.abcnews.go.com/wire/Living/ap20040221_768.html. February 21; Accessed February 23, 2004.

28. The Institute of Medicine (2002). *Immunization Safety Review: Hepatitis B Vaccine and Demyelinating Neurological Disorders.* Washington DC: Author.

29. The Institute of Medicine (2002). *Immunization Safety Review: Multiple immunizations and Immune Dysfunction.* Washington, DC: Author.

30. The Institute of Medicine (2003). *Immunization Safety Review: Vaccinations and Sudden Unexpected Death in Infancy.* Washington DC: Author.

31. Offit PA and Jew R (2003). Addressing parents' concerns: Do vaccines contain harmful preservatives, adjuvants, additives, and residuals? *Pediatrics* 112(6): 1394-1401.

32. Hogenesch H, Azcona-Olivera J, Scott-Moncrieff C, Snyder PW, Glickman LT. (1991). Vaccine-induced autoimmunity in the dog. *Advances in Vet Med* 41:733-747.

33. Kelly WN, Hogenesch H, and Chen RT (2004). Antibody response to impurities in human vaccines. Presented at the Mercer University Health Science Center Research Conference. Macon, GA, March 4.

34. Chen RT (1999). Vaccine risks: Real, perceived and unknown. *Vaccine* 17:S41-S46.

35. Plotkin SA (2001). Lessons learned concerning vaccine safety. Presented at the Europe Vaccine Manufacturer's Meeting. Lucerne, March 22.

36. A guide to locating information on vaccine safety (1998). *Pediatric Annals* 27(7):459-464.

37. American Academy of Pediatrics, Pennsylvania Chapter (2004). Immunization education program: Evaluating anti-vaccine claims. http://paaap.org.immunize/course/slide57.html. Accessed February 19, 2004.

38. Centers for Disease Control and Prevention (2004). Vaccine safety. http://www.cdc.gov/nip. Accessed February 19, 2004.

Chapter 9

1. Cherry DK and Woodwell DA (1998). National ambulatory medical care survey: 2000 summary. *Vital Health Stat* 300:1-16.

2. Clause SL (2003). Patient-safety mandates in ambulatory care. *Am J Health-Syst Pharm* 60:2368-2369.

3. Kuznets N (2002). Spotlight on ambulatory care patient safety. *Focus on Patient Safety* 5(4):1-2.

4. Forster AJ, Murff HJ, Peterson JF, Gandhi TK, Bates DW (2003). The incidence and severity of adverse events affecting patients after discharge from the hospital. *Ann Intern Med* 138:161-167.

5. Gandhi TK, Weingart SN, Borus J, Seger AC, Peterson J, Burdick E, Seger DL, Shu K, Federico F, Leape LL, Bates DW (2003). Adverse drug events in ambulatory care. *N Engl J Med* 348(16):1556-1564.

6. Hutchinson TA, Flegel KM, Kramer MS, Leduc DG, Kong HH. (1986). Frequency, severity, and risk factors for adverse drug reactions in adult out-patients: A prospective study. *J Chron Dis* 39(7):533-542.

7. Gurwitz JH, Field TS, Harrold LR, Rothschild J, Debellis K, Seger AC, Cadoret C, Fish LS, Garber L, Keleher M, Bates DW (2003). Incidence and preventability of adverse drug events among older persons in the ambulatory setting. *JAMA* 289(9):1107-1116.

8. Classen D (2003). Medication safety. Moving from illusion to reality. *JAMA* 289(9):1154-1156.

9. Sinkovitis HS, Kelly MW, and Ernst ME (2003). Medication administration in day care centers for children. *J Am Pharm. Assoc* 43(3):379-382.

10. Kozma CM (2000). Medication administration practices of school nurses. *J School Health* 70(9):371-376.

11. Rupp MT, DeYoung M, and Schondelmeyer SW (1992). Prescribing problems and pharmacist interventions in community pharmacy. *Medical Care* 30 (10):926-940.

12. Goulding MR (2004). Inappropriate medication prescribing for elderly ambulatory care patients. *Arch Intern Med* 164:305-312.

13. Allan EL, Barker KN, Malloy MJ, and Heller WM (1995). Dispensing errors and counseling in community practice. *American Pharmacy* NS35(12):25-33.

14. Flynn EA, Barker, KN, and Carnahan BJ (2003). National observational study of prescription dispensing accuracy and safety in 50 pharmacies. *J Am Pharm Assoc* 43(2):191-200.

15. Whitney HAK (1989). Errors as a way of life. *Pharm Tech* 5:1-2.

16. Kuyper AR (1993). Patient counseling detects prescription errors. *Hosp Pharm* 28:1180-1181, 1184-1189.

17. Kistner UA, Keith MR, Sergeant KA, and Hokanson JA (1994). Accuracy of dispensing in a high-volume outpatient pharmacy. *Am J Hosp Pharm* November 15, 57(22): 2793-2797.

18. Friedman R (2002). Pharmacist-made products prone to error, FDA finds. *Reuters Health.* http://www.drbobmartin.com/2002k_09_24news08.html. September 9. Accessed February 9, 2004.

19. Spencer J and Matthews AW (2004). As druggists mix customized brews, FDA raises alarm. *The Wall Street Journal* (p. 1), February 27.

20. Hall L (1999). Medication compliance. *Am J Nursing* 99(7):14.

21. Clinite JC and Kabat HF (1969). Errors during self-administration. *J Am Pharm Assoc* NS9:450-452.

22. Liberman P and Swartz AJ (1972). Prescription dispensing to the problem patient. *Am J Hosp Pharm* 29:163-166.

23. Aparasu RR and Helgeland DL (2000). Visits to hospital outpatient departments in the United States due to adverse effects of medications. *Hosp Pharm* 35(8):825-831.

24. Johnson JA and Bootman LJ (1995). Drug-related morbidity and mortality: A cost-of-illness model. *Arch Intern Med* 155(18):1949-1956.

25. Ernst FR and Grizzle AJ (2001). Drug-related morbidity and mortality: Updating the cost-of-illness model. *J Am Pharm Assoc* 41(2):192-199.

26. Goulding MR (2004). Inappropriate medication prescribing for elderly ambulatory care patients. *Arch Intern Med* 164:305-312.

27. Young D (2002, January 25). Many consumers misuse nonprescription drugs. *ASHP News*. http://www.ashp.org/news/showArticle.cfm?cfid=69635&CFToken=91512427&id=2776. Accessed on January 24, 2004.

28. Wolfe SM, Sasich LD, Hope RE, and the Public Citizen's Health Research Group (1999). *Worst Pills, Best Pills*. New York: Pocket Books.

29. Cohen JS (2001). *Overdose—The Case Against the Drug Companies*. New York: Penguin Putnam, Inc.

30. Lazarou J, Pomeranz BH, and Corey PN (1998). Incidence of adverse drug reactions in hospitalized patients: A meta-analysis of prospective studies. *JAMA* 279(15):1200-1205.

31. Kelly WN (2001). Potential risks and prevention, part 1: Fatal adverse drug events. *Am J Health-Sys Pharm* 58(14):1317-1324.

32. Kelly WN (2001). Potential risks and preventions, part 2: Drug-induced permanent disabilities. *Am J Health-Sys Pharm* 58(14):1325-1329.

33. Kelly WN (2001). Potential risks and prevention, part 3: drug-induced threats to life. *Am J Health-Sys Pharm* 58(15):1399-1405.

34. Simoni-Wastila L and Stricker G (2004). Risk factors associated with problem use of prescription drugs. *Am J Pub Health* 94(2):266-269.

35. Bond CA and Raehl CL (2001). Pharmacists' assessment of dispensing errors: risk factors, practice sites, professional functions, and satisfaction. *Pharmcotherapy* 21(5):614-626.

36. Naik RM and Kelly WN (2003). The identification and documentation of significant patient risk problems in Florida pharmacies. *Florida Pharmacy Today* (pp. 19-19-22, 26), June/July.

37. Raschke CG, Hatton RC, Weaver SJ, and Belgado BS (2003). Evaluation of electronic databases used to identify solid oral dosage forms. *Am J Health-Syst Pharm* 60:1735-1740.

38. Over-the-counter drugs: How safe? (2001). *Consumer Reports on Health* 13(8):1-4.

39. Boodman SG. (2003). Consumers face a baffling wall of choices—and a surprising number of serious risks—when they seek relief from minor pains and illnesses at the drugstore. *The Washington Post*, (HE01), February 11.

40. Schiff GD and Rucker TD (1998). Computerized prescribing: Building the electronic infrastructure for better medication usage. *JAMA* (13):1024-1029.

41. Center for Information Technology Leadership (2003). Current research topic: CPOE in ambulatory care. http://www.citl.org/research/currentTopic.htm. Accessed October 6, 2003.

42. Honigman B, Lee J, Rothschild J, Light P, Pulling RM, Yu T, Bates DW (2001) Using computerized data to identify adverse drug events in outpatients. *J Am Med Informatics Assoc* 8:254-266.

43. Koecheler JA, Abramowitz PW, Swim SE, and Daniels CE (1998). Indicators for the selection of ambulatory patients who warrant pharmacist monitoring. *Am J Hosp Pharm* 46:729-732.

44. Rucker NL (2003). Risk, respect, responsibility: Educational strategies to promote safe medicine use. *J Med Sys* 27:519-530.

45. NCC MERP (2003). Medication error prevention council releases recommendations to reduce medication errors in the non-health care settings. Rockville, MD. http://nccmerp.org/council2003-06-20.html. Accessed January 2006.

Chapter 10

1. Bates DW, Boyle DL, Vander Vliet MB, Schneider J, Leape L (1995). Relationship between medication errors and adverse drug events. *J Gen Intern Med* 10(4):199-205.

2. *Doe vs Overdose*. Antibiotic gentamicin causes destruction of patient's vestibular system—$800,000 settlement in Ohio (2003). *Medical Malpractice, Verdicts, Settlements, and Experts* 19(4):25-26.

3. *Betsinger vs Fontana, Al-Hussaini, Werner and Beaufort Memorial Hospital*. Use of cytotec during labor despite lack of FDA approval for this use—VBAC uterine rupture—Failure to perform timely cesarean results in quadriplegia and non-cognitive developmental impairments in infant—$6.258 million guaranteed payout settlement in South Carolina. (2003). *Medical Malpractice, Verdicts, Settlements and Experts* (5):36-37.

4. *RO Braaten vs Walgreen Co*. Man given doxepin instead of doxycycline. Hospitalized twelve days and then requires nursing home care until death. $400,000 Illinois verdict (2002). *Medical Malpractice, Verdicts, Settlements and Experts* 18(12):44.

5. *Monte vs Crittenton Hospital*. Medication error causes injury during inpatient care: anoxic brain injury, shock, and heart failure: $75,000 verdict in Michigan. (2002). *Medical Verdicts, Settlements and Experts* 18(10):52.

6. *Grecco vs Unnamed Hospital*. Medication error in child with urea cycle syndrome results in excessive blood ammonia levels and brain damage. $2.5 million settlement in New Jersey (2002). *Medical Verdicts, Settlements and Experts* 18(11): 26-27.

7. *Anon. Brain Damaged Twin Infant vs Anon Hosp*. Dopamine administered into artery rather than vein of premature newborn—below the knee amputation of one leg with global development delays and bowel/bladder dysfunction—$4.5 million settlement in Michigan (2003). *Medical Verdicts, Settlements and Experts* 19(5):31.

8. *Molina vs V Zaharia and Anon*. Administration of adriamycin for chemotherapy causes extravasation—scaring, carpal tunnel syndrome.—$612,500 in New York (2003). *Medical Malpractice, Verdicts, Settlements and Experts* 19(4)26.

9. *Anon. Plaintiff vs Anon Defendant Physician and Anon Defendant Nursing Home*. Failure to monitor for gentimicin toxicity causes renal failure and death of

resident—$600,000 settlement in Maryland (2003). *Medical Malpractice, Verdicts, Settlements and Experts* 19(5):33.

10. Runciman WB, Merry AF, and Tito F (2003). Error, blame, and law in health care—An antipodean perspective. *Ann Intern Med* 138:974-979.

11. Smetzer J and Cohen MR (1998). Lesson from the Denver medication error/criminal negligence case: Look beyond blaming individuals. *Hosp Pharm* 33 (6):640-657.

12. Channel 1 Communications (2004). Plaintiff's issues in drug product liability. http:// www.channel1.com/users/medlaw/legal/plaint.htm. Accessed March 14, 2004.

13. Abood RB (2001). Pharmacist malpractice liability and risk management strategies. In *Pharmacy Practice and the Law*, Fourth Edition (pp. 313-364). Gaithersburg, MD: Aspen Publications.

14. Mills DH (ed). (1977). Report on medical insurance feasibility study. San Francisco: California Medical Association.

15. Danzon PM (1985). *Medical malpractice: Theory, evidence, and public policy.* Cambridge, MA: Harvard University Press.

16. Kelly WN (2005). The role of pharmacoepidemiology and expert testimony in drug injury. In *Drug Injury: Liability, Analysis, and Prevention,* Second Edition (pp. 151-163). James T. O'Donnell (Ed). Tucson, AZ: Lawyers and Judges Publishing Company, Inc.

17. Ubell E (1993). When should a doctor pay for a mistake? *Parade Magazine* (pp. 17, 19), September 12.

18. Fink JL (1983). Liability claims based on drug use. *Drug Intell Clin Pharm* 17:667-670.

19. General Accounting Office (1987, April). Medical malpractice. Characteristics of claims closed in 1984. GAO/HRD-87-55. Washington, DC: Author.

20. Leape LL, Brennan TA, Laird N, Lawthers AG, Localio AR, Barnes BA, Hebert L, Newhouse JP, Weiler PC, Hiatt H (1991). The nature of adverse events in hospitalized patients: Results of the Harvard Medical Practice Study II. *N Engl J Med* 324(6):377-384.

21. Conlan MF (1993). Medication errors a concern to physician insurers. *Drug Topics* 137(15):41.

22. Rothschild JM, Federico FA, Gandhi TK, Kaushal R, Williams DH, Bates DW (2002). Analysis of medication-related malpractice claims: Causes, preventability, and costs. *Archives of Intern Med* 162(21):2414-2420.

23. Fitzgerald WL and Wilson DB (1998). Medication errors: Lessons in law. *Drug Topics* 142:84-93.

24. Kelly WN (2001). Potential risks and prevention, part 4: Reports of significant adverse drug events. *Am J Health-Syst Pharm* 58:1406-1412.

25. Jury Verdict Research (2000). *Current Awards Trends for Personal Injury.* Horsham, PA: LRP Publications.

26. Brushwood DB and Mullan K (1996). Corporate pharmacy's responsibility for a dispensing error. *Am J Hosp Pharm* 53:668-670.

27. Large verdict for a dispensing error. (2000). *Managed Care Interface* 13 (July):37.

28. Baker KR and Mondt D (1994). Risk management in pharmacy: Preventing liability claims. *Am Pharmacy* NS34(10):60-72.

29. Williams KG (1992). Pharmacists' duty to warn of drug interactions. *Am J Hosp Pharm* 49:2787-2789.

30. Wakefield V and Bryant-Friedland B (1999). Prescription for trouble. *The Florida Times-Union* (p. 1), August 31.

31. American Society for Pharmacy Law (1993). Physician/pharmacist standoff. *Legal Lessons for the Hospital Pharmacist,* 2(1):3. Clifton, NJ: Medical Legal Lessons Publications.

32. Brushwood DB (1993). Duty to warn? Yes and no! But mostly yes. *Georgia Pharm J* (November):24-25.

33. Brushwood DB (1994). Expanding liability: Is *The Wall Street Journal* right? *Georgia Pharm J* (April):25.

34. Brushwood DB (1994). A new legal precedent for duty to warn. *Georgia Pharm J* (May):24.

35. Georgia case focuses on duty to warn (1994). *Georgia Pharm J* (August):23.

36. Brushwood DB (1994). Hospital pharmacists' duty to question clear errors in prescriptions. *Am J Hosp Pharm* 51:2031-2033.

37. Cacciatore GG (1994). Pharmacist's duty to warn. *Am J Hosp Pharm* 51:2824-2826.

38. Brushwood DB (1995). Limits to pharmacists' duty to warn. *Am J Health-Syst Pharm* 52:1337-1339.

39. Chernin T (2001). Legal panel offers script for safe drug dispensing. *Drug Topics* 145:16.

40. Agency on Healthcare Research and Quality (2003). Fear of lawsuits may make physicians reluctant to disclose medical errors to patients. *Research Activities* 273(May):12.

41. Thompson CA (2003). Getting practical about patient safety. *Am J Health-Syst Pharm* 60:1229-1232.

Chapter 11

1. Kelly WN (2003). The quality of published adverse drug event reports. *Ann Pharmacotherapy* 37:1-5.

2. Rosenberg JM, Natan JP, and Cicero LC (1999). Pharmacist operated drug information centers in the United States: A directory of centers that meet listed criteria-1999. *Hosp Pharm* 34(7):797-810.

3. Miwa LJ, Jones JK, Pathiyal A, and Hatoum H (1997). Value of epidemiologic studies determining the true incidence of adverse events: The nonsteroidal anti-inflammatory drug story. *Arch Intern Med* 157(18):2129-2136.

4. Evidence-Based Medicine Working Group (1992). Evidence-based medicine: A new approach to teaching the practice of medicine. *JAMA* 268:2420-2425.

5. Last JM (2000). *A Dictionary of Epidemiology,* Fourth Edition. New York: Oxford University Press.

6. Verhagen AP, de Vet HC, de Bie RA, Kessels AG, Boers M, Bouter LM, Knipschild PG (1998). The Delphi list: A list for quality assessment of randomized clinical trials for conducting systematic reviews developed by Delphi consensus. *J Clin Epidemiology* 51(12):1235-1241.

7. Altman DG, Decks JJ, Clarke M, and Cates C (2000). The quality of systematic reviews. High quality reporting of both randomized trials and systematic reviews should be priority. *BMJ* 320(7234):537-540.

8. Khalid K, Daya S, Jadad A (1996). The importance of quality of primary studies in producing unbiased systematic reviews. *Arch Intern Med* 156(6):661-666.

9. International Society for Pharmacoepidemiology (2002). Guidelines for good epidemiology practices for drug, device, and vaccine research in the United States. http://www.pharmacoepi.org/resources/goodprac.htm. Accessed November 25, 2002.

10. Writing Group for the Women's Health Initiative (2002). Risks and benefits of estrogen plus progestin in healthy postmenopausal women. *JAMA* 288:321-333.

11. Levine M, Walter S, Lee H, Haines T, Holbrook A, Moyer V. (1994). Users' guides to the medical literature IV. How to use an article about harm. Evidence-Based Medicine Working Group. *JAMA* 271(20):1615-1619.

12. Hill AB (1965). The environment and disease: Association or causation? *Proc R Soc Med* 58:295-300.

13. Naranjo CA, Busto U, Sellers EM, Sandor P, Ruiz I, Roberts EA, Janecek E, Domecq C, Greenblatt DJ (1981). A method for estimating the probability of adverse drug reactions. *Clin Pharm Ther* 30(2):239-245.

14. Hansten PD and Horn JR (1998). *Hansten's and Horn's Drug Interactions Analysis and Management.* Vancouver, WA: Applied Therapeutics.

Chapter 12

1. Benichou C (1994). Could it be drug-related? In *Adverse Drug Reactions. A Practical Guide to Diagnosis and Management* (p. viii), Benichou, C. (Ed.). New York: John Wiley and Sons.

2. Naranjo CA, Busto U, Sellers EM, Sandor P, Ruiz I, Roberts EA, Janecek E, Domecq C, Greenblatt DJ (1981). A method for estimating the probability of adverse drug reactions. *Clin Pharm Ther* (2):239-245.

3. Hansten PD and Horn JR (1998). *Hansten's and Horn's Drug Interactions Analysis and Management.* Vancouver, WA: Applied Therapeutics.

4. Bates D (2002). Using information technology to screen for adverse drug events. *Am J Health-Syst Pharm* 59:2317-2319.

5. Murff HJ, Forster AJ, Peterson JF, Fiskio JM, Heiman HL, Bates DW (2003). Electronically screening discharge summaries for adverse medical events. *J Am Med Informatics Assoc* 10:339-350.

6. Kaushal R (2002). Using chart review to screen for medication errors and adverse drug events. *Am J Health-Syst Pharm* 59:2323-2325.

7. Dean B and Barber N (2001). Validity and reliability of observational methods for studying medication administration errors. *Am J Health-Syst Pharm* 58:54-59.

8. Barker KN, Flynn EA, and Pepper GA (2002). Observation method of detecting medication errors. *Am J Health-Syst Pharm* 59:2314-2316.

9. Barker KN and McConnell WE (1962). The problems of detecting medication errors in hospitals. *Am J Hosp Pharm* 19:360-369.

10. Bates DW (2002). Using information technology to screen for adverse drug events. *Am J Health-Syst Pharm* 59:2317-2319.

11. Miller AS (2002). Implementing the rules engine. *Hosp Pharm* 37(4):413-417.

12. Bailey TC (2000). Real-time notification of medication errors. *Health Management Technology* 21:24,26.

13. Brown D (2001). A new prescription for medical errors. *The Washington Post* (A-3), March 18.

14. Electronic system alerts pharmacists to potential adverse drug events (2001). *Am J Health-Syst Pharm* 58(24):2362, 2365.

15. Jha AK, Kuperman GJ, Teich JM, Leape L, Shea B, Rittenberg E, Burdick E, Seger DL, Vander Vliet M, Bates DW (1998). Identifying adverse drug events: Development of a computer-based monitor and comparison with chart review and stimulated voluntary report. *J Am Med Informatics Assoc* 5(3):305-314.

16. Classen DC, Pestotnik SL, Evans RD, and Burke JP (1991). Computerized surveillance of adverse drug events in hospital patients. *JAMA* 266:2847-2878.

17. Brennan TA, Localio AR, Leape LL, Laird NM, Peterson L, Hiatt HH, Barnes BA (1990). Identification of adverse events occurring during hospitalization: A cross-sectional study of litigation, quality assurance, and medical records at two teaching hospitals. *Ann Intern Med* 112(3):221-226.

18. Fisher S (1995). Patient self-monitoring: A challenging approach to pharmacoepidemiology. *Pharmacoepdi and Drug Safety* 4:359-378.

19. Hanlon JT (2001). Comparison of methods for detecting potential adverse drug events in frail elderly inpatients and outpatients. *Am J Health-Syst Pharm* 58:1622-1626.

20. Gibb IA, Miller K, Veltri JC, Page BA, Charlesworth A, Kellett N (2001). *Using community pharmacies to evaluate the safety of prescription only medicine (POM) in an OTC environment: A unique study method in Europe.* Presented at the 17th International Conference on Pharmacoepidemiology. Toronto, Ontario, Canada. August 24, 2001.

21. van Grootheest K, de Graaf L, de Jong-van Berg LT (2003). Consumer adverse drug reaction reporting: A new step in pharmacovigilance? *Drug Safety* 26(4):211-217.

22. Schiff GD (1990). Using a computerized discharge summary data base check box for adverse drug reaction monitoring. *Quality Review Bulletin* 16(4):149-155.

23. Are you tracking medication-related incidents? (2003). *Healthcare Financial Management* 57:118.

24. Housely SC and Kelly WN (2003). Drug-interaction monitoring: Good, bad, and ugly. *Drug Topics* 147(17):41-42.

25. Hartwig SC, Denger SD, and Schneider PJ (1991). Severity-indexed, incident report-based medication error-reporting program. *Am J Health-Syst Pharm* 48:2611-2616.

26. Davis NM (1994). Avoid point-rating system. *Am J Nursing* 94(8):18.

27. Naik RM and Kelly WN (2003). The identification and documentation of significant patient risk problems in Florida pharmacies. *Florida Pharmacy Today* 67:19-22, 26.

28. Steele DR and Kelly WN (2004). Documenting errors benefits patients, pharmacies. *Drug Topics* 148(2):66, 71.

Chapter 13

1. Naik RM and Kelly WN (2003). The identification and documentation of significant patient risk problems in Florida pharmacies. *Florida Pharmacy Today* 67:19-22.

2. JCAHO (2004). Sentinel events. http://www.jcaho.org/accredited+organizations/hospitals/sentinel+events/index.htm. Accessed October 1, 2004.

3. JCAHO (2004). Sentinel events. http://www.jcaho.org/accredited+organizations/ambulatory+care/sentinel+events/rc+of+medication+errors.htm. Accessed October 1, 2004.

4. Donnelly P and Alteri D (2001). Anatomy of an error. *Am J Health-Syst Pharm* 58:977-985.

5. American Society of Consultant Pharmacists (2004). Appendix A. Medication system: Potential breakdown points. http://www.ascp.com/public/pr/guidelines/appendixa.shtml. Accessed February 12.

6. National Coordinating Council for Medication Error Reporting and Prevention (2004). NCC MERP Taxonomy of Medication Errors. http://www.nccmerp.org/pdf/taxo2001-07-31.pdf. Accessed May 4, 2004.

7. Chiles JR (2001, 2002). *Inviting Disaster: Lessons from the Edge of Technology*. London: Harper Collins Publishers.

8. National Coordinating Council for Medication Error Reporting and Prevention (2004). Index for categorizing medication errors. http://www.nccmerp.org/pdf/indexBW2001-06-12.pdf. Assessed May 11.

9. Hartwig SC, Denger SD, and Schneider PJ (1991). Severity-indexed, incident report-based medication error-reporting program. *Am J Hosp Pharm* 48:2611-2616.

10. Schneider PJ and Hartwig MS (1994). Use of severity-indexed medication error reports to improve quality. *Hosp Pharm* 29:205, 208-211.

11. Cobb MD (1986). Evaluating medication errors. *Hosp Pharm* 21:925-929.

12. Davis NM (1994). Avoid point-rating systems. *Am J Nursing* 94(8):8.

13. Oberg KC (1999). Adverse drug reactions. *Am J Pharm Ed* 63:199-204.

14. National Coordinating Council for Medication Errors Reporting and Prevention (2003). NCC MERP approves principles for patient safety reporting programs. Press release dated November 25.

15. Steele DR and Kelly WN (2004). Documenting errors benefits patients, pharmacists. *Drug Topics* 148(2):66:71.

16. U.S. Department of Health and Human Services. Food and Drug Administration (2002). Report to the Nation: Improving Public Health Through Human Drugs. http://www.fda.gov/cder/reports/rtn/2002/rtn2002.htm. Accessed May 10, 2004.

17. Cowley E, Williams R, and Cousins D (2001). Medication errors in children: A descriptive summary of medication error reports submitted to the United States Pharmacopeia. *Curr Ther Res* 62:627-640.

18. USP. (2003, March 12). USP identifies leading medication errors in hospital emergency departments. News release. Rockville, MD: USP.

19. Kelly WN (2003). The quality of published adverse drug event reports. *Ann Pharmacotherapy* 37:1774-1778.

20. Fracica PJ (2002). *The use of technology to enhance ADE reporting, intervention, and safety improvement.* Presented at Measuring Medication Safety in Hospitals: An Invitational Conference Sponsored by the ASHP Research and Education Foundation and the Latiolais Leadership Program of the Ohio State University, held in Tucson, AZ, on April 8-9, 2002.

21. Schiff GD (1990). Using a computerized discharge summary database check box for adverse drug reaction monitoring. *Quality Review Bulletin* 16(4):149-155.

22. National Coordinating Council for Medication Error Reporting and Prevention (2004). Use of medication error rates to compare health care organizations is of no value. http://www.nccmerp.org/council/council2002-06-11.html. Accessed May 11.

Chapter 14

1. U.S. Department of Health and Human Services, Center for Drug Evaluation and Research, U.S. Food and Drug Administration. (2004). CDER Report to the Nation: 2003. http://www.fda.gov/cder/reports/rtn/2003/rtn2003.htm. Accessed June 7.

2. Pharmacy computer systems need major work in order to detect medication errors (1999). *Health Care Strategic Management* 17(4):8.

3. Ringold DJ, Santell JP, and Schneider PJ (2000). ASHP national survey of pharmacy practice in acute care settings: Dispensing and Administration—1999. *Am J Health-Syst Pharm* 57:52-68.

4. Bates DW, Miller EB, Cullen DJ, Burdick L, Williams L, Laird N, Peterson LA, Small SD, Sweitzer BJ, Vander Vliet M, Leape LL (1999). Patient risk factors for adverse drug events in hospitalized patients. *Arch Intern Med* 159(21):2553-2560.

5. Pearson TF, Pittman DG, Longley JM, Grapes ZT, Vigliotti DJ, Mullis SR (1994). Factors associated with preventable adverse drug reactions. *Am J Hosp Pharm* 51(18):2268-2272.

6. Kelly WN (2001). Potential risks and prevention, part 4: Reports of significant adverse drug events. *Am J Health-Syst Pharm* 58:1406-1412.

7. Park BK, Pirmohamed M, and Kitteringham NR (1992). Idiosyncratic drug reactions: A mechanistic evaluation. *Br J Clin. Pharmac* 34:377-395.

8. Hutchinson TA, Flegel KM, Kramer MS, Leduc DG, Kong HH (1986). Frequency, severity, and risk factors for adverse drug reactions in adult out-patients: A prospective study. *J Chron Dis* 39(7):533-542.

9. Field TS, Gurwitz JH, Avorn J, McCormick D, Jain S, Eckler M, Benser M, Bates DW (2001). Risk factors for adverse drug events among nursing home residents. *Arch Intern Med* 161(13):1629-1634.

10. Hoigne R, Maibach R, Maurer P, Jaeger MD, Egli A, Galeazzi R, Hess T, Muller U, Kuenzi UP (1991). Risk factors for adverse drug reactions communication of the CHDM. *Bratislavske Lekarske Listy* 92(11):564-567.

11. Gurwitz JH and Avorn J (1991). The ambiguous relation between aging and adverse drug reactions. *Annals of Internal Med* 114(11):956-966.

12. Montastruc JM, Lapeyre-Mestre M, Bagheri H, Fooladi A (2002). Gender differences in adverse drug reactions: Analysis of spontaneous reports to a regional

pharmacovigilance centre in France. *Fundamental and Clinical Pharmacology* 16(5):343-346.

13. Smith JW, Seidl LG, and Cluff LE (1966). Studies on the epidemiology of adverse drug reactions. *Ann Intern Med* 65(4):629-640.

14. Kelly WN (2001). Potential risks and prevention, part 1: Fatal adverse drug events. *Am J Health-Syst Pharm* 58:1317-1324.

15. Lesar TS, Lomaestro BM, and Pohl H (1997). Medication-prescribing in a teaching hospital. *Arch Intern Med* 157:1569-1576.

16. Saltsman CL and Hamilton RA (1999). Risk factors for patient hospitalization. *Am J Health-Syst Pharm* 56:450-732.

17. Lesar TS, Briceland L, and Stein DS (1997). Factors related to errors in medication prescribing. *Am J Health-Syst Pharm* 277:312-317.

18. Landfield CS, McQuire E, III, and Rosenblatt MW (1990). A bleeding risk index for estimating the probability of major bleeding in hospitalized patients starting anticoagulant therapy. *Am J Med* 89:569-578.

19. Gail MH, Brinton LA, Byar DP, Corle DK, Green SB, Schairer C, Mulvihill JJ (1989). Projecting individualized probabilities of developing breast cancer for white females who are being examined annually. *J Natl Cancer Inst* 81(24):1879-1886.

20. Benichou J, Gail MH, and Mulvihill JJ (1996). Graphs to estimate individualized risk of breast cancer. *J Clin Oncology* 14(1):103-110.

21. Bondy ML, Lustbader ED, Halabi S, Ross E, Vogel VG (1994). Validation of a breast cancer risk assessment model in women with a positive family history. *J Natl Cancer Inst* 86(8):620-625.

22. Spiegelman D, Colditz GA, Hunter D, Hertzmark E (1994). Validation of the Gail et al. model for predicting individual breast cancer risk. *J Natl Cancer Inst* 86(8):600-607.

23. Rockhill B, Spiegelman D, Byrne C, Hunter DJ, Colditz GA (2001). Validation of the Gail et al. model of breast cancer risk prediction and implications for chemoprevention. *J Natl Cancer Inst* 93(5):358-366.

24. Gail MH and Costantino JP (2001). Validating and improving models for projecting the absolute risk of breast cancer. *J Natl Cancer Inst* 93(5):334-335.

25. Walter LC, Brand RJ, Counsell SR, Palmer RM, Landefeld CS, Fortinsky RH, Covinsky KE (2001). Development and validation of a prognostic index for 1-year mortality in older adults after hospitalization. *JAMA* 285(23):2987-2994.

26. Young WW, Bell JE, Bouchard VE, Duffy MG (1974). Clinical pharmacy services: Prognostic criteria for selective patient monitoring, part 1. *Am J Hosp Pharm* 31:562-568.

27. Young WW, Bell JE, Bouchard VE, Duffy MG (1974). Clinical pharmacy services: Prognostic criteria for selective patient monitoring, part 2. *Am J Hosp Pharm* 31:667-676.

28. Koecheler JA, Abramowitz PW, Swim SE, Daniels CE (1989). Indicators for the selection of ambulatory patients who warrant pharmacist monitoring. *Am J Hosp Pharm* 46(4):729-732.

29. Tschepik W, Segal R, Sherrin TP, Schneider DN, Hammond RL (1990). Therapeutic risk-assessment for identifying patients with adverse drug reactions. *Am J Hosp Pharm* 47(2):330-334.

30. Benichou J and Gail MH (1995). Methods of inference for estimates of absolute risk derived from population-based case control studies. *Biometrics* 51:182-194.

31. Guzey C and Spigset O (2002). Genotyping of drug targets: A method to predict adverse drug reactions? *Drug Safety* 25(8):553-560.

32. Hellmold H, Nilsson CB, Schuppe-Koistinen I, Kenne K, Warngard L. (2002). Identification of end points relevant to detection of potentially adverse drug reactions. *Toxicol Lett* 127(1-3):239-243.

33. Morse ML (2002). The empowerment of pharmacogenomics by pharmaco-epidemiology. Presented at the 18th International Conference on Pharmacoepidemiology. Edinburgh, Scotland, August 20, 2002.

34. Wilkins MR (2002). What do we want from proteomics in the detection and avoidance of adverse drug reactions? *Toxicol Lett* 127(1-3):245-249.

35. Nebert DW, Jorge-Nebert L, and Vesell ES (2003). Pharmacogenomics and "individualized drug therapy": High expectations and disappointing achievements. *Am J Pharmacogenomics* 3(6):361-370.

36. Waters R (2004). Making medicine safe. *Reader's Digest,* 115-120, May.

Chapter 15

1. Covey SR (1986). *The 7 Habits of Highly Effective People.* New York: Fireside.

2. Agency for Healthcare Research and Quality. (2001, July). Evidence Report/Technology Assessment, No. 43. Making health care safer: A critical analysis of patient safety practices. Part III. Patient safety practices and targets. Rockville, MD. http://www.ahrq.gov/clinic/ptsaftety. Accessed October 30, 2001.

3. Doolan DF and Bates DW (2002). Computerized physician order entry systems in hospitals: Mandates and incentives. *Health Affairs* 21(4):180-188.

4. Schiff GD and Rucker D (1998). Computerized prescribing. Building the electronic infrastructure for better medication usage. *JAMA* 279(13):1024-1029.

5. Schiff GD (2002). Computerized prescriber order entry: Models and hurdles. *Am J Health-Syst Pharm* 59:1456-1460.

6. eHealth Initiative (2004, April 14). Electronic prescribing: Toward maximum value and rapid adoption. Washington, DC. April 14; Accessed June 15, 2004.

7. Schiff GD, Klass D, Peterson J, Shah G, Bates DW (2003). Linking laboratory and pharmacy. *Arch Intern Med* 163(8):893-899.

8. Randolph AG, Haynes RB, Wyatt JC, Cook DJ, Guyatt GH (1999). Users' guides to the medical literature: XVIII. How to use an article evaluating the clinical impact of a computer-based clinical decision support system. *JAMA* 282(1):67-74.

9. Miller AS (2002). Implementing the rules engine. *Hosp Pharm* 37(4):413-417.

10. Winterstein AG, Hatton RC, Gonzalez-Rothi R, Johns TE, Segal R (2002). Identifying clinically significant preventable adverse drug events through a hospital's database of adverse drug reaction reports. *Am J Health-Syst Pharm* 59(18): 1742-1749.

11. Hunt DL, Haynes RB, Hanna SE, Smith K (1998). Effects of computer decision support systems on physician performance and patient outcomes: A systematic review. *JAMA* 280(15):1339-1346.

12. Classen DC (1998). Clinical decision support systems to improve clinical practice and quality of care. *JAMA* 280(15):1360-1361.

13. Kauschal R and Bates DW (2001). Computerized physician order entry (CPOE) with clinical decision support systems (CDSSs). In *Making Healthcare Safer: A Critical Analysis of Patient Safety Practices* (pp. 59-70), Markowitz AJ (Ed.). Rockville, MD: Agency for Healthcare Research and Quality.

14. Gandi TK and Bates DW (2001). Computer adverse drug event (ADE) detection and alerts. In *Making Healthcare Safer: A Critical Analysis of Patient Safety Practices* (pp. 79-86), Markowitz AJ (Ed.). Rockville, MD: Agency for Healthcare Research and Quality.

15. Chaffee BW (2003). Developing and assessing requirements for clinical decision support. *Am J Health-Syst Pharm* 60:1875-1879.

16. Kaushal R, Shojania K, and Bates DW (2003). Effects of computerized physician order entry and clinical decision supports systems on medication safety: A systematic review. *Arch Intern Med* 163(12):1409-1416.

17. Raschke RA, Gollihare B, Wunderlich TA, Guidry JR, Leibowitz AI, Peirce JC, Lemelson L, Heisler MA, Susong C (1998). A computer alert system to prevent injury from adverse drug events. *JAMA* 280(15):1317-1320.

18. Bates DW, Teich JM, Lee J, Seger D, Kuperman GJ, Ma'Luf N, Boyle D, Leape L (1999). The impact of computerized physician order entry on medication error prevention. *J Am Med Informatics Assoc* 6(4):313-321.

19. Teich JM, Merchia PR, Schmiz JL, Kuperman GJ, Spurr CD, Bates DW (2000). Effects of computerized physician order entry on prescribing practices. *Arch Intern Med* 160:2741-948.

20. Potts, AL, Barr FE, Gregory DF, Wright L, Patel NR (2004). Computerized physician order entry and medication errors in a pediatric critical care unit. *Pediatrics* 113(1):59-63.

21. Monane M, Matthias DM, Nagle BA, Kelly MA (1998). Improving prescribing patterns for the elderly through an online drug utilization review intervention: A system linking the physician, pharmacist, and computer. *JAMA* 280(14):1249-1252.

22. Center for Information Technology Leadership (2003). The value of computerized provider order entry in ambulatory care. http://www.citl.org/research/current Topic.htm. Accessed October 6-7, 2003.

23. Bates DW, Leape LL, Cullen DJ, Laird N, Petersen LA, Teich JM, Burdick E, Hickey M, Kleefield S, Shea B, Vander Vliet M, Seger DL (1998). Effect of computerized physician order entry and a team intervention on prevention of serious medication errors. *JAMA* 280(15):1311-1316.

24. Senholzi C and Gottlieb J (2003). Pharmacist interventions after implementation of computerized prescriber order entry. *Am J Health Syst Pharm* 60:1880-1882.

25. Anderson JG, Jay SJ, Anderson M, Hunt TJ (1997). Evaluating the potential effectiveness of using computerized information systems to prevent adverse drug events. *Proc/AMIA Annual Fall Symposium* 228-232.

26. Ash JS, Gorman PN, Seshadri V, Hersh WR (2004). Computerized physician order entry in U.S. Hospitals: Results of a 2002 survey. *J Am Med Informatics Assoc* 11(2):95-99.

27. Ten community hospitals find success with CPOE: Facilities offer strategies to gain physician support (2003). *Hospital Pharmacy Regulation Report,* September 1.

28. Top-priority actions for preventing adverse drug events in hospitals (1996). *Am J Health-Syst Pharm* 53:747-751.

29. Gunasekaran S, Knecht K, and Garets D (2003). To HYPE is human. *Healthcare Informatics* 20(8):49-50.

30. Berger RG (2004). Computerized physician order entry: Helpful or harmful? *J Am Med Informatics Assoc* 11(2):100-103.

31. Leapfrog Group (2004). Patient safety. http://www.leapfroggroup.org/safety. htm. Accessed June 16, 2004.

32. Berman J (2004). CPOE most popular California app in reducing errors. 2003. http://www.imaknews.com/health-itworld/e_article000198601.cfm. Accessed June 16, 2004.

33. CPOE could reduce errors, cut costs in California (2004). http://www.ihealth beat.org/index.cfm?action=chcflogin&RDaction=dspItem&redirect=102042. Accessed June 16, 2004.

34. Shane R (2003). CPOE: the science and the art. *Am J Health-Syst Pharm* 60:1273-1276.

35. Krizner K (2002). Technology is the right prescription for minimizing medical errors. *Managed Healthcare Executive* 12(9):44-45.

36. Gouveia WA, Shane R, and Clark T (2003). Computerized prescriber order entry: Power, not panacea. *Am J Health-Syst Pharm* 60:1838.

37. Grissinger M and Globus NJ (2004). How technology affects your risk of medication errors. *Nursing* 34(1):36-41.

38. Ballentine AJ (2003). Prescription errors occur despite computerized prescriber order entry (Letter). *Am J Health-Syst Pharm* 60:708-709.

39. Farbstein K (2002). Computerized physician order entry: Getting started. *Briefings on Patient Safety* 3(9):11.

40. Miller AS (2000). Prescriber computer order entry: Team structure and physician impact. *Hosp Pharm* 35(8):822-824.

41. Young D (2003). CPOE takes time, patience, money and teamwork. *Am J Health-Syst Pharm* 60:635, 639-640, 642.

42. Miller AS (2000). Prescriber computer entry: A work in progress. *Hosp Pharm* 35(7):714-720.

43. CPOE, bedside technology, and patient safety: A roundtable discussion. (2003). *Am J Health-Syst Pharm* 60:1219-1228.

44. GroupPOE (2004). Landmines and pitfalls of computerized prescriber order entry. htpp:/www.ismp.org. Accessed May 11, 2004.

45. Leape LL, Bates DW, Cullen DJ, Cooper J, Demonaco HJ, Gallivan T, Hallisey R, Ives J, Laird N, Laffel G, et al. (1995). Systems analysis of adverse drug events. *JAMA* 274:35-43.

46. Murray MD and Shojania KG (2001, July). Unit-dose drug distribution. *Making Healthcare Safer: A Critical Analysis of Patient Safety Practices* (pp. 101-

110), Markowitz AJ (Ed.). Rockville, MD: Agency for Healthcare Research and Quality.

47. Hynniman CE, Conrad WF, Urch WA, Rudnick BR, Parker PF (1970). A comparison of medication errors under the University of Kentucky unit dose system and traditional drug distribution systems in four hospitals. *Am J Hosp Pharm* 27:803-814.

48. Means BJ, Derewicz HJ, and Lamy PP (1975). Medication errors in a multidose and computer-based unit dose drug distribution system. *Am J Hosp Pharm* 32:186-191.

49. Bar coding: Tops for reducing med errors (2003). *NCPA Newsletter* 125:1.

50. A cure for drug ills (2004). *USA Today.* Section 12A, March 16.

51. Medication errors reduced by 87 percent with new tool (2002). *Drug Week,* 33-34, December 20.

52. Putting safety first (2002). *Health Management Technology* 23(5):38-39.

53. Grotting JB (2002). Reducing medication errors at the point of care. *Trustee* (2):21.

54. Thielke TS, Perini VJ, Gates DM, Baker, LE (1993). Impact of robotic medication dispensing, checking, and inventory control system on hospital pharmacy drug distribution system. ASHP Annual Meeting. MCS-33. June.

55. Thielke TS, Perini VJ, Klauck JA, Gates DM (1993). Impact of a robotic medication dispensing, checking, and inventory control system on a hospital pharmacy drug distribution system. ASHP Midyear Clinical Meeting. 28:MCS-29. December.

56. Klein EG, Santora JA, Pascale PM, Kitrenos JG (1994). Medication cart-filling time, accuracy, and cost with an automated dispensing system. *Am H Health-Syst Pharm* 51(9):1193-1196.

57. Barker KN, Pearson RE, Hepler CD, Smith WE, Pappas CA (1984). Effect of an automated bedside dispensing machine on medication errors. *Am J Hosp Pharm* 41(7):1352-1358.

58. Borel JM and Rascati KL (1995). Effect of an automated, nursing unit-based drug-dispensing device on medication errors. *Am J Health-Syst Pharm* 52:1875-1879.

59. Schwartz HO and Brodowy BA (1995). Implementation and evaluation of an automated dispensing system. *Am J Health-Syst Pharm* 52:823-828.

60. Murray MD (2001, July). Automated medication dispensing devices. In *Making Healthcare Safer: A Critical Analysis of Patient Safety Practices* (pp. 127-140), Markowitz AJ (Ed.). Rockville, MD: Agency for Healthcare Research and Quality.

61. Oren E, Shaffer ER, and Gugliemo BJ (2003). Impact of emerging technologies on medication errors and adverse drug events. *Am J Health-Syst Pharm* 60:1447-1458.

62. Kaushal R and Bates DW (2001). The clinical pharmacist's role in preventing adverse drug events. In *Making Healthcare Safer: A Critical Analysis of Patient Safety Practices* (pp. 71-78), Markowitz AJ (Ed.). Rockville, MD: Agency for Healthcare Research and Quality.

63. Folli HL, Poole RL, Benitz WE, Russo JC (1987). Medication error prevention by clinical pharmacists in two children's hospitals. *Pediatrics* 79(5):718-722.

64. Scarsi KK, Fotis MA, and Noskin GA (2002). Pharmacist participation in medical rounds reduces medication errors. *Am J Health-Syst Pharm* 59:2089-2092.

65. Kucukarslan SN, Peters M, Mlynarek M, Nafziger DA (2003). Pharmacists on rounding teams reduce preventable adverse drug events in hospital general medicine units. *Arch Intern Med* 163(17):2014-2018.

66. Leape LL, Cullen DJ, Clapp MD, Burdick E, Demonaco HJ, Erickson JI, Bates DW (1999). Pharmacist participation on physician rounds and adverse drug events in the intensive care unit. *JAMA* 282(3): 267-270.

67. Lee AJ, Boro MS, Knapp KK, Meier JL, Korman NE (2002). Clinical and economic outcomes of pharmacist recommendations in a Veterans Affairs medical center. *Am J Health-Syst Pharm* 59:2070-2077.

68. Rupp MT. (1992). Value of community pharmacists' interventions to correct prescribing errors. *Ann Pharmacotherapy* 26:1580-1584.

69. Gandi TK, Shojania KG, and Bates DW (2001, July). Protocols for high risk drugs: Reducing adverse drug events related to anticoagulants. In *Making Healthcare Safer: A Critical Analysis of Patient Safety Practices* (pp. 87-100), Markowitz AJ (Ed.). Rockville, MD: Agency for Healthcare Research and Quality.

70. Shojania KG, Duncan BW, McDonald KM, Wachter RM (2002). Safe but sound: patient safety meets evidenced-based medicine. *JAMA* 288(4):508-513.

71. Leape LL, Berwick DM, and Bates DW (2002). What practices will most improve safety? Evidence-based medicine meets patient safety. *JAMA* 288(4):501-507.

72. Grotting JB (2002). Reducing medication errors at the point of care. *Trustee* 55(2):21.

73. Cohen MR and Smetzer JL (2004). New models of accountability. *Hosp Pharm* 39(6)515-516.

74. Davis NM (2002). *Medical Abbreviations: 24,000 Conveniences at the Expense of Communications and Safety.* Philadelphia: Neil M. Davis Associates.

75. Spielberg SP (1993). Populations at risk: Predicting and preventing drug-induced disease. *Pharmacoepi and Drug Safety* 2:S31-S36.

76. Fortescue EB, Kaushal R, Landrigan CP, McKenna KJ, Clapp MD, Federico F, Goldmann DA, Bates DW (2003). Prioritizing strategies for preventing medication errors and adverse drug events in pediatric inpatients. *Pediatrics* 111(4):722-729.

77. Goulding MR (2004). Inappropriate medication prescribing for elderly ambulatory care patients. *Arch Intern Med* 164:305-312.

78. Jameson J and VanNoord G (1995). The impact of pharmacotherapy consultation on the cost and outcome of medical therapy. *J Family Practice* 41(5):469-472.

79. Farrell VM, Hill VL, Hawkins JB, Newman LM, Learned RE Jr. (2003). Clinic for identifying and addressing polypharmacy. *Am J Health-Syst Pharm* 60(18):1830, 1834-1835.

80. Senders JW and Senders SJ (2000). Failure mode and effects analysis in medicine. In *Medication Errors: Causes, Prevention, and Risk Management* (pp. 3.1-3.8), Michael R. Cohen (Ed.). Boston: Jones and Barlett Publishers.

81. William E and Talley R (1994). The use of failure mode effect and critically analysis in a medication error subcommittee. *Hosp Pharm* 29(4):331-332, 334-337.

82. Cohen MR, Senders J, and Davis, NM (1994). Failure mode and effects analysis: A novel approach to avoiding dangerous medication errors and accidents. *Hosp Pharm* 29(4):319-330.

83. Anderson HH (2003, February). How to make pharmacy safe now and in the future. *Florida Pharmacy Today,* 10-17.

84. Cohen MR and Smetzer JL (2000). Risk analysis and treatment. In *Medication Errors: Causes, Prevention, and Risk Management* (pp. 20.1-20.34), Michael R. Cohen (Ed.). Boston: Jones and Barlett Publishers.

85. USP. (2003, November 18). Summary of information submitted to MEDMARX in the year 2002. Rockville, MD.

86. Spalding BJ (1990). What is a safe dispensing speed? *American Druggist* 201(6):22-24.

87. Only 4 of 10 patients report receiving pharmacist counseling on outpatient prescriptions (1991). *Am J Hosp Pharm* 51:3020.

88. Marcellino K (2001). What do Georgia's patients expect from their pharmacist? *Georgia Pharmacy J* 23(10):22-23.

89. Kuyper AR (1993). Patient counseling detects prescription errors. *Hosp Pharm* 28(12):1180-1181,1184-1189.

90. Young D (2002, January 25). Many consumers misuse nonprescription medication. *ASHP News.* http:/www.ashp.org/news/showArticle?cfid=69635&CF Token=91512427&id=2776. Accessed January 24, 2004.

91. Medication safety: New technology helps reduce medication errors (2003). *Medical Devices and Surgical Technology Week* (September):124.

92. NCC MERP (2004). Medication error prevention council releases recommendations to reduce medication errors in non-health care settings. http://www. nccmerp.org/council/council2003-06-20.html. Accessed June 26, 2004.

93. Wright C (2002, April 9). E-scripts are just a click away at Giant Food and Pharmacy. http://www.giantfood.com/company_press_article.cfm?press_id=119. Accessed April 11, 2002.

94. Velasco P and Whittemore K (2002, October 16). Two-thirds of chain pharmacy market commits to SureScripts to deliver prescribing connectivity to 21,000 pharmacies. http://www.surescript.com/oct16htm. Accessed October 31, 2002.

95. E-prescribing technologies may improve efficiency and safety while lowering costs for three billion prescriptions a year (2002, November 12). http://www. chef.org/press/view.cfm?itmeID=20190. Accessed January 2006.

96. Boston area physicians embrace e-prescribing technology as a tool to improve healthcare: Docs say paperless prescribing prevents errors (2003). http:// newswatch.cnn.com.content.php?page=AllArticleXml&feed=bizwire&type=xml&s . . . Accessed February 7, 2003.

97. Giant pharmacies expands e-script service through partnership with DrFirst (2003). http://newswatch.cnn.com/content.php?page=AllArticleXml&feed=prnews andtypc=xml&s. . . Accessed February 20, 2003.

98. Vaczek D (2003). Preparing for e-prescribing. *Pharmac Times* 69(1):48-52.

99. It's time for standards to improve safety with electronic communication of orders. (2003). ISMP. http://www.ismp.org/MSAarticles/ improve.htm. Accessed May 11, 2004.

100. Schneider PJ (2002). Applying human factors in improving medication-use safety. *Am J Health-Syst Pharm* 59:1155-1159.

101. Weinger MB, Pantiskas C, Wiklund ME, Carstensen P (1998). Incorporating human factors into the design of medical devices. *JAMA* 280:1484. Letter.

102. Daniels J, Kelly WN, and Malone JT (2004). Managing behavior can reduce medical and medication errors. In press 2005.

Chapter 16

1. Robert Caswell. *The Doctor.* Touchstone Pictures (1991). Based on the 1998 novel *A Taste of My Own Medicine: When the Doctor is the Patient* by Edward E. Rosenbaum. MD. New York: Random House.

2. American Society of Health-System Pharmacists (2002, July 17). Survey reveals patient concerns about medication-related issues. http://www.ashp.org/news/showArticle.cfm?cfid=2628430&CFToken=25465950&id=2996.

3. Santell JP and Camp S (2004). Better communication may reduce med errors in the home.www.rnweb.com.67(6):75.

4. Marcellino, K (2001). What do Georgia's patients expect from their pharmacist?" *Georgia Pharmacy Journal* 23(10):22-23.

5. Drane JF (1998). Becoming a good doctor: The place of virtue and character in medical ethics. The Catholic Health Association. Kansas City: Sheed and Ward Publishers.

6. Rucker NL (2003). Risk, respect, responsibility: Educational strategies to promote safe medicine use. *J Med Systems* 27(6):519-529.

7. Gardner M, Boyce RW, and Herrier RN (1993). Pharmacist-Patient Consultation Program PPC-Unit 1. Pfizer, National Healthcare Operations, New York.

8. Geller ES, Perdue SR, and French A (2004). Behavior-based safety coaching. *Professional Safety* 49(7):42-49.

9. Awe C and Lin S-J (2003). A patient empowerment model to prevent medication errors. *J Med Systems* 27(6):503-517.

10. Hussey TC (2000). Including patients in medication error reduction. *Pharmacy Times* 66:22, 24.

11. Wiegman SA, and Cohen MR (2000). The patient's role in preventing medication errors. In *Medication Errors: Causes, Prevention, and Risk Management* (pp. 14.1-14.12), MR Cohen (Ed.). Boston: Jones and Barlett Publishers.

Chapter 17

1. Kohn LT and Donaldson MS (Eds.) (1999). *To Err is Human—Building a Safer Health System.* Institute of Medicine. Washington DC: National Academy Press.

2. Institute of Medicine. (2001). *Crossing the Quality Chasm—A New Health System for the 21st Century.* Washington, DC: The Committee on Quality of Health Care in America, National Academy Press.

3. Aspden P, Corrigan JM, Wolcott J, and Erickson SM (2004). *Patient Safety—Achieving a New Standard for Care.* Institute of Medicine. Washington, DC: National Academy Press.

4. McDonald CJ, Weiner M, Hui SL (2000). Deaths due to medical errors are exaggerated in Institute of Medicine Report. *JAMA* 284:93-97.

5. Kimmel KC and Sensmeier J (2002). A technological approach to enhancing patient safety. A White Paper. *Healthcare Information and Management System Society.* http://www.himss.org/content/files/whitepapers/patient_safety.pdf. Accessed July 22, 2004.

6. American Hospital Association (2004). Pathways for medication safety: Leading a strategic planning effort. www.medpathways.info. Accessed July 24, 2004.

7. Greiner AC, Knebe E, and the Committee on the Health Professions Education Summit (2003). *Health Professions Education: A Bridge to Quality.* Washington DC: The National Academies Press.

8. Study tells of medical mistakes (2004). *The Atlanta Journal-Constitution* (p. A6), July 28.

9. The Health Information and Management Systems Society (2004, July 21). 2004 HIMSS national health information infrastructure survey finds industry supports NHII, but challenges remain. *HIMSS News.* http://www.himss.org/ASP/ContentRedirector.asp?ContentID=52470. Accessed July 22, 2004.

10. The Health Information and Management Systems Society (2003, April). Position statement on national health information infrastructure (NHII). http://www.himss.org/content/files/positionstatements/NHIIPositionStatement.pdf.

11. Schneider PJ (2001). Pharmacists building a safer health system. *Am J Health-Syst Pharm* 58:66-68.

12. DeJoy DM, Gershon RM, and Schaffer BS (2004). Safety climate—assessing management and organizational influences on safety. *Professional Safety* 49 (7):50-57.

13. Conway JB (2002). Preserving and restoring patient trust. *Healthcare Executive* 17(2):72-73.

14. Gandhi TK, Graydon-Baker E, Barnes JN, Neppl C, Stapinski C, Silverman J, Churchill W, Johnson P, Gustafson M (2003). Creating an integrated patient safety team. *Joint Commission J on Quality and Safety* 29(8):383-390.

15. Covey SR (1989). *Seven Habits of Highly Effective People.* New York: Fireside Books.

16. Schneider PJ (2002). Using technology to enhance measurement of drug safety. *Am J Health-Syst Pharm* 59:2330-2332.

17. American Society of Health-System Pharmacists. (2003). Pharmacy-nursing shared vision for safe medication use in hospitals: Executive session summary. *Am J Health-Syst Pharm* 60:1046-1052.

18. Kelly WN (1986). Strategic planning for clinical services: Hamot Medical Center. *Am J Hosp Pharm.* 43(9):2159-2163.

19. Dunham RB (2004). Nominal group technique: A users' guide. http://instruction.bus.wisc.edu/obdemo/readings/ngt.html. Accessed July 28, 2004.

20. MEDSTAT (2004). Patient safety organizational Readiness Tool. http://www.medstat.com. Accessed July 27, 2004.

21. Voelker R (2001). Hospital collaborative creates tools to help reduce medication errors. *JAMA* 286:3067-3069.

22. Ukens C (2001). Improve your safety with this new self-assessment tool. *Drug Topics* 145:30.

23. Diane DeMichele Cousins (Ed.) (2004). *Advancing Patient Safety in U.S. Hospitals,* Rockville, MD: United States Pharmacopeia.

24. Silverman JB, Stapinski CD, Churchill WW, Neppl C, Bates DW, Gandhi TK (2003). Multifaceted approach to reducing preventable adverse drug events. *Am J Health-Syst* 60:582-586.

25. Rozich JD (2001). Medication safety: One organization's approach to the challenge. *J Clin Outcomes Management* 8(10):27-34.

Chapter 18

1. Rucker TD (1987). Prescribed medications: System control or therapeutic roulette? IFAC monograph. In *Control Aspects of Biomedical Engineering*, Nalecz Maciej (ed). Oxford: Permamon Press, 167-175.

2. Kohn LT, Corrigan JM, and Donaldson MS (2000). *To Err is Human: Building a Safer Health System*. Washington, DC: National Academy Press.

3. Kelly WN (2004). Medication errors: Lessons learned and actions needed. *Professional Safety* July:35-41.

4. Cohen JS (2001). *Overdose—The Case Against Drug Companies*. New York: Jeremy P. Tarcher/Putnam.

5. Raschke CG, Hatton RC, Weaver SJ, Belgado BS (2003). Evaluation of electronic databases used to identify solid oral dosage forms. *Am J Health-Syst Pharm* 60:1735-1740.

6. Villanueva P, Peiro S, Librero J, Pereiro I (2003). Accuracy of pharmaceutical advertisements in medical journals. *The Lancet* 361(9351):10-11, 27-32.

7. Drug maker admits misleading doctors (2004). *The Atlanta Journal-Constitution* (p. A-11), July 25.

8. Judd J (2004). Truth in advertising? http://www.ABCNews.com. FDA calls prescription drug advertising misleading. Accessed August 8, 2004.

9. Milloy S (2004). Beware drug company marketing. FOXNews.com/Views-Junk Science—Beware Drug Company Marketing. Accessed August 8, 2004.

10. Moore T (1999). Prescription for error. *The Boston Globe* (p. D-1), December 5.

11. Findlay S (2004). Pill-popping replaces health habits. *USA Today* (p. 15-A), February 5.

12. Editorial (2004). One firm's bold step helps doctors, patients avoid errors. *USA Today* (p. 10-A), August 10.

13. Relman AS and Angell M (2002). America's other drug problem. *The New Republic* 227(5):27-41.

14. Rucker TD (2003, March 18). Drug policy as prescribed by doctors Relman and Angell: Therapeutic dose or sub optimal treatment? (The escapades of Brer Rabbit in the Drug Policy Arena). Unpublished. Used by permission.

15. Davis NM (1998). The FDA has awesome responsibilities: Let it err on the side of conservatism. *Hosp Pharm* 33(10): 1153.

16. Hilts PJ (2003). *Protecting America's Health: The FDA, Business, and One Hundred Years of Regulation*. New York: Knopf, Borzoi Publishers.

17. Avorn J (2004). *Powerful Medicines: The Benefits, Risks, and Costs of Prescription Drugs*. New York: Alfred A. Knopf.

18. Pomper S (2000, May). Drug rush: Why the prescription drug market is unsafe at high speeds. *The Washington Monthly*. http://www.washingtonmonthly.com/features/2000/0005.pomper.html. Accessed November 12, 2003.

19. Moore TJ (2000). FDA in crisis. Adapted from the *Boston Globe* Sunday Focus Section of April 2, 2000. http:/www.thomasmoore.com/pages/fda_crisis.html. Accessed June 25, 2000.

20. Farewell to ephedra (2004). *St. Petersburg Times* (p. 12A), January 2.

21. Staff and wire reports (2004). Epehdra to be off shelves by April 12. *USA Today* (p. 4-D), February 9.

22. New York outlaws OTC sales of ephedra (2003). *USA Today* (p. 7D), November 4.

23. Elias M (2004). Add suicide warnings to antidepressant labels, FDA asks. *USA Today* (p. 7D), March 25.

24. Leinwand D (2003). Latest trend in drug abuse: Youths risk death for cough-remedy high. *USA Today* (p. 1A), December 29.

25. Sharav VH. (2004). FDA's neglect of safety concerns ignores duty to "do no harm." *USA Today* (p. 20A), June 21.

26. The Associated Press Wire Service. (2003, May 22). FDA: Half of companies promises follow-up drug studies not begun yet.

27. Petersen M (2003, June 29). Who's minding the drugstore? *The New York Times.*

28. Moore TJ (2000). What you don't know. *The Washingtonian,* 35(10):31-35.

29. Millenson ML (1997, 1999). *Demanding Medical Excellence.* Chicago, IL: The University of Chicago Press.

30. Wood AJ, Stein C, and Woolsley R (1998). Making medicines safer—the need for an independent drug safety board. *N Eng J Med* 25:339.

31. Institute of Medicine (2003, July 31). Key capabilities of an electronic health record system. http://www.iom.edu/report.asp?id=14391. Accessed October 10, 2003.

32. eHealth Initiative. (2004, April 14). Electronic prescribing: Toward maximum value and rapid adoption. Washington, DC. http://www.ehealthinitiative.org/iniatives/erx/. Accessed January 2006.

33. Medical paper-pushers resist opportunity to improve care (2004). *USA Today* (p. A-21), May 13.

34. Schmidt J and Appleby J (2004). Report to promote e-records for health care. *USA Today* (p. 3-B), July 21.

35. Schiff G and Rucker TD (1998). Computerized prescribing: Building the electronic infrastructure for better medication usage. *JAMA* 279(13): 1024-1029.

36. Medicare program shortchanges seniors and soaks taxpayers (2004). *USA Today* (p. 14-A), July 12.

37. Rx import foes seek support on capital hill (2004).*Pharmacy Times* 70:7, 14.

38. Associated Press (2004). Bogus drugs raise alarm. Cheap Mexican counterfeits don't work, Americans told. *The Atlanta-Journal Constitution* (p. A-18), July 31.

39. Rudolf PM and Bernstein BG (2004). Counterfeit drugs. *N Eng J Med* 350:1384-1386.

40. Appleby J (2004). Some Internet drug sales put buyers at risk. *USA Today* (p. 3-B), June 18.

41. Young D (2004). GAO details perils of Internet drug buying. *Am J Health-Syst Pharm* 61:1526, 1528, 1530.

42. Young D (2003). Experts warn drug industry, government about weaknesses in drug supply chain. *Am J Health-Syst Pharm* 60:2176, 2180, 2184.

43. Wittingham RB (2003). *The Blame Machine*. Burlington, MA: Elsevier Butterworth-Heinemann.

44. American Medical Association (2004, July 22). Senate passage of patient safety bill victory for America's patients and physicians. Press release. http://www.ama-assn.org/ama/pub/article/print/1617-8719.html. Accessed July 25, 2004.

45. Institute for Medicine (2003, November 4). Keeping patients safe: Transforming the work environment of nurses. http://www.iom.edu/report.asp?id=16173. Accessed August 9, 2004.

46. Rogers AE, Hwang WT, Scott LD, Aiken LH, Dinges DF (2004). The working hours of hospital staff nurses and patient safety. *Health Affairs* 23(4):202-212.

47. Turner R. (2004). A high dose of tech. *U.S. News and World Reports* (pp. 47-50, 52, 56, 60), August 2.

48. Rucker TD (1976). Drug information for prescribers and dispensers: Toward a model system. *Medical Care* 14(2):156-164.

49. Teng J, Song CK, Williams RL, Polli JE (2002). Lack of medication dose uniformity in commonly split tablets. *J Am Pharm Assoc* 42(2):195-199.

50. Reinberg S (2004, August 9). Many older patients on risky drugs. *USA Today.Com*. http://www.healthscout.com/channel/68/1001/main.html. Accessed August 10, 2004.

51. O'Briant D (2003). When drugs collide. *The Atlanta Journal-Constitution* (p. E-1), October 7.

52. Bero LA, Lipton HL, and Bird JA (1991). Characterization of geriatric drug-related hospital readmissions. *Medical Care* 29(10):989-1003.

53. McCoy K and Hansen B (2004). Havens for elderly may expose them to deadly risks. *USA Today* (p. 1-A), May 25.

54. Gurwitz J and Rochon P (2002). Improving the quality of medication use in the elderly patients: A not-so simple prescription. *Arch Intern Med* 162(15):1670-1672.

55. Johnson MS, Latif DA, and Gordon B (2002). Medication error instruction in schools of pharmacy curricula: a descriptive study. *Am J Pharm Ed* 66:364-371.

56. Why do so many still die needlessly in hospitals? (2004). *USA Today* (p. 14-A), August 5.

57. Schiff GD (2002). Computerized order entry: Models and hurdles. *Am J Health-Syst Pharm* 59: 1456-1460.

58. McDonald CJ, Weiner M, and Hui SL (2000). Deaths due to medical errors are exaggerated in Institute of Medicine report. *JAMA* 284: 93-97.

59. Traynor K (2003). Physicians, public not overly concerned about medical errors. *Am J Health-Syst Pharm* 60: 116, 122.

60. Pomper, S (2000, May). Drug rush. *The Washington Monthly*. http://www.washingtonmonthly.com/features/2000/0005.pomper.html. Accessed June 20, 2004.

61. Gladwell M (2002). *The Tipping Point—How Little Things Can Make a Big Difference*. New York: Little, Brown and Company.

62. Lawrence D (1999). *Is medical care obsolete?* A presentation to the National Press Club. Washington, DC, July 14.

63. Broder DS (2004). U.S. health system care system terminally ill. *St. Petersburg Times* (p. 18-A), July 16.

64. Silverman JB, Stapinski CD, Huber C, Ghandi TK, Churchill WW (2004). Computer-based system for preventing adverse events. *Am J Health-Syst Pharm* 61:1599-1603.

65. Leatherman S, Berwick D, lles D, Lewin LS, Davidoff F, Nolan T, Bisognano M (2003). The business case for quality: case studies and analysis. *Health Affairs* 22(2):17-23.

Index

Page numbers followed by the letter "f" indicate figures; those followed by the letter "t" indicate tables.